Modules for Basic Nursing Skills   Volume 1

Modules   6+7 - Sept. 4 - 8:00

Modules   4, 12, 13, 14, 2X   Sept. 11 10:00

Houghton Mifflin offers two other books for introductory nursing, which can be used either in conjunction with the present volume or independently.

Ellis/Nowlis: Nursing: A Human Needs Approach presents the theory and rationale that underlie nursing practice.

Ellis/Nowlis/Bentz: Modules for Basic Nursing Skills, Second Edition, Volume 2, contains the following skill topics: Common Laboratory Tests; Gastric Intubation; Tube Feeding; Ostomy Care; Administering Oxygen; Inspection, Palpation, Auscultation, and Percussion; Respiratory Care Procedures; Preoperative Care; Postoperative Care; Sterile Technique; Surgical Asepsis (Scrubbing, Gowning, and Gloving); Irrigations; Catheterization; Sterile Dressings; Oral and Nasopharyngeal Suctioning; Tracheostomy Care and Suctioning; Administering Oral Medications; Administering Topical Medications; Giving Injections; Preparing and Maintaining Intravenous Infusions; Administering Intravenous Medications; and Starting Intravenous Infusions.

Modules for Basic Nursing Skills   Volume 1

Second Edition

Janice Rider Ellis, R.N., M.N.

Elizabeth Ann Nowlis, R.N., M.N.

Patricia M. Bentz, R.N., M.S.N.

Shoreline Community College

Houghton Mifflin Company   Boston
Dallas   Geneva, Illinois   Hopewell, New Jersey
Palo Alto   London

Cover photo by Fredrik D. Bodin

Illustrations by Jeremy Elkin and Richard Spencer

Printed in the U.S.A.

Library of Congress Catalog Card Number: 79-89521

ISBN: 0-395-28654-9

Contents

List of Skills

The following skills are included in this volume. For easy reference, a module number and page number are provided for each skill.

To the Instructor

Modules for Basic Nursing Skills, Second Edition, is a two-volume text designed to teach beginning nursing students how to perform basic skills and procedures. It can be used in the clinical practice laboratory of an introductory nursing course or in any other suitable setting.

Skills are arranged in a progression from simple to complex throughout the two volumes, but each skill module is self-contained to permit instructors to omit or reorder skills according to the needs of their own programs. In the second edition, we have doubled the number of skills covered in the first edition and now present forty-eight modules in two volumes. Volume 1 contains the most basic skills and may be appropriate by itself for some courses enrolling LPN/LVN students, as well as for courses for nursing aides and nursing assistants. Volumes 1 and 2 together may be most useful in programs for RN students. Because programs vary considerably from state to state and from institution to institution, we have tried to make our second edition as adaptable as possible to many different programs by offering comprehensive coverage of nursing skills.

The format of the modules focuses on the student's practice and mastery of skills and procedures. It is designed for independent learning and self-instruction. Each module contains a main objective, a rationale, a list of prerequisites, specific learning objectives, a set of learning activities, a vocabulary list, a core of background and step-by-step instructions with carefully chosen photographs and illustrations, a performance checklist, and a quiz. These parts are described in detail in the next section entitled "To The Student." At the back of each volume of modules, we have given a glossary containing definitions of the words in the vocabulary lists and answer keys to the quizzes. The two volumes are three-hole punched with perforated pages, so students can tear out pages

and hand them in or keep the modules in notebooks.

Modules for Basic Nursing Skills, Second Edition, Volumes 1 and 2 can be used in conjunction with the text by Ellis and Nowlis, *Nursing: A Human Needs Approach,* which treats the theory behind nursing practice. The two volumes of modules are designed to stand alone, however, and can be used by themselves in a course addressing nursing skills. *Modules for Basic Nursing Skills* can also be used in conjunction with any other text covering nursing theory or fundamentals.

We would like to thank the following individuals for their reviews of our manuscript at various stages and their many useful suggestions: the late Susan T. Reynolds, Bryn Mawr Hospital; Joan Long, University of North Carolina; Ramona Gonzales, College of Santa Fe; Betty Fallath, Community College of Baltimore; Teresa Gherkin, Montgomery County Community College; Martha Worthington, St. Petersburg Junior College; Marilee Creelan, Isabelle Firestone School of Nursing, Akron City Hospital; the late Dorothea T. Schmidt Penta, Middlesex Community College, Massachusetts; and Elizabeth Winning, R.N., Group Health Cooperative of Puget Sound, Seattle, Washington. We are especially grateful to our students and colleagues who have worked with the modules as they were originally written, through the changes made for the first published edition, and in planning for this revision. Their constant feedback has been essential to us.

To the Student

This set of modules is designed to enable you to learn the procedures basic to your role as a nurse. Each module has the following parts, unless they are not applicable to a particular skill:

Main Objective   A general statement of the basic skill that is taught in the module.

Rationale   The reason why you need to learn the skill.

Prerequisites   A list of specific skills or abilities needed to master the new skill. Also listed are other modules whose contents are necessary for an understanding of the skill.

Specific Learning Objectives   A table that breaks down the basic skill you are studying into specific subskills that you can test yourself on after completing the module.

Learning Activities   Activities designed to help you progress safely and gradually into carrying out the new skill. Practice, in whatever setting is available, is essential to skillful performance. Different students will need differing amounts of practice, depending on their manual dexterity and previous experience. Your school may provide audiovisual aids to use with the module. If so, view them after reading the module but before going on to actually practice the skill. Do not hesitate to contact your instructor if you encounter difficulties.

Vocabulary   A list of special terms used in the module. The glossary will give the definitions of most. Some terms will be best understood in the context of the module itself.

Module Core   Necessary background information and a step-by-step guide to performing the skill, including photographs and illustrations where necessary.

Performance Checklist   A brief guide both to use while you are practicing the skill and to judge your performance by.

Quiz   A brief review for self-testing.

Key   The answers at the back of the text allow you to score yourself.

Glossary   At the end of the volume, a glossary provides definitions for the key vocabulary terms.

There are, of course, many advanced nursing procedures not covered in the modules, but the skills that are included are basic to the educational preparation of the nurse.

As authors, we hope you will find gaining these essential skills to be a satisfying endeavor, and we wish you our best as you begin your studies.

Janice Rider Ellis
Elizabeth Ann Nowlis
Patricia M. Bentz

Module 1 Assessment

MAIN OBJECTIVES

To perform a beginning-level assessment of individual patients, collecting data for all pertinent areas and using all senses through a systematic method.

To identify simple patient problems from the data collected.

RATIONALE

A major responsibility of the registered nurse is to assess patients. In every nursing care setting, the nurse is called on to gather data in order to determine patients' problems, establish priorities in treating them, and plan their care. A systematic method of assessment provides a framework to do this in an orderly, comprehensive way. Without some type of system, significant areas may be omitted accidentally. This module provides only a beginning framework; experience and further education will refine it.

PREREQUISITES

None

SPECIFIC LEARNING OBJECTIVES

	Know Facts and Principles	Apply Facts and Principles	Demonstrate Ability	Evaluate Performance
1. *Sources of assessment data*	State four sources of assessment data	Given a list of information needed, identify appropriate source for that information	Gather assessment data using all four sources	
2. *Areas of assessment*	Using the human needs approach, list and define ten areas to be assessed. Using the body systems approach, list and define nine areas to be assessed.	Given patient data, determine to what areas data are pertinent	Gather assessment data in all areas	Evaluate own performance using Assessment Guide
3. *Identification of problems* *a. Objective data (signs or objective symptoms)* *b. Subjective data (symptoms or subjective symptoms)*	Differentiate between objective and subjective data	Given data and their source, identify them as subjective or objective	Include and appropriately identify both subjective and objective information	Evaluate differentiation of data with instructor
4. *Statement of problems*	Define nursing problem	Given a list of assessment data, identify problem area and state problem in concrete, patient-centered terms	In clinical setting, correctly identify simple problem and state problem on patient's record in concrete, patient-centered terms	Verify accuracy of problem identification with instructor

LEARNING ACTIVITIES

1. Review the Specific Learning Objectives.
2. Read the chapter on the nursing process and the section on interviewing in Ellis and Nowlis, *Nursing: A Human Needs Approach,* or comparable material in another textbook.
3. Read through the module.
4. Review the format of the Assessment Guide, pages 10-11.
5. Arrange to practice the following activities with a partner:
   a. Select an assessment approach and write its assessment categories on one side of a blank piece of paper.
   b. Observe each other without speaking or touching. Write all the data you can gather for each area. You may use the module as a reference while observing each other.
   c. Compare your lists. Discuss the differences and similarities of the data collected. Go through your lists together and star each item that is truly objective.
   d. Show your lists to your instructor for suggestions or corrections.
   e. Next, gather additional data without speaking but using touch and contact. Compare your lists again, discuss the data collected, and star objective data. Show your lists to your instructor again for suggestions or corrections.
   f. As a final step, interview each other to gather further data in each area.
   g. Discuss these data. What data gathered by interview would cue you to make further observations? Also, what data gathered by observation over a longer period of time might be needed? What data are unique and obtainable only by interview? Underline the subjective data.
   h. Show these lists of data to your instructor.

6. In the clinical setting:
   a. Again, select an assessment approach and write its assessment categories on one side of a blank piece of paper.
   b. Consult with your clinical instructor before choosing a patient to observe. Choose a patient who will not be upset or disturbed by your visit.
   c. When you are with the patient, explain your task in a way that will make him or her feel comfortable. You can simply say that you are trying to improve your observational skills. Observe the patient for five or ten minutes. Write all data gathered by observation. You may socialize with the patient during this time, but do not interview him or her. At the end of the time period, excuse yourself and look over your list. You may complete this activity with a partner if that does not upset the patient. In that instance, you could compare lists.
   d. Consult with your instructor regarding the data collected. If you or your instructor feel it would be beneficial to you, repeat this activity with another patient.
7. Look at an available clinical record. From the record, gather only what you feel to be pertinent assessment data. List the data under appropriate assessment areas. Mark each item *O* for objective or *S* for subjective. From this assessment data, identify and write what you consider the patient's problems to be. Consult with your instructor regarding your determination.
8. For a patient assigned in the clinical area, use the Assessment Guide to gather data from all four sources. Have your instructor review this assessment.
9. Continue to use the guide to assess all patients assigned in the clinical area.

ASSESSMENT

Assessment involves gathering all possible
data regarding patients in order to identify
problems. Data are gathered in a variety of
ways from four primary sources or modes:
(1) the patient's record, (2) an interview,
(3) general observation, and (4) physical
examination.

The Patient's Record

A patient's record provides essential data
relative to his or her identified problems.
Consult the physician's history and physical
examination records, the results of laboratory and diagnostic studies, the various
nursing records, and the records of other
specialists working with the patient. It is not
always possible to completely review a
record before your initial patient contact,
but a thorough nursing assessment cannot
be made without reference to the data
contained in the record.

Interview

As you make general observations and do a
nursing physical examination, you also must
interview the patient. Ask specific questions
about the patient's health status, health
history, and responses to illness. The information gained from an interview is *subjective data*. These data may lead you to further observation or examination of the
patient. Note that your nursing history is a
formalized tool for interviewing patients.

General Observation

Observational skills improve with experience.
Whenever you contact a patient, be sure to
observe him or her very carefully, paying
close attention to detail.

When we speak of general observation,
we think of what is *seen, heard,* and *smelled.*
Look at both the patient and his or her
environment. (Maintaining an environment
that is therapeutic for the patient is a nurs-

ing responsibility.) Note the general symmetry of the body, posture, and movement,
as well as facial expressions and gestures,
which are especially important. Listen for
the characteristic sounds of ordinary life,
among them the sound of breathing. Check
out any differences from the norm thoroughly. Smells are often difficult to describe,
but comparing them to something familiar
can help. For example, there are odors
associated with wounds and drainage, with
the breath, and sometimes with the body
itself. Be familiar with these smells; they
are all important.

Physical Examination

After you have made a general survey, perform a physical examination. Take temperature and blood pressure; measure height,
weight, and fluid intake and output; palpate,
count, and describe the pulse.

You will need a stethoscope for *auscultation* (listening to body sounds) from the
lungs, the bowel, and other organs. Although
at first you may not recognize what you
hear, you will quickly learn to identify
normal sounds; then you can consult
someone else when you hear a sound that is
abnormal. Palpate soft areas of the body to
check for solid masses or abnormal rigidity.
(See Volume 2, Module 32, for specific
information on auscultation and palpation.)

Some parts of a nursing physical examination can be done while bathing a patient or
during other contact. You can examine the
skin closely, check any dressings, and observe the patient's response to activities. All
information gathered by observation and
examination is *objective data.*

A physical examination is a complex task,
involving many components, and here too
experience improves skills. Still, as you
begin, you can identify normal and abnormal characteristics in general ways. Then,
as you study each system of the body in
physiology and learn disease entities and
nursing care, you will develop new skills to
use in physical examinations.

An Assessment Guide

The Assessment Guide on pages 10-11 gives you a basic systematic way to approach assessment. Still, it is only a tool and should not become too confining. You should fill in the major categories of assessment in their order of importance for the individual patient.

As you study the physiology and pathophysiology related to each category below, you will recognize the complexity of assessment. This discussion does not begin to cover all the data relating to specific areas; rather, it is an outline of major components to give you a beginning framework. Some components relate to skills and knowledge you have now; others require skills you will learn in the weeks ahead. As you learn, you will add more and more detail to your assessments of patients.

Because people are whole entities, not simply a collection of parts, you may find it difficult to determine whether certain data are more applicable to one area than to another. In this case, note the data under two or more categories. At other times, the problem may be very clear, in which case list the data in the area that pertains to the known problem. Remember that the location of data is not so critical as is your ability to relate facts to one another in order to recognize problems.

Two systems for organizing your assessment will be presented. It is important to understand that the *total patient* is to be assessed, whichever system you use. The same data are required in both, but the organization will differ. The differences in the assessment systems are based on differing approaches to organizing concepts regarding people and nursing. Your instructor may specify that you are to use a particular assessment system. In that instance, you may not need to read the section on the other system. If you are to choose your own assessment system, read through both, comparing and contrasting the terminology and the organization of the data. Be aware that identical information is contained in both sections; it is the organization of that information which differs. Consider both systems in the light of your own approach to nursing and to people, and identify which will work more comfortably for you.

Human Needs Approach

This system for assessment is based on an understanding of the person as oriented around human needs. It is used most often by those who approach nursing from a viewpoint of meeting human needs or preventing interference with the meeting of needs. The physiologic needs are identified separately and the psychosocial needs are grouped together.

ACTIVITY AND REST

This component pertains to the patient's ability to move and exercise for optimal functioning. Consider the patient's usual exercise at home, diversional choices, and the effects of exercise. Any recent variation from the norm, such as joint or muscle pain or disability, is important. The individual's posture and positioning and the level of activity ordered by the physician are other items of concern. Note the pathophysiology of bones, joints, and muscles, as well as the use of traction, bedboards, or assistive devices. Note also any medications prescribed for the patient that relate to this area. Sleep patterns and the need for rest are considered here.

CIRCULATION

Under this category, collect all data that relate to the delivery of nutrients and oxygen to the cells and the removal of wastes from the cells. Objective data include pulse and blood pressure; color of the skin; medications taken for heart, blood pressure, or other cardiovascular problems; as well as any symptoms the patient has that are specific to cardiovascular problems. Include laboratory data that relate to hematology and blood chemistry in this category.

Fluid and electrolyte balance are very important components of circulatory data. List intravenous fluids being given and the status of any site of entry into the circulatory system.

During your interview, try to elicit the patient's perception of any current cardiovascular problem and his or her understanding of previous problems.

COMFORT

The comfort component includes the nature of pain and its location, the duration of pain, the patient's perception of its intensity, the pathophysiology involved, the time pain has been present, and all medications used for its control. Sometimes it is more appropriate to list pain under another area, for example, when the pain is known to relate to a specific problem.

ELIMINATION

This category pertains to the excretion of wastes from the large intestine and the urinary system. Observe the patient's bowel habits and the type and frequency of stools. Listen for bowel tones. Ask about the patient's normal pattern of bowel movements and characteristics of the stool, noting those that are unusual. Elicit any history of constipation or diarrhea, along with pertinent information about medication. Be aware of the pathophysiology of the GI system, as well as of any relevant medications or laboratory tests ordered by the physician.

The urinary system pertains to the excretion of waste products by the kidneys via the urethra and bladder. Note usual patterns of urination and the appearance and odor of the urine. Consider the presence of a catheter of any kind or a problem with incontinence. Measure urinary output and compare it to fluid intake. Note any urinary pathophysiology and medications taken for urinary problems.

NUTRITION

This category deals with getting nutrients into the body. Observe the patient's eating habits (the amount of food taken and the kinds of foods preferred). Ask the patient about food likes and dislikes, dietary modification, and history in regard to food intake. Consider the patient's knowledge of proper nutrition as well as his or her understanding of any special dietary restrictions. Also, you may have to note the patient's fluid intake in terms of both content and quantity.

OXYGENATION

This category includes all data concerned with getting oxygen into the lungs and carbon dioxide out of the lungs. Gather information on breathing patterns and/or changes in breathing patterns, including rate, depth, and rhythm of respirations. Check breath sounds. Look for indications of impaired airways or signs or symptoms of difficulty in respiration. Note the patient's need for oxygen: coughing, suctioning, medications used at home as well as currently, and pathophysiology, if any, are important factors.

PSYCHOSOCIAL DATA

These data include the patient's ability to communicate, level of understanding, educational background, socioeconomic and occupational factors that could influence health status (for example, health insurance and job security), and previous hospitalizations or contacts with nurses and responses to them. Note the effects of family problems and relationships, including age, marital status, and sex, on the nursing needs of the patient. The patient's response to care, behavioral manifestations of anxiety, and feelings regarding his or her status are also important considerations.

SAFETY

These data include the total environment and its effect on the patient. Consider the environment both in light of the patient's ability to respond to it and in terms of safety from microorganisms for the patient as well as for others. Include data concerning the position of side rails, procedures for handwashing, provisions for isolation, and care of equipment. Consider also such factors as room temperature, cleanliness, drafts, lighting, and noise. Note whether the patient is able to reach the call light. Also note the accommodations (private or nonprivate room), the impact of other patients on your patient, and the location of the patient's room in relation to the nurses' station.

Include levels or states of consciousness and sleep patterns in these data. Note visual and auditory acuity or lack of it, and sensitivity to touch or lack of it. Be sure to include the pathophysiology of the nervous system (unconsciousness, tremor, and the like), and any related observations you have made.

SEXUALITY

Gather information about sexual difficulties, menstruation, and menopause. Note medications taken or pathophysiology that relates to the reproductive system.

SKIN INTEGRITY AND HYGIENE

The condition of the skin—its turgor, hydration, color, lesions, wounds, rashes, scars, tattoos, and needle injection scars—should be noted. It is also important to list any sensitivity of the skin to soaps or lotions. Finally, include hygienic needs, among them the care of mouth, hair, and nails.

Body Systems Approach

The body systems approach to assessment is based on organizing data according to the anatomic-physiologic divisions of the body. It is often favored by those who see it as more easily fitting into the systems used by other health care professionals; data, therefore, are more easily communicated through-

out the health care system. This approach to nursing is based on dealing with imbalances or disturbances in basic body systems. In order to encompass the whole person, psychosocial concerns and the patient's environment are included.

CIRCULATORY DATA

Under this category, collect all data that relate to the delivery of nutrients and oxygen to the cells and the removal of wastes from the cells. Objective data include pulse and blood pressure; color of the skin; medications taken for heart, blood pressure, or other cardiovascular problems; as well as any symptoms the patient has that are specific to cardiovascular problems. Include laboratory data that relate to hematology and blood chemistry in this category.

Fluid and electrolyte balance are very important components of circulatory data. List intravenous fluids being given and the status of any site of entry into the circulatory system.

During your interview, try to elicit the patient's perception of any current cardiovascular problem and his or her understanding of previous problems.

ENVIRONMENTAL DATA

These data include the total environment and its effect on the patient. Consider the environment both in light of the patient's ability to respond to it and in terms of safety from microorganisms for the patient as well as for others. Include data concerning the position of side rails, procedures for handwashing, provisions for isolation, and care of equipment. Consider also such factors as room temperature, cleanliness, drafts, lighting, and noise. Note whether the patient is able to reach the call light. Also note the accommodations (private or nonprivate room), the impact of other patients on your patient, and the location of the patient's room in relation to the nurses' station.

GASTROINTESTINAL DATA

This category deals with getting nutrients into the body and excreting wastes from the large intestine. Observe the patient's eating habits (the amount of food taken and the kinds of foods preferred). Interview the patient about food likes and dislikes, dietary modification, and history in regard to food intake. Observe the patient's bowel habits and the type and frequency of stools. Listen for bowel tones. Ask about the patient's normal pattern of bowel movements and characteristics of the stool, noting those that are unusual. Elicit any history of constipation or diarrhea, along with pertinent information about medication. Be aware of the pathophysiology of the GI system, as well as of any relevant medications or laboratory tests ordered by the physician.

GENITO-URINARY DATA

This approach combines the genital and urinary systems because of their close proximity in the female and their interrelationship in the male. In terms of the genital or reproductive area, gather information about sexual difficulties, menstruation, and menopause. Note medications taken or pathophysiology that relates to the reproductive system.

The urinary system pertains to the excretion of waste products by the kidneys via the urethra and bladder. Note usual patterns of urination and the appearance and odor of the urine. Consider the presence of a catheter of any kind or a problem with incontinence. Measure urinary output and compare it to fluid intake. Note any urinary pathophysiology and medications taken for urinary problems.

INTEGUMENTARY DATA

Integument concerns the condition of the skin and mucous membranes. The condition of the skin—its turgor, hydration, color, lesions, wounds, rashes, scars, tattoos, and needle injection scars—should be noted. It is also important to list any sensitivity of the skin to soaps or lotions. Finally, include hygienic needs, among them the care of mouth, hair, and nails.

MUSCULOSKELETAL DATA

This component pertains to the patient's ability to move and exercise for optimal functioning. Consider the patient's usual exercise at home, diversional choices, and the effects of exercise. Any recent variation from the norm, such as joint or muscle pain or disability, is important. The individual's posture and positioning and the level of activity ordered by the physician are other items of concern. Note the pathophysiology of bones, joints, and muscles, as well as the use of traction, bedboards, or assistive devices. Note also any medications prescribed for the patient that relate to this area.

NEURAL DATA

The nervous system includes all characteristics associated with both the central nervous system and the autonomic nervous system, including special senses and pain. Levels or states of consciousness and sleep patterns are included in these data. Special senses include visual and auditory acuity or lack of it, and sensitivity to touch or lack of it. The pain component includes the nature of pain and its location, the duration of pain, the patient's perception of its intensity, the pathophysiology involved, the time pain has been present, and all medications used for its control. Sometimes it is more appropriate to list pain under another area, for example, when the pain is known to relate to a specific problem. Be sure to include the pathophysiology of the nervous system (unconsciousness, tremor, and the like) and any related observations you have made.

PSYCHOSOCIAL DATA

These data include the patient's ability to communicate, level of understanding, educational background, socioeconomic and occupational factors that could influence health status (for example, health insurance and job security), and previous hospitalizations or contacts with nurses and responses to them. Note the effects of family problems and relationships, including age, marital status, and sex, on the nursing needs of the patient. The patient's response to care, behavioral manifestations of anxiety, and feelings regarding his or her status are also important considerations.

RESPIRATORY DATA

This category includes all data concerned with getting oxygen into the lungs and carbon dioxide out of the lungs. Gather information on breathing patterns and/or changes in breathing patterns including rate, depth, and rhythm of respirations. Check breath sounds. Look for indications of impaired airways or signs or symptoms of difficulty in respiration. Note the patient's need for oxygen: coughing, suctioning, medications used at home as well as currently, and pathophysiology, if any, are important factors.

Identifying the Patient's Problem

Once the data are gathered, review them and identify any problems that exist. You will begin with simple, clear-cut deviations from the norm. As you understand more of the pathophysiological and psychosocial aspects of care, you will become more adept at identifying covert problems.

An important aspect of problem identification is that the problem be related to the patient at the moment. For example:

Data
1. Skin over coccyx is red.
2. Patient complains of tenderness over coccyx.
3. Patient does not turn in bed at all. Lies on back continuously.

Problem
Beginning skin breakdown on coccyx due to immobility

This statement of the problem clearly points out the current situation.

Another important aspect of problem identification is that the statement describe the actual problem and underlying causes. Don't state the problem in terms of something a person needs. For instance, using the example above, the problem should not be stated: "Needs to move about more in bed." This statement does not identify what is wrong; it only identifies a possible solution.

ASSESSMENT GUIDE

Patient's Initials _____   Age _____   Date of Admission _____

Student's Name _____

Diagnosis _____

Operation and Date _____

Assessment Category	Data from Patient's Record	Interview	Physical Examination	General Observations	Nursing Problem Identified

QUIZ

Short-Answer Questions

For questions 1–3, provide answers for (a) the human needs approach and (b) the body systems approach.

1. Respiratory rate is included in which assessment category?

    a. _____

    b. _____

2. Chest pain could be listed under which assessment category?

    a. _____

    b. _____

3. A patient tells you he or she can breathe comfortably at night only if resting on two pillows. Under which assessment category should this information be listed?

    a. _____

    b. _____

Multiple-Choice Questions

For questions 4–6, notate (a) patient's record, (b) interview, (c) general observation, or (d) physical examination, whichever applies.

_____ 4. The best source to learn whether a patient has had a bowel movement during your shift.

_____ 5. The best source to learn whether a patient is developing edema (tissue swelling from retained fluid).

_____ 6. For a night nurse, the best source to learn the sleeping patterns of a patient.

For questions 7–10 mark O if the data are objective and S if they are subjective.

_____ 7. The patient says he or she has severe nausea.

_____ 8. After ambulation, the patient is pale and has a pulse rate of 100.

_____ 9. The patient feels depressed.

_____ 10. The patient is breathing shallowly at a rate of 30 respirations per minute.

Module 2 Charting

MAIN OBJECTIVES

To use patients' records to communicate effectively with other health care team members.

   To provide a legal record of the nursing aspect of patients' care.

RATIONALE

The chart, or patient's record, is used by all members of the health care team to follow the patient's progress and to learn what is being done concerning that progress by other members of the team. Entries into the record must be clear. The chart serves as a legal record of care and is used to determine the quality of care being given; therefore accuracy, legibility, and clarity are very important. Finally, each health care facility establishes its own format for patients' records. This format must be used for all charting in the facility.

PREREQUISITES

Successful completion of the following module:

VOLUME 1
Assessment

SPECIFIC LEARNING OBJECTIVES

	Know Facts and Principles	Apply Facts and Principles	Demonstrate Ability	Evaluate Performance
1. Purposes	Explain rationale for use of chart as a legal record, for determining quality of care, and for communication	Given a situation in which someone wants information from a chart, determine whether that should be permitted.	Maintain privacy of patient's record. Use record to gain information regarding patient.	Evaluate own performance
2. Content	List types of information to be recorded. Give rationale for use of objective terminology. State situations in which subjective terminology is appropriate.	Given a situation, do sample charting containing all appropriate information. Given a situation, describe it in objective terminology.	Record all needed information as outlined on Performance Checklist. Use objective terminology for all observations. Identify subjective material clearly. State problems clearly. Describe nursing actions taken. Record evaluation of patient response.	Evaluate own performance using Performance Checklist
3. Styles of charting	List two major styles of charting. List information common to both styles. State information recorded that is unique to POMR.	Given a situation, chart information in both styles	Chart in style appropriate to the facility	Evaluate charting style with instructor

4. Mechanics of charting	Identify special forms used on chart. State the purpose of special forms. State appropriate resource for abbreviations.	Given a situation, state which special form would be used for charting data	Use correct special forms when charting in the clinical areas. Use ink. Indicate date and time on entries. Indicate errors correctly. Complete charting promptly. Maintain privacy of chart. Use correct abbreviations.	Evaluate own performance using Performance Checklist

LEARNING ACTIVITIES

1. Review the Specific Learning Objectives.
2. Review the abbreviations in Ellis and Nowlis, *Nursing: A Human Needs Approach*, or those in the procedure manual of your facility.
3. Read the section on written communication in Ellis and Nowlis, *Nursing: A Human Needs Approach*, or comparable material in another textbook.
4. Look up the module vocabulary terms in the glossary.
5. Read through the module.
6. If samples of charting are available in your practice setting, review them.
7. Practice charting using the situations provided in the module. Make a sample form for practice charting that is similar to the one used in your facility.
8. Exchange your practice charting with another student and check each other's work. Review and rewrite your own charting based on this critique.
9. Have your instructor review your practice charting.
10. Review your instructor's comments and rewrite your practice charting if necessary.
11. Chart data regarding a patient to whom you are assigned. Make a first draft on a piece of paper and have it reviewed by your clinical instructor before you write in the patient's record.
12. Continue to chart on patients assigned in the clinical area. Have your first draft reviewed before writing in the patients' records until your instructor directs you to do otherwise.

VOCABULARY

assessment
data
excretion
flow sheet
graphic
infused
ingested
legibility
military (24-hour) clock
narrative charting
objective
problem-oriented medical record (POMR)
subjective

CHARTING

Charting Content

In order to provide a complete record, you must determine what information to include in your charting. This is a complex responsibility, and one in which you will become more skilled with experience. Basically, you should try to provide a clear and concise record of the nursing process in relation to the individual patient. This includes aspects of assessment, planning, intervention, and evaluation.

Assessment data include both subjective and objective information. Again, you will have to decide which assessment data are relevant in a particular situation. As a general guideline, record assessment data when they reflect (1) findings that relate to the patient's reason for being hospitalized, (2) any abnormal findings, and (3) normal findings that relate to previously noted problems. In addition to these data, you also must record any new problems that you have identified.

Depending on the policies of your facility, *planning data* may or may not be included in the chart. In some institutions, planning is recorded on a separate nursing care plan, which is then included with the rest of a patient's record at the time of discharge.

Intervention data include nursing actions that are taken in response to an existing problem, as well as measures that are planned to prevent problems. Even actions that are part of routine care, such as those related to hygiene, are usually noted in some manner.

Evaluation data, which gauge the effectiveness of nursing actions and therapies, are also important. They are a vital aspect of planning future care.

Styles of Charting

In traditional charting, all these items were written out in prose paragraphs. This was inefficient for both writer and readers. Therefore, most facilities began to alter the system.

Currently, patients' records are organized in two major ways: the narrative style and the problem-oriented medical record (POMR or POR). Both styles of charting contain the following elements:

1. *Data base* This includes the initial history and physical examination, original laboratory and diagnostic test results, the social and financial data, and the admission nursing interview. The particular term *data base* may not be used, but this type of information will be part of the record.
2. *Flow sheets* These are charts or graphs which allow information to be recorded quickly and progress to be monitored with ease. Some facilities use many different flow sheets; others, only a few. Usually, you will use flow sheets to record vital signs, intake and output, medications given, and routine nursing care, although a more-complex parameter such as patient teaching may also be recorded on flow sheets. Again, the term *flow sheet* may not be used, but you will easily recognize the charts and graphs that compose this element.
3. *Progress notes* The most important difference between the two styles of charting is in the structure of their progress notes. In narrative charting, these are often separated: one form for the physician's progress notes, another for nurses' notes, and still others for health care groups (physical therapy, respiratory therapy, occupational therapy). Since narrative charting tends to use few flow sheets, most information is included in the various progress notes. In the POMR style, all progress notes (from all sources) use the same form. The notes have a formal, specific structure (page 22), which makes them easier to use in finding information.

A fourth feature—the problem list—is unique to POMR; it is not found in the narrative style of charting. This list serves as a combination table of contents and index to the patient's condition and progress. Each problem is numbered and titled for easy reference. The date when the problem was initially identified is included and, once the problem is resolved, that fact and the date of resolution are added.

Mechanics of Charting

LEGAL STANDARDS

As a legal record, a chart must conform to certain legal standards. All entries must be in ink so that changes are noticeable and the record is permanent. Your facility may specify that a particular color of ink be used. If it has no policy, remember that black or dark blue ink reproduces especially well on microfilm. *Legibility* is critical: obviously statements that are not legible are not usable.

Errors   If you make an error, draw a line through the incorrect entry so that it remains legible. In the space above, notate "error" and your initials. This practice is traditional. Recently, attorneys have recommended that a brief note as to the nature of the error would be helpful if the chart were needed in a legal proceeding. In that case, you might write "charted on wrong page" and your initials. Either of these notations is legally correct, so follow the policy of your facility. If it has no policy, we recommend the second type of notation.

Spaces   If you are using the narrative form of charting, do not leave blank spaces. Draw a straight line through any empty space to prevent later entries from being made in front of your signature.

Signature   When you sign a notation on a patient's record, use your first initial and full last name followed by the abbreviation of your position. If you were a student nurse named Jane Smith, you would sign the record "J. Smith SN" (unless your facility requires that you sign your full name). Traditionally, student nurses have used the abbreviation *SN* (student nurse) to designate their position. In some areas,

the current practice is to use the abbreviation *NS* (nursing student). Your instructor will indicate the preferred notation in your facility.

You must use the designation appropriate to your current position. For instance, a licensed practical nurse who is currently enrolled in a program preparing registered nurses would use the SN or NS designation while working as a student; the LPN designation would be used only in an LPN working situation.

Time   Notations of time and date are important for health care reasons as well as for legal reasons. Time sequences can be crucial in certain problems.

You can note time in conventional notation or according to the 24-hour clock, or *military clock*. The 24-hour clock works as follows: when the time reaches 12:00 noon (or 1200), instead of returning to 1:00 p.m., the clock goes on to 1300, continuing until 2400 is reached, at midnight. The hours before noon are recorded as 0100, 0200, 0300, and so on. The 24-hour clock eliminates confusion as to whether something took place before noon (a.m.) or after noon (p.m.). In some facilities this confusion is lessened by using different colors of ink for different shifts or different times of the day. This method is quite effective in the original, but when records are photocopied or microfilmed the color distinction is lost and certain colors do not reproduce as well as others.

Right to Privacy   A chart is a legally protected, *private* record of a patient's care. Access to a chart is restricted to those in the facility using it for care and, in some instances, for research or teaching. A chart may not be photocopied except through careful procedures designed to protect the patient's privacy. If, as a student, you are using a chart as a learning tool, it is your responsibility to protect the privacy of the patient by not using his or her name or any identifying statements in any notations you make. Papers or case studies based on a patient's care should likewise protect the anonymity of the patient.

The patient's access to his or her own record is currently a matter of debate. In some places patients have access to their records, in others access is only available through court action, and in still others only certain professional persons (attorneys, doctors) are given access to records on behalf of patients.

SPECIAL TERMINOLOGY AND ABBREVIATIONS

Traditionally, a great deal of specialized medical terminology has been used in charting. In addition, there are traditional patterns of word usage. As a beginner, concentrate on describing what you see. Even if you do not know the medical terminology, you will be understood if you *clearly describe* the situation.

As you progress in your nursing and related studies, you will pick up a large medical vocabulary. Then, you must be careful to use this vocabulary effectively and correctly, as needed. For example, a false belief is called a *delusion*. Rather than chart that a patient has a delusion, chart the exact nature of his or her belief, which is certainly more informative to others using the chart. (It also can save you from jumping to conclusions: sometimes that which appears to be a false belief is true.)

Abbreviations are used in charting to save time and space. Most nursing texts include a list of common abbreviations; and health care facilities often have a list of approved abbreviations. Although certain abbreviations are used standardly, others are used only in one geographic area. When in doubt, use the full term, which will be understood regardless of local custom. This is particularly true for simple initial-type abbreviations.

Sentences are typically reduced to their essential components in charting. Thus articles (a, an, the) and even verbs may be omitted. Because the entire chart is about an individual patient, the subject of a sentence is omitted when it represents the patient (See Example 1.) Do not omit the subject if it represents someone other than the patient. Also, be careful when you omit words that your meaning remains clear.

CHART FORMS

Many different chart forms are in use. It is important that you become familiar with all of the forms used in your facility, so that you know where to look for information you need as well as where to record your own data. The ones to concentrate on initially are those that are the nurses' responsibility to maintain. These usually include a graphic chart for vital signs, an intake and output record, a checklist for routine care, a medication record, and the nursing progress notes. Other forms that may be your responsibility are the parenteral fluid record, the diabetic record (for recording urine testing, blood sugar results, and insulin given), the blood pressure graph, and the patient teaching flow sheet.

Writing Progress Notes

NARRATIVE CHARTING   Narrative charting, as the name indicates, is a narration or telling, of information. Most narrative charting is time sequenced. You begin your statement with data that were observed or that occurred first and move forward in time. This type of narration is easy to follow, and most persons find that it traces thought patterns well. There can be difficulty, however, in trying to find relevant data regarding a single problem, since a great deal of material must be read to gather a small amount of data. Thus, individual hospitals have made some modifications of narrative charting. Checklists and graphs are sometimes used for routine information; and the narration itself may be organized according to anatomical systems or assessment categories. In this case, you would chart, in a time sequence, all the information available on one area before going on to another category. (See Examples 2–4.)

Example 1   Using a Minimum Number of Words

Thought: The patient ate all of the soft diet.
Charted: Ate all of soft diet.

Thought: Bedbath was given to the patient by the nurse.
Charted: Bedbath given.

Example 2   Simple Narrative Charting

1/1/80

7:00 a.m.	a.m. care. Up in chair c̄ assistance. IV running @ 22 gtt/min. Drsg. dry.
7:30 a.m.	Ate all of soft diet.
8:00 a.m.	Returned to bed. 250 ml clear straw-colored urine. Moderate-sized, soft, dark brown BM. Pain medication given for abd. incisional pain. Relief in 15 min.
8:30 a.m.	Complete bedbath given. ROM done.
9:00–10:30 a.m.	Rested quietly in bed. No c/o pain. J. Jones RN

Example 3   Modified Narrative Charting

1/1/80

7:00–10:30 a.m.   Hygiene: a.m. care ā bkfst. Complete bedbath.
Activity: Up in chair c̄ assistance for bkfst. ROM p̄ bath. Rested in bed p̄ bath.
Nutrition: Ate all of soft diet.
Elimination: Voided clear amber urine—250 ml @ 8:00. BM—moderate, soft, dark brown @ 8:00.
Pain: c/o abd. incisional pain @ 8:00. Pain med. given. Relief in 15 min. No further pain in a.m.
Fluid & Elec.: IV @ 22 gtt/min.   J. Jones RN

Example 4   Modified Narrative Charting

1/1/80

7:00–10:30 a.m.   Circ.: IV @ 22 gtt/min. Drsg. dry.
GI: Ate all of soft diet. Mod. am't soft, dark brown BM @ 8:00
GU: Urine—voided 250 ml, clear amber, @ 8:00.
Musc-Skel.: Up in chair c̄ assistance. ROM p̄ bath. Rested p̄ bath.
Neur.: c/o incisional pain @ 8:00. Pain med. given. Relief in 15 min. No further pain in a.m.   J. Jones RN

PROBLEM-ORIENTED MEDICAL RECORDS

In this style, progress notes are written for significant data regarding any problem; and detailed data may be entered by any member of the health care team. Use the following format *(sometimes all components are not included)*:

Problem   Identified by number and title
Subjective data   The patient's perception or statements regarding the problem
Objective data   Your observation regarding the problem and data from the chart that are relevant (for example, temperature and blood pressure)
Assessment   Your interpretation of the meaning of the data (This is a slightly different meaning for *assessment* than we commonly use. Some persons call this *analysis*.)
Plan   Your plan of action to deal with the problem

This format is commonly called *SOAP notation,* and the process has been called *SOAPing* (see Examples 5–7), from the terms *S*ubjective, *O*bjective, *A*ssessment, and *P*lan. SOAPing may be used for progress notes even when the entire record is not a POMR.

On occasion, facilities modify the POMR and use a more traditional style for progress notes. It is also common for facilities to make individual modifications in charting style.

Charting Procedure

When you are ready to chart, review all the activities in which you have engaged and the assessments you have made. Consider your plans for the future and your evaluation of the patient's response to care. Be sure to consider such things as drainage and excretions; substances ingested or infused; the condition of all devices, tubes, and dressings; the feelings and concerns of the patient; and all the patient's activities.

Example 5   POMR Progress Note (SOAPing)

4. Abdominal pain
S States pain relieved by passing flatus but has not been able to pass flatus.
O Abd. feels tense and hard. Guards when moving.
A Has retained gas.
P Increase ambulation. Encourage movement in bed.   J. Jones RN

Example 6   POMR Progress Note (SOAPing)

3. Dyspnea on exertion
S States cannot walk farther than doorway without shortening of breath. Feels as if cannot get enough air.
O Resp. 24, shallow, rales over both lung bases. Became cyanotic when moving to chair.
A Fluid in lungs causing decreased aerating surface. Not enough O_2 exchange for activity.
P Minimize activity. Provide supportive care to lessen O_2 need. Encourage coughing and deep breathing and turning to remove secretions.
                                                   J. Jones RN

Example 7   Sample SOAPing Notation for POMR

8/10/80
1600   Temporary problem: Missing hearing aid
S Wife thought it was with patient when he entered through Emergency Room.
O Hearing aid not listed in initial personal effects list and not found in belongings.
A ———————
P 1. Emergency room to be contacted
    2. Wife to search at home for hearing aid
    3. Recheck tomorrow evening when wife visits
                                                   J. Jones RN

8/11/80
1700   Temporary problem: missing hearing aid, resolved: Wife brought in hearing aid this evening.   J. Jones RN

8/11/80
2000   3. Urinary incontinence
S States: "I think I'm doing better. I was only wet once today."
O Voiding when offered urinal on q2h schedule. See flow sheet.
A ———————
P Continue bladder rehab. program without change.
                                                   J. Jones RN

Start with the specialized checklists and graphs in the chart. Fill each one in appropriately. The forms will help you to remember what data need to be recorded. Go over each form thoroughly to make sure you have not forgotten anything. Then, sign each form as required by your facility.

Next, turn to the form on which you will record your nursing progress notes (the nurses' notes or progress notes). Chart your relevant assessment data, both objective and subjective, and new problems. Then, using the narrative style, record actions you have taken, something not necessarily done in the POMR style. Using the POMR style, record future plans in the chart. Using the narrative style, consider where plans are recorded (perhaps in a separate nursing care plan) and make a note to yourself to add to or alter the nursing plan. Record your evaluation of the patient's response to care. Be sure that you organize your information in the style required by your facility. Do not duplicate information already recorded on a checklist or flow sheet unless your facility expressly requires duplication. Duplicating records not only wastes time, it also makes the record more cumbersome. Finally, sign your charting as required.

After you have finished, go back and double-check all that you have done to make sure that dates, times, and signatures are present and correct. Reread your progress notes to make sure that they are legible and understandable. Although as a student you will be expected to write out your charting on separate paper for approval before putting it in the actual record, you should develop the habit of double-checking yourself. It is very easy to forget a time or signature. Although it might make the record less neat in appearance, correcting errors or adding information that was omitted may be essential to the accuracy and clarity of the record.

PRACTICE CASES

Case 1

You worked as a student nurse from 7:00 a.m. until 10:30 a.m. During that time you cared for Mr. Oscar Johanson. He is sixty-six years old and is in the hospital for bronchial pneumonia. This is his third hospital day. You assisted him with a bedbath; you washed his back and legs and he did the rest. He sat in a chair while you made his bed. At the end of 15 minutes, he felt tired and asked to return to bed. For breakfast he was served and ate hot cereal with cream, toast with butter and jelly, orange juice, and coffee. His blood pressure was 146/84, his pulse was 78, and his respirations were 22. He coughed intermittently, but the cough was nonproductive.

Case 2

You worked as a student nurse from 4:30 p.m. to 8:30 p.m., caring for Mrs. Effie Sturdevan. She is forty-five years old and had a hysterectomy five days ago. Her post-op course has proceeded smoothly. She had a soft diet for dinner and had a large, soft bowel movement after dinner. She complained of abdominal pain and was given a pain pill by the medication nurse at 7:00 p.m. During visiting hours her husband and daughter were present. After they left you observed that she was quiet, did not speak, and had tear-stained cheeks. You helped her to ambulate at 4:30 p.m. and again at 8:00 p.m. Then you helped her get ready for bed and gave her a back rub. While you were giving her the back rub, she said that she knew the surgery had been necessary but she somehow felt like a different person. After you had listened to her for ten minutes she seemed more relaxed and said she felt she would be able to sleep.

Case 3

You worked as a student nurse from 0700 to 1200, caring for Mr. John Steiner, age thirty-six. He is recovering from surgery to repair a right inguinal hernia. This is his second post-op day, and you helped him bathe himself and gave him back care. For breakfast he ate one egg and a slice of toast, and drank a cup of coffee. You assisted him in ambulating the length of the hall and back, after which he asked for and was given his pain medication. His vital signs were T, 98^8 (o); P, 78; R, 14; BP, 134/86. His pulse and respiration were unchanged after ambulation.

Case 4

During clinical laboratory practice, from 1300 to 1600, you cared for Mrs. Jennie Johnson, age seventy-seven. She had a mild stroke two weeks ago, has some difficulty speaking, and cannot use her right arm. You washed her hair and set it, read a newspaper article to her, and helped her select her menu for the next day. She understood what you asked her about the menu and nodded yes or no about food selection. She could not comb her hair with her left hand; she held the comb awkwardly and kept dropping it. Her speech was not clear, but with enough time, she made some appropriate verbal responses. She said, "Toilet," and urinated when taken to the bathroom. Her right arm was in a supportive sling. When you took her arm out to exercise it, her elbow flexed easily but her shoulder was stiff.

Case 5

Your clinical time was from 0700 to 1100. You were assigned to care for Mrs. Dorothy Wu, age eighty-eight. Mrs. Wu was transferred from a nursing home for diagnostic studies. She is totally dependent and on complete bed rest. You did complete morning hygiene, including a bedbath and oral, nail, and hair care. You turned her every two hours and gave her a back massage each time you turned her. At 0800 you fed her breakfast. She took a bowl of oatmeal, a dish of applesauce, and a glass of milk (240 ml.); she would not take coffee and could not chew toast because she had no dentures. She was incontinent of urine twice and had an incontinent stool after breakfast.

Case 6

Between the hours of 3:00 p.m. and 7:00 p.m., you cared for Mr. Joseph Gonzales, age thirty-eight. He had surgery for repair of a right inguinal hernia at 8:00 a.m. today. He returned to the surgical nursing unit from the postanesthesia room at 12:00 noon.

You took his blood pressure, pulse, and respiration every two hours, and they were as follows: 4:00 p.m. 130/82, 68, 14; 6:00 p.m. 128/82, 66, 16. He took 200 ml liquid during the four hours you were present and had no nausea. You helped him to walk to the bathroom to stand to void. He voided 150 ml. When you examined his dressing you noted that there was no drainage and the dressing was clean. He had pain in the incisional area and you gave him Demerol 50 mg IM at 6:00 p.m. He stated this relieved his pain. He moved about in bed with ease and deep-breathed well when directed to do so.

PERFORMANCE CHECKLIST

Mechanics	Unsatisfactory	Needs more practice	Satisfactory	Comments
1. Ink used				
2. Legible				
3. No erasures—errors drawn through and identified				
4. Dated				
5. Time noted				
6. Signed				
7. Material not unnecessarily duplicated				
8. Brief				
9. Correct abbreviations used				
10. Signature				
Type of charting				
1. Correct style of charting used				
2. Correct location or form used for each category of information				

Content	Unsatisfactory	Needs more practice	Satisfactory	Comments
1. Data clear to another person				
2. Terms used are objective, descriptive				
3. Subjective material clearly identified as such				

4. All appropriate data included
   a. Assessment
     (1) Complete assessment for initial data base
        if needed				

(2) Assessments related to presenting or existing problem				
(3) Drainage and excretions				
(4) Substances ingested or infused				
(5) Condition of all devices, tubes, and dressings				
(6) Feelings and concerns of patient				
(7) Activities of patient				
b. Identification of problems				
c. Nursing actions taken				
d. Evaluation of effectiveness of nursing actions				
e. Routine items noted (baths and the like) (1) Checklist (if applicable)				
(2) On notes (if applicable)				

QUIZ

Multiple-Choice Questions

_____ 1. Ink is used for all charting because (1) it looks neater; (2) it is more permanent; (3) changes or erasures can be seen; (4) it is a custom.

   a. 1 and 2
   b. 2 and 3
   c. 3 and 4
   d. 1 and 4

_____ 2. If a 24-hour clock is in use, the correct term for 4:00 p.m. would be

   a. 0400.
   b. 0800.
   c. 1600.
   d. 2000.

_____ 3. In problem-oriented medical records, the progress notes are often written in a standard form. This form is abbreviated

   a. SOAP.
   b. SOLD.
   c. COAP.
   d. PROP.

Short-Answer Questions

4. What are the two major styles of charting?

   a. _____

   b. _____

5. Why should objective terminology be used in charting? _____

6. In the following sample, underline the subjective terms:

   Is depressed and crying. Upset over
   upcoming surgery. Paced the room for
   an hour before bedtime.

7. On the following charting sample an error was made in the quantity of urine. The correct amount was 175 ml. Correct the sample as if it were a real chart.

   Up in chair for 30 min. No sign of fatigue. Assisted to BR to urinate. 225
   ml. clear yellow urine.

8. Who may legally read a patient's chart? _____

Module 3 Medical Asepsis

MAIN OBJECTIVE

To apply principles of medical asepsis when practicing all aspects of nursing, with particular emphasis on handwashing.

RATIONALE

Persons who have health problems are frequently more susceptible to infections than are those who do not. In addition, more pathogenic strains of microorganisms are found in hospitals than anywhere else.

Because the nurse may be in contact with a number of patients during any given day, it is especially important to be aware of the principles of medical asepsis, to avoid transferring microorganisms from a patient to the nurse, from the nurse to a patient, from the nurse to a co-worker, or from one patient to another. Microorganisms can also be transferred from equipment.

PREREQUISITES

None

SPECIFIC LEARNING OBJECTIVES

	Know Facts and Principles	Apply Facts and Principles	Demonstrate Ability	Evaluate Performance
1. *Movement of microorganisms*	State five ways micro-organisms move from one area to another	Given a situation, state methods to prevent micro-organisms from moving from dirty to clean items or areas		
2. *Personal hygiene* *a. Hair* *b. Fingernails* *c. Jewelry*	State personal hygiene guidelines related to hair, fingernails, and jewelry	Describe manner of fixing own hair that conforms to guidelines given	Wear hair short or restrained. Keep fingernails clean and trimmed. Do not wear jewelry in clinical facility.	Evaluate own performance with instructor using Performance Checklist
3. *Handwashing*	State when handwashing is indicated	State rationale for washing hands before and after each patient contact, before handling food, after using toilet, after blowing nose or sneezing, and after touching hair	Wash hands at appropriate times	Evaluate own performance with instructor using Performance Checklist
4. *Procedure* *a. Friction* *b. Running water* *c. Cleansing agents*	State effect of friction, running water, and cleansing agents on handwashing. Describe correct handwashing techniques.	State rationale for use of friction, running water, and cleansing agents during handwashing	Employ friction, running water, and cleansing agent when washing hands, using correct handwashing techniques	Evaluate own performance with instructor using Performance Checklist
5. *Medical asepsis related to general nursing* *a. Handling linens* *b. Disposition of soiled articles*	State medical asepsis guidelines related to handling linens and disposition of soiled articles	State rationale for holding linen away from uniform, not shaking or tossing linen, keeping clean items separate from dirty items	Hold linen away from uniform. Do not shake or toss linen Keep clean items separate from dirty items.	Evaluate own performance with instructor using Performance Checklist

LEARNING ACTIVITIES

1. Review the Specific Learning Objectives.
2. Read the section on asepsis (in the chapter on infection), in Ellis and Nowlis, *Nursing: A Human Needs Approach,* or comparable material in another textbook.
3. Look up the module vocabulary terms in the glossary.
4. Read through the module.
5. Arrange for time to practice handwashing techniques.
6. In the practice setting, practice safe handwashing techniques using the procedure as a guide and the Performance Checklist as an evaluation tool. When you are satisfied with your ability, have your instructor evaluate you.
7. In the clinical setting, demonstrate handwashing to your clinical instructor.

VOCABULARY

bacteria
barrier
contaminate
droplet nuclei
friction
medical asepsis
microorganism
pathogenic organism

MEDICAL ASEPSIS

How Microorganisms Spread

Microorganisms move through space on air currents. Because of this movement, avoid shaking or tossing linens, motions that create air currents on which microorganisms can be transported. For this reason, most hospitals are built so that the ventilation system does not circulate air from one section to another. Be sure that all doors leading to isolation rooms are kept closed to stop air currents.

Microorganisms are transferred from one surface to another whenever one object touches another. There are both clean and dirty items in a hospital. Even among ostensibly clean items, some are more clean than others. When a clean item touches a less-clean item, it becomes "dirty," because microorganisms (which are not visible) are transferred to it. Therefore, keep your hands away from your own hair and face, keep linens away from your uniform, and always keep clean items separate from dirty ones. If you drop anything on the floor, consider it dirty.

Proper handwashing removes many of the microorganisms that would be transferred by the hands from one item to another. Therefore, wash your hands, not only when they are soiled, but whenever you move from one patient to another, or from patient contact to contact with the general environment or vice versa.

Microorganisms move from one object to another as a result of gravity when one item is held above another. Avoid passing dirty items over clean items or areas because it is possible for microorganisms to drop off onto a clean item or area. When storing items in a bedside stand, place clean items on upper shelves and potentially dirty items, such as bedpans, on lower shelves.

Microorganisms are released into the air on droplet nuclei whenever a person breathes or speaks. Coughing or sneezing dramatically increases the number of microorganisms released from the mouth and nose. Avoid having a patient breathe directly into your face, and avoid breathing directly into a patient's face. Whenever you have coughed, sneezed, or blown your nose, wash your hands before touching anything else. If you handle tissues that a patient has used when coughing or sneezing, always wash your hands thoroughly.

Microorganisms move slowly on dry surfaces but very quickly through moisture. For this reason, use a dry paper towel when you turn off faucets, and dry a bath basin before you return it to a bedside stand for storage.

Handwashing

One of the most effective methods to prevent the transfer of bacteria is correct and frequent handwashing. Properly done, handwashing protects the patient, your coworkers, and you and your family as well.

For medical aseptic purposes, we recommend that a 2-minute handwashing procedure be carried out at the beginning of every work shift and after each situation in which you might have been in contact with pathogenic organisms (for example, after handling urine, stool, or sputum specimens, or after working in an isolation situation). At other times, a more abbreviated, but still complete, procedure can be used.

Friction, running water, and a cleansing agent are necessary to remove microorganisms and/or other material that may be present on the hands. A deep sink with controls that can be operated by foot, leg, or elbow is ideal for handwashing. In situations where faucets are operated by hand, it is common practice to use a dry paper towel as a barrier in turning the water *off* because a dirty hand was used to turn it on. Because the handwashing procedure causes microorganisms to accumulate in the sink, it is important that you avoid touching the sink as you wash and also avoid splashing dirty water on your uniform.

HANDWASHING PROCEDURE

1. Roll your sleeves above your elbows and remove your watch. If your watch has an expansion band, you may simply move it up above your elbow.
2. Turn on the water and adjust the temperature. Warm water removes fewer oils from the skin than does hot water, and it is more effective in removing microorganisms than is cold water.
3. Dispense liquid or powdered soap, preferably with a foot control. Bar soap is not recommended because it may harbor microorganisms. If only bar soap is available, lather and rinse the bar thoroughly to remove the outside layer of soap before you use it.
4. Lather your hands and arms well.
5. Clean your fingernails as needed with a nail file or orange stick. (If these utensils are not provided, do this before you leave home.)
6. Wash your hands and arms up to your elbows, adding soap as needed to maintain a lather. Keep your hands lower than your elbows at all times.
   a. Use a rotary motion (as opposed to back and forth) and friction.
   b. Pay particular attention to the areas between your fingers and to your knuckles.
7. Holding your hands and forearms lower than your elbows, rinse thoroughly, starting at one elbow and moving down the arm. Then repeat this step for the other arm. This position prevents microorganisms from being rinsed up your arms.
8. Repeat steps 4, 6, and 7.
9. Dry your hands thoroughly. Most facilities provide paper towels for this purpose. Blotting, rather than rubbing, with a paper towel is easier on the skin.
10. Use a dry paper towel to turn off the faucet if it is hand operated.
11. Use lotion if needed to maintain your skin condition. In some settings you may be asked not to use lotion because it can be an excellent medium for bacterial growth.

ABBREVIATED HANDWASHING PROCEDURE

This procedure is frequently used during the care of a single patient or when moving from relatively clean tasks to new tasks. The differences are minimal.

1. Wash well above the wrists; washing up to the elbows is not usually necessary.
2. Do not clean nails routinely.
3. Lather and rinse only once instead of twice.

Personal Hygiene

Obviously, in order to enhance medical asepsis, you must practice good personal hygiene. Also, it is much more pleasant for patients to be near someone who smells fresh and who is wearing a clean uniform. Use the following important guidelines for personal hygiene:

1. Style hair in such a way that it does not fall forward when you lean forward (as for example, when you examine a patient). When hair falls over an area, microorganisms can drop from the hair (by gravity) onto the patient, or the hair itself may fall onto trays or wounds. Keep your hair short or restrain it in some way so that it does not fall forward. Also avoid any style in which you are constantly brushing your hair out of your eyes. Your hair is usually less clean than your hands because it is not washed as frequently. In addition, if your hands have been contaminated by contact with a patient, you will transfer microorganisms from them to your hair and near your face, where they remain until your next shampoo.
2. Keep your fingernails clean and trimmed or filed short, so as not to endanger patients by scratching them or by harboring bacteria. If you use polish, it

must be intact; chipped polish is also a place for bacteria to lodge.

3. Jewelry, too, is a place for microorganisms to lodge; therefore, wear only a minimum. Plain studs or posts for pierced ears and plain wedding bands are the most jewelry you should wear in a clinical setting. Necklaces and large hoop or dangling earrings are not only a hazard in terms of medical asepsis; a patient can grab them and hurt both you and the jewelry.

These guidelines often are not enforced by the employing agency; therefore, your knowledge of the rationale for such guidelines and your conscience must guide your actions.

PERFORMANCE CHECKLIST

Medical asepsis related to general nursing	Unsatisfactory	Needs more practice	Satisfactory	Comments
1. Hold linen away from uniform.				
2. Do not shake or toss linen.				
3. Keep clean items separate from dirty ones.				

Handwashing

1. Roll sleeves above elbows and remove watch.				
2. Do not touch outside or inside of sink.				
3. Turn on water and adjust temperature.				
4. Lather hands and arms well using rotary motion.				
5. Clean fingernails.				
6. Hold hands and forearms lower than elbows. Wash with running water, using rotary motion and giving special attention to areas between fingers. Leave water running during entire procedure.				
7. Wash hands and arms to elbows twice.				
8. Rinse thoroughly, keeping hands lower than elbows.				
9. Dry hands thoroughly.				
10. Turn off water with paper towel if faucet is hand operated.				

Personal hygiene

1. Keep hair restrained.				
2. Keep fingernails clean and short.				
3. Do not wear jewelry.				

QUIZ

Multiple-Choice Questions

_C_ **1.** How long should you wash your hands at the beginning of a work shift to provide for medical asepsis?

    a. 30 seconds
    b. 1 minute
    c. 2 minutes
    d. 4 minutes

_D_ **2.** Which of the following are essential components of the handwashing procedure? (1) friction; (2) running water; (3) foot-operated water controls; (4) cleansing agent

    a. 1 only
    b. 1 and 4
    c. 2, 3, and 4
    d. 1, 2, and 4

_D_ **3.** Which of the following areas should the nurse _not_ touch during the handwashing procedure? (1) the inside of the sink; (2) the outside of the sink; (3) a hand-controlled faucet; (4) own hair

    a. 1 only
    b. 2 only
    c. 1, 2, and 3
    d. All of these

_B_ **4.** Which of the following should receive attention during the handwashing procedure? (1) palms; (2) elbows; (3) spaces between the fingers; (4) fingernails

    a. 1 and 4
    b. 1, 3, and 4
    c. 2, 3, and 4
    d. All of these

Module 4 Basic Body Mechanics

MAIN OBJECTIVE

To apply the principles of good body mechanics so as to conserve energy and decrease the potential for strain, injury, and fatigue for the nurse, and to promote the safety of patients.

RATIONALE

A nurse engaged in clinical practice daily performs a variety of physical tasks, including reaching, stooping, lifting, carrying, pushing, and pulling. Practiced incorrectly, any of these has the potential to cause strain, fatigue, or injury to the nurse and/or to threaten the safety of patients. Practiced correctly, using the principles of body mechanics, the nurse will move smoothly and surely, minimizing personal strain and enhancing the safety, comfort, and confidence of patients.

PREREQUISITES

None

41

SPECIFIC LEARNING OBJECTIVES

	Know Facts and Principles	Apply Facts and Principles	Demonstrate Ability	Evaluate Performance
1. *Principles of body mechanics*	State principles of body mechanics	Given a situation, correctly identify which principles could apply and state why	In the clinical setting, apply principles of body mechanics correctly	Evaluate own performance with instructor using Performance Checklist

LEARNING ACTIVITIES

1. Review the Specific Learning Objectives.
2. Read the section on posture and body mechanics for the nurse (in the chapter on activity and rest) in Ellis and Nowlis, *Nursing: A Human Needs Approach,* or comparable material in another textbook.
3. Look up the module vocabulary terms in the glossary.
4. Read through the module.
5. In the practice setting, with a partner observing:
    a. Stand with your weight balanced over your base of support.
    b. Stand 3 feet from a table or counter. Try to place a book on the table without enlarging your base of support. Return to where you started and place the book on the table using an enlarged base of support. Compare your stability in the two situations.
    c. Stand in a normal position. Have your partner take your arms and pull until you begin to tip forward. Using the same base of support, squat low and have your partner pull again. Compare the force needed to disrupt your stability in the two positions.
    d. Stand with your feet 8 inches apart, but side to side, and try to push a bed. Now enlarge your base of support in the direction toward which you are pushing and note the difference.
    e. Practice tightening your abdominal muscles upward and your gluteal muscles downward. Relax. Tighten the muscles again. Do this before you attempt any task.
    f. Pick an object up from the floor or other low surface by bending the knees and keeping the back straight.
    g. With your partner as your assistant, try to move another person up in bed with the head of the bed at a 30-degree angle. Now, place the bed in a flat position and repeat the activity.

Compare the amount of energy required. Have your "patient" evaluate his or her experience.

    h. Again, with your partner as your assistant and with the bed in a flat position, move your "patient" up in bed without a turn sheet and against a wrinkled bottom sheet. Now, tighten the bottom sheet and use a turn sheet for the same activity. Compare the experiences. Ask your "patient" to comment.
    i. Hold a 10-pound object (brick, book) with both hands directly in front of and close to your body for three minutes. Now, do the same thing except hold the object at arm's length from your body. Compare the amount of energy required for each task.
    j. With a turn sheet, turn your "patient" from a supine position to a lateral position, using your weight as a counterbalance. Note the ease with which you can do this.
    k. When you feel you have practiced enough, perform all the above tasks *correctly* for your instructor, using your partner as a "patient" as necessary.
6. In the clinical setting, apply basic body mechanics whenever possible. If you are unsure or need help, consult your instructor.

VOCABULARY

base of support
body mechanics
center of gravity
internal girdle
torsion

BASIC BODY MECHANICS

The following principles of body mechanics have been selected because of their applicability to commonly encountered nursing situations. Examples of how they can be applied are included to facilitate your understanding.

1. *Weight is balanced best when the center of gravity is directly above the base provided by the feet.* In this position, you can maintain balance and stability with the least amount of effort. When this posture is *not* maintained, the potential for strain, fatigue, and poor stability is increased (Figure 4.1).

2. *Enlarging the base of support increases the stability of the body.* (Changes in position should not cause the center of gravity to fall beyond the edge of the base.) Therefore, when you assist a patient to move, you will be more stable if your feet are apart than if they are close together.

3. *A person or an object is more stable if the center of gravity is close to the base of support.* Apply this principle by bending at the knees and keeping your back straight (thus keeping the center of gravity directly above and close to the base of support), rather than by bending forward at the waist.

4. *Enlarging the base of support in the direction of the force to be applied increases the amount of force that can be applied.* Place one foot forward when you push a heavy object (such as a bed with a patient in it), or place one foot back when moving a patient toward the side of the bed.

5. *Tightening of the abdominal muscles upward and the gluteal muscles downward before undertaking any activity decreases the chance of strain or injury.*

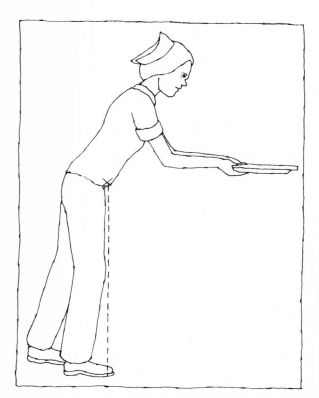 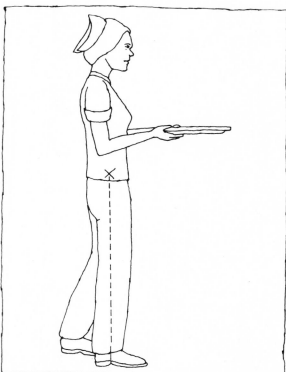

FIGURE 4.1   USING THE BASE OF SUPPORT   *Left:* Center of gravity *(X)* not over base of support (incorrect). *Right:* Center of gravity *(X)* over base of support (correct).

It also protects ligaments and muscles from strain or injury. (We call this putting on the "internal girdle.") If you practice this continually, you will eventually do it automatically when you prepare for any activity.

6. *Facing in the direction of the task to be performed and turning the entire body in one plane (rather than twisting) lessens the susceptibility of the back to injury.* Also, the spine functions less effectively when it is twisted (Figure 4.2).

7. *Lifting is better undertaken by bending the legs and using leg muscles rather than by using the back muscles.* Because large muscles tire less quickly than small muscles, you should use the large gluteal and femoral muscles rather than the smaller muscles of the back (Figure 4.3).

8. *It is easier to move an object on a level surface than to move it against the force of gravity, for example, on a slanted surface.* Therefore, you will need less effort to move a patient up in bed if you first lower the head of the bed.

9. *Less energy is required to move an object when friction between the object and the surface on which it rests is minimized.* Because friction opposes motion, you can make the task of moving a patient in bed easier by working on a smooth surface.

10. *It takes less energy to hold an object close to the body than at a distance from the body; it is also easier to move an object that is close.* This is because the muscles are strongest when contracted and weakest when stretched. Therefore, hold heavy objects close to your body, and move the patient near to your side of the bed (for bathing, for example) to conserve energy.

11. *The weight of the body can be used to assist in lifting or moving.* When you help a patient to stand, you can use the weight of your body by rocking back,

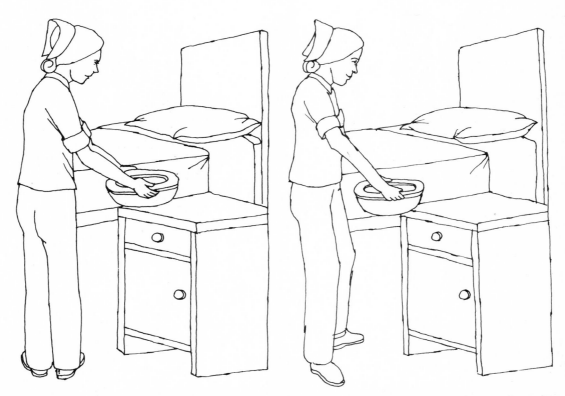

FIGURE 4.2 AVOID TORSION OF THE SPINE *Left:* Nurse twisting to lift basin from bed to table (incorrect). *Right:* Nurse turning whole body to lift basin from bed to table (correct).

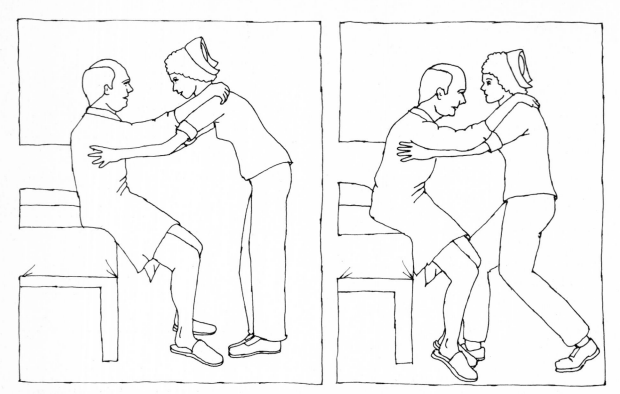

FIGURE 4.3   LIFTING WITH THE LEG MUSCLES   *Left:* Nurse assisting patient to stand, hands under patient's arms, body bent over from waist (incorrect). *Right:* Nurse assisting patient to stand, hands under patient's arms, back straight, knees flexed (correct).

counterbalancing the patient's weight, as illustrated in Figure 4.3. You can use the patient's weight by placing his or her legs in a knees-up position before moving from back to side.

12. *Smooth, rhythmical movements at moderate speed require less energy.* Smooth, continuous motions also are more accurate, safer, and better controlled than sudden, jerky movements.

13. *When a soft object is pushed, it absorbs part of the force being exerted, leaving only a part available to do the moving. When a soft object is pulled, all of the force exerted is available for the task of moving.* Think of patients to be moved as soft objects, and try to use a pulling motion whenever possible.

PERFORMANCE CHECKLIST

	Unsatisfactory	Needs more practice	Satisfactory	Comments
1. Keep weight balanced above base of support.				
2. Enlarge base of support as necessary to increase body's stability.				
3. Lower center of gravity toward base of support as necessary to increase body's stability.				
4. Enlarge base of support in direction in which force is to be applied.				
5. Tighten abdominal and gluteal muscles in preparation for all activities.				
6. Face in direction of task and turn body in one plane.				
7. Bend hips and knees (rather than back) when lifting.				
8. Move objects on level surface when possible.				
9. Slide (rather than lift) objects on smooth surface when possible.				
10. Hold objects close to body and stand close to objects to be moved.				
11. Use body's weight to assist in lifting or moving when possible.				
12. Carry out tasks using smooth motions and reasonable speed.				

QUIZ

True-False Questions

_True___ **1.** The body is less stable when the center of gravity falls beyond the edge of the base of support.

_True___ **2.** Stability is increased when the center of gravity is close to the base of support.

_False__ **3.** Facing in the direction of the task to be performed is not recommended.

_False__ **4.** Friction enhances movement.

_True___ **5.** It takes less energy to hold an object close to the body than at a distance from the body.

_False__ **6.** When carrying out a task, the faster one moves, the better.

Module 5 Feeding Adult Patients

MAIN OBJECTIVE

To feed hospitalized patients who are unable to feed themselves independently.

RATIONALE

The body, during illness, trauma, or wound healing, demands more nutrients than are usually needed. Many patients, because of illness and immobility, are unable to feed themselves all or part of a meal. To ensure the patient's adequate nutrition, the nurse must be knowledgeable and skillful in carrying out the feeding procedure. To promote the patient's well-being, the nurse must also consider the psychological response to being fed.

PREREQUISITES

1. Successful completion of the following modules:

   VOLUME 1
   Assessment
   Charting
   Medical Asepsis

2. Familiarity with the basic diets used in most institutions
3. Knowledge of the five major nutrients needed by all individuals

SPECIFIC LEARNING OBJECTIVES

	Know Facts and Principles	Apply Facts and Principles	Demonstrate Ability	Evaluate Performance
1. *Nutrition*	Name five major categories of nutrients needed by all individuals	When presented with sample diet, ascertain nutritional value in terms of five major categories	If patient's capacity for intake is limited, select most nutritious items for feeding	Determine if nutritional needs are met for particular meal
2. *Diets (routine)*	List diets and their consistency from clear liquid to regular	Choose, from several diets offered, proper diet for particular category	In the clinical setting, check special diet against order before feeding patient	Instructor evaluates accuracy
3. *Preparation* a. *Environment* b. *Patient (physical and psychological)*	List factors in environment that might affect appetite. Describe optimum position for comfort and ease of eating and discuss possible modifications. Discuss emotional needs and responses related to eating.	When at patient's bedside, recognize items to be removed and prepare patient for meal	Carry out preparation	Evaluate own performance regarding patient's satisfaction
4. *Adaptations of procedure*	List factors that often make adaptations to procedure necessary	Assess muscular difficulties, including swallowing problems, and emotional reactions	When feeding patient in the clinical setting, vary the procedure appropriately	Review performance with instructor, considering patient's satisfaction
5. *Retention and tolerance*	List untoward reactions to feeding	Know problems most commonly experienced by patients in care	When caring for patient in the clinical setting, assess afterward for specific responses unique to patient	Share problems with instructor
6. *Recording*	State importance of monitoring food intake of ill patient	Be familiar with portions of food items and terms used. Describe amount of food taken and responses.	After feeding an individual patient, properly record amounts taken and pertinent observations	Show recording to instructor

LEARNING ACTIVITIES

1. Review the Specific Learning Objectives.
2. Read the section on nutrition (in the chapter on nutrition) in Ellis and Nowlis, *Nursing: A Human Needs Approach,* or comparable material in another textbook.
3. Look up the module vocabulary terms in the glossary.
4. Read through the module.
5. Review the steps of the procedure in the Performance Checklist.
6. In the practice setting:
   a. Have a classmate feed you lunch. Try eating half in a recumbent position (lying down) and half in a sitting position in bed. Close your eyes for three minutes while being fed. At this point, have your classmate describe the food to you. Now answer the following questions:
      (1) What was pleasant about the experience?
      (2) What was unpleasant?
   b. Repeat a, only this time you feed your classmate. Discuss the questions from your point of view as the one administering the feeding.
   c. Examine the pictures of feeding aids on page 56. These aids can be purchased commercially or simply made by members of the patient's family or by the physical therapy department.
7. In the clinical setting:
   a. Observe a patient being fed. What was done that was helpful to the patient? What improvements could have been made?
   b. Review the following questions. Now feed a patient an entire meal. Note the time when you begin and end the procedure. Answer the questions for your own learning or discuss them with your instructor.
      (1) How long did the feeding procedure take?
      (2) What conclusions can you draw from the timing?
      (3) What were some of the blocks you encountered to effective feeding?
      (4) What went well?
      (5) Were you uncomfortable at any point?
      (6) Did the patient appear to be uncomfortable at any point?
      (7) Did you use all the steps of the procedure?
      (8) Did you have to make adaptations? If so, in what way?
      (9) Why were adaptations made?
   d. Record, on a piece of paper, observations you would make on the amount of food taken and the response of the patient. Share your notes with your instructor.

VOCABULARY

agility
anorexia
body language
condiments
dysphagia
ethnic
ingestion
regurgitate
respite
stereotype
tremor

FEEDING ADULT PATIENTS

Psychological Overtones

To human beings, eating is ultimately more than taking in food for purposes of vital bodily function and metabolism. At times the meal is a ritual, a celebration, a habit, and, importantly, a social event.

The psychological aspects of feeding an adult patient are formidable. Supplying food for someone is a satisfying experience for most persons. Many mothers and fathers enjoy providing healthful, attractive diets for their young children. And preparing a festive meal for guests or for a special family occasion is a delight to most homemakers. In the same way, helping a patient eat a meal can be equally challenging and satisfying for you.

To the institutionalized person, the meal takes on new meaning. It may well be the high point of the day, often punctuating an otherwise long, weary day of immobilization. In having the meal fed, the patient may have the nurse at the bedside for a longer time span than at any other period in the nursing day. However, it is crucial to remember that being fed can be degrading to some patients and might give them a feeling that they are now dependent persons, unable to carry out for themselves such a simple task as spooning their own food into their mouths.

Influences on Eating Habits

What affects the manner in which a person eats? At first glance, this seems to be a simple question; however, watching people eat in a restaurant proves otherwise. We can observe in a restaurant that persons select very different foods, use condiments in various ways, and show different kinds of "body language" while eating.

There are many factors that influence eating. For example, eating habits have been affected by rocketing food prices during the last few years. Although you must recognize individual differences and not contrive stereotypes, ethnic backgrounds also must be considered. More often than not, people of the same ethnic heritage enjoy the foods that were prevalent in their family groups. However, not all blacks like "soul food," nor do all Germans relish sauerbraten.

Age is another important factor. Watching teenagers wolf down two large hamburgers, fries, and large shakes and then rush off to other activities is a totally different experience from joining an elderly couple who linger before a TV set with a prepackaged dinner on a tray.

Also, the nature of the patient's illness is important. Remember that illness interferes with both body and mind, and every illness produces a degree of anxiety within the individual that may cause decreased eating, increased eating, or erratic eating. An understanding attitude on your part, taking into account all these factors, will promote a more satisfying outcome to the eating-feeding experience.

Assessment During Feeding

Being with the patient during a meal and entering directly into his or her care also gives you time for several of your most basic and important functions: observing, assessing, and recording. Some patients have dysphagia, or difficulty swallowing. You can easily and accurately assess the patient's muscular agility, mental status, and feelings at this time; and signs such as skin color, respiratory rate, and the presence or absence of tremor can also be assessed during feeding. Recording the success of the meal, including the patient's response and abilities of ingestion, is one of your essential duties.

Feeding patients has been considered less than a professional skill, often relegated to aides or volunteers. You should welcome this extended interaction with patients for many of the reasons outlined. As with all skills and procedures, whether performed by the professional or the paraprofessional, time and caring are essential components.

Feeding Techniques

Communication is a skill basic to all inter-action with patients, and feeding is no exception. Telling the patient he or she *must* eat in order to get well is, in reality, not helpful and seldom elicits cooperation. It is better to approach the meal as an enjoyable experience, both for yourself as a sharer of time and conversation and for the patient as a respite from painful experiences that may take place during the day. A more positive approach is an expectation on your part that the patient will join in the procedure willing-ly and benefit from it. Do not discuss stress-ful events at mealtime; it has been shown that digestion is better when a patient is not emotionally upset. Try to create a sharing, lighthearted atmosphere.

The elderly patient who has difficulty eating due to poorly fitting dentures often prefers to mix eggs, fruit, cereal, and toast together. Although this may strike you as unappetizing, affably feeding this mixture to the patient serves to develop a good nurse-patient relationship. Do not feel compelled to change long-standing eating habits, although your long-term goal, for example, may be to fit the patient with comfortable dentures.

With any patient, it would be preferable if the meal could be served at approximately the same time as he or she usually eats at home, but this is often impossible to ar-range in an institution.

Try to provide an environment for the patient that is as clean and attractive to the individual as possible. Pleasant surroundings promote good appetite. Control or elim-inate odors that are unpleasant, replace linens that are soiled, and remove offending equipment. Look at the environment from the patient's view. An empty syringe on the bedside table may not be distasteful to you, but it can prove stressful to the patient.

It is good practice to wash a patient's face and hands before a meal; this activity pro-vides comfort and approximates normal preparation for a meal. As the food handler, your hands must be meticulously washed.

Utensils are not always selected for con-venience. For example, the fluid "bottle" feeders are fast, convenient facilitators of the feeding process, but they often convey to the patient, "We are treating you like a baby." It is far better to have a few spots of spilled food on the bedding than to diminish, even unintentionally, a patient's dignity. Other utensils, such as those shown in Figure 5.1, foster self-esteem by allowing patients who are partially disabled to feed themselves.

When feeding a patient, *involve* him or her as much as possible. This can be done best if you work from the unaffected side (the side of the patient least affected by the disease process). In this way, the patient gains a sense of participation. Place the tray in such a way that the patient can see the food that is being offered. If the patient is sightless, describing what is on the meal tray is both necessary and helpful. If possible, find out from the patient what food sequence is preferred. If this is not possible, feed the items in the order that you would choose to eat them. This is good practice because it affords the patient a variety of tastes, which is usually the most pleasant way to eat a meal.

Patients have few choices available when they are in the hospital. If a patient is able to specify a particular choice (likes or dis-likes) in menu, communicate this informa-tion to the dietician. To the well individual, this may appear unimportant; but to the incapacitated person, it says, "I am still a person," "This nurse cares what I think," "I still have some control." If the patient does not respond to being given a choice, feed the more nutritious items of the diet first, in case the patient's intake capacity is limited. For example, if the choice is be-tween broth and tea; broth, which is high in protein, would be preferable.

Many disabled patients can hold and enjoy feeding themselves pieces of bread or

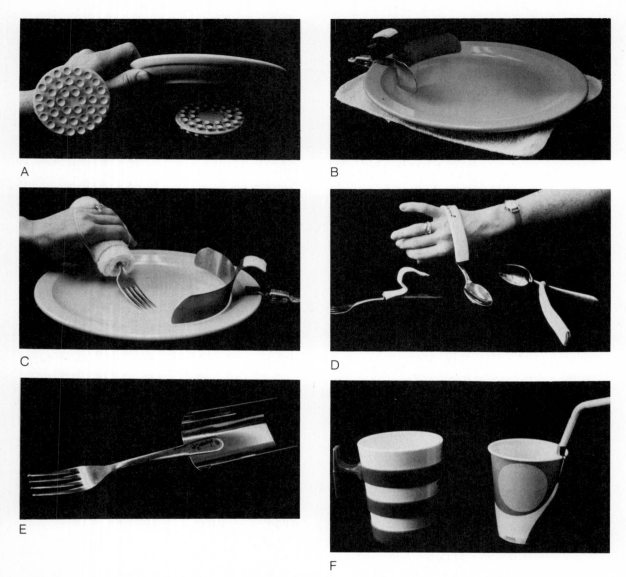

FIGURE 5.1   FEEDING UTENSILS   *A:* "Octopus" suction cups for securing plates; *B:* plate secured by wet washcloth, metal food guard attached to keep food on plate; *C:* washcloth in handroll for easy grip; *D and E:* modified handles; *F:* cup handle and straw secured with pen clip.
Courtesy Florence E. Smith

toast during the meal. Managing their own napkins also offers them some degree of independence.

Never hurry a patient's eating. This can make the patient uncomfortable and fearful of taking up your time. Feeding, if performed properly, is a time-consuming task, but it can give satisfaction to you and to the patient as well.

Feeding Procedure

Assume, for purposes of the lesson, that trays are prepared for patients' specific conditions and by order in a central kitchen area, and are then delivered to the floors at the proper temperature.

1. Prepare the patient's room by removing

all unsightly equipment, replacing soiled linens, and arranging the bedside table.

2. Greet the patient and explain *what you are going to do;* that is, you are going to help with the meal.

3. Offer the patient a bedpan or a urinal, so you will not have to interrupt the meal later.

4. Make a final check of the tray, making sure it is indeed the correct tray for that particular patient.

5. Position the patient comfortably in mid- or high-Fowler's if possible (see Module 12).

6. With a warm cloth, wash the patient's face and hands.

7. Be sure the patient has dentures or eyeglasses in place if either are worn.

8. Arrange the tray so that it can be seen by the patient.

9. Protect the bedclothing by using appropriate linen. Avoid using the word bib, which may be a humiliating term to the patient. Place a colorful napkin, if available, over the protecting linen for attractiveness.

10. Position yourself at the patient's eye level by sitting if at all possible. This establishes an unhurried atmosphere.

11. Allow the patient to determine the sequence and size of bites of food as fully as possible. If the patient can use the larger muscles and hold toast or bread, encourage him or her to do so.

12. Feed solid and liquid food alternately.

13. Take care to keep communications nonstressful during the meal.

14. Allow the patient to determine when he or she has consumed enough of the items on the tray.

15. Remove the tray and provide hygiene as needed.

16. Reposition the patient.

17. Provide quiet so that the patient may relax after the meal, which promotes good digestion.

18. Wash your hands.

19. Record the food that was taken, either by using the checklist the institution provides or by charting in more detail on the progress notes, depending on the situation. If food intake has previously presented problems, it is more accurate to chart the specific food items and the amounts taken.

20. If there is a history of digestive problems, check back with the patient to be sure regurgitation has not taken place.

PERFORMANCE CHECKLIST

	Unsatisfactory	Needs more practice	Satisfactory	Comments
1. Straighten room and remove unsightly equipment.				
2. Greet the patient and explain what you plan to do.				
3. Offer bedpan or urinal.				
4. Wash patient's hands and face.				
5. Check and arrange tray.				
6. Position patient.				
7. Supply dentures or eyeglasses.				
8. Feed patient following the guidelines on pages 56–57.				
9. Remove tray and provide hygiene.				
10. Reposition patient and provide quiet.				
11. Wash your hands.				
12. Record procedure.				
13. Check back with patient for problems of digestion.				

QUIZ

Short-Answer Question

1. List four factors that can influence a patient's eating abilities.

   a. _____

   b. _____

   c. _____

   d. _____

Multiple-Choice Questions

_____ 2. Every feeding situation presents which of the following opportunities for the nurse?

   a. Time for health teaching
   b. Determination of the medical diagnosis
   c. Time for nursing assessments to be made
   d. Repositioning of the patient

Situation: Mr. Swenson, a sixty-three-year-old Scandinavian with a right-sided hemiplegia (paralysis on the right side of the body) has been in the hospital for ten days. The patient's chart states that a soft diet has been ordered and that he is allowed up in a chair q.d. (once daily).

Lunch trays will be arriving in 20 minutes, and you have been assigned to feed Mr. Swenson. As you enter his room you see a denture cup sitting on the bedside table and glasses lying on the overbed table. A urinal is on the floor. Questions 3–10 refer to Mr. Swenson.

_____ 3. From the data given, you determine that Mr. Swenson's feeding problem is

   a. lack of ability to swallow food.
   b. not evident from the information available.
   c. lack of ability to use small-muscle groups to feed himself.
   d. depression brought on by dependency.

_____ 4. Your *first* action in the above situation should be to

   a. introduce yourself and give the reason for your presence.
   b. empty and put away the urinal.
   c. encourage Mr. Swenson to discuss his feelings about being dependent.
   d. reposition Mr. Swenson in a high-Fowler's position for lunch.

_____ 5. If Mr. Swenson must be fed his meal, you should stand on

   a. his left side.
   b. his right side.
   c. either side.

_____ 6. Mr. Swenson's speech is unclear and difficult to understand. Which action should you take?

    a. Don't speak so that he won't feel embarrassed knowing he has to reply.
    b. Carry on a one-sided conversation so that mealtime isn't silent.
    c. Take as much time as necessary and encourage him to speak and repeat until you understand him.
    d. Only make brief comments that require yes or no answers, so that his energy can be devoted to eating.

True-False Questions

_____ 7. Mr. Swenson should be encouraged to talk about his anxieties while you are at his bedside feeding him.

_____ 8. Because Mr. Swenson is Scandinavian, he will certainly enjoy the fish on the lunch menu.

_____ 9. The goal for Mr. Swenson in regard to self-feeding this meal should be established only after you check to see what his previous ability has been.

_____ 10. Mr. Swenson ate only half of his meal. This means your feeding plan was unsuccessful.

Module 6 Bedmaking

MAIN OBJECTIVE

To make beds correctly for hospitalized patients.

RATIONALE

One of the most important parts of the environment of hospitalized patients is the bed. Knowing how to make various types of beds and how to modify them for special situations is of paramount importance for the nurse. A wrinkle-free bed that remains intact when a patient moves around does a great deal for the patient's physical and psychological comfort.

PREREQUISITES

Successful completion of the following modules:

> **VOLUME 1**
> Medical Asepsis
> Basic Body Mechanics

SPECIFIC LEARNING OBJECTIVES

	Know Facts and Principles	Apply Facts and Principles	Demonstrate Ability	Evaluate Performance
1. *Related principles* a. *Medical asepsis* b. *Body mechanics*	State principles of medical asepsis and body mechanics related to bedmaking	Apply principles of medical asepsis and body mechanics when making beds	Use principles of medical asepsis and body mechanics in making hospital beds	Evaluate own performance with instructor
2. *Types of beds* a. *Closed* (*unoccupied*) b. *Open* c. *Occupied* d. *Post-op*	Describe types of beds	Given a patient situation, identify appropriate type of bed to be made	In the clinical setting, identify type of bed to be made for particular patient	Evaluate own performance with instructor
3. *Linen*	Identify individual pieces of linen used in making hospital beds	Given a patient situation, identify appropriate pieces of linen to use in correct order	In the clinical setting, identify appropriate pieces of linen to use in correct order for particular patient	Evaluate own performance with instructor
4. *Procedures* a. *Closed* (*unoccupied*) b. *Open* c. *Occupied* d. *Post-op*	Describe correct procedures for making closed (unoccupied), open, occupied, and post-op beds	Initiate appropriate bedmaking activities in patient settings	Demonstrate ability to correctly make closed (unoccupied), open, occupied, and post-op beds	Evaluate own bedmaking ability with instructor using Performance Checklist
5. *Accessory devices* a. *Cradle* b. *Footboard* c. *Bedboard*	Identify cradle (Anderson frame), footboard, and bedboard	Given a patient situation, identify appropriate accessory device to use	Initiate use of accessory devices in appropriate situations	Evaluate appropriateness of choice with instructor

LEARNING ACTIVITIES

1. Review the Specific Learning Objectives.
2. Read the section on care of the patient's bed (in the chapter on hygiene) in Ellis and Nowlis, *Nursing: A Human Needs Approach,* or comparable material in another textbook.
3. Look up the module vocabulary terms in the glossary.
4. Read through the module.
5. In the practice setting:
   a. Identify the various pieces of linen used in making beds in the facility to which you are assigned.
   b. Make a closed bed using the Performance Checklist as a guide. When you are satisfied with your performance, have a fellow student evaluate you. Compare your own evaluation with that of the other student. Perfect your technique. Have your instructor evaluate your performance.
   c. Demonstrate how to make an open bed from a closed bed.
   d. Demonstrate how to make a post-op bed from a closed bed.
   e. Make an occupied bed using a fellow student as a patient. Pretend that it is a real situation, complete with patient explanation. Have the student comment on his or her comfort. When you are satisfied with your performance, have your instructor evaluate you.
   f. Identify the bedboard, footboard, and cradle, and incorporate them in the making of an unoccupied bed.
6. In the clinical setting:
   a. Make an unoccupied bed, an occupied bed, and a post-op bed to your instructor's satisfaction.

VOCABULARY

bedboard
cradle
edema
fan-fold
footboard
footdrop
mitered corner
toe pleat

BEDMAKING

Asepsis in Bedmaking

Apply these principles of asepsis to all
bedmaking procedures:

1. Wash your hands before you begin
   bedmaking.
2. Handle linen carefully; avoid shaking it,
   tossing it into the laundry hamper (it
   should be *placed* in the hamper), or
   throwing it on the floor.
3. Hold both dirty and clean linen away
   from your uniform.
4. Wash your hands after you finish bedmaking.

Body Mechanics in Bedmaking

Apply these principles of body mechanics to
all bedmaking procedures:

1. Raise the bed (if possible) to an appropriate height for you before you
   begin. Lock the wheels.
2. When you must bend, bend your knees,
   not your back. (See Figure 6.1.)

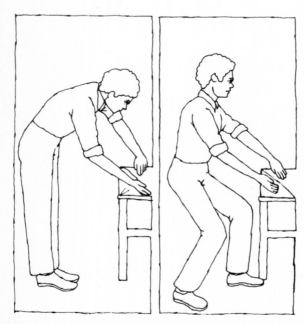

FIGURE 6.1 POSTURE FOR BEDMAKING
Left: Back bent over to reach bed (incorrect).
Right: Back straight, knees bent (correct).

3. Point your toes and face in the direction that you are moving. Avoid twisting.
4. Conserve steps by making as few trips
   around the bed as possible.

Stripping the Bed

You will need a laundry hamper or a bag.

1. Remove attached equipment (call light,
   waste bag, personal items). Side rails
   should be in the down position.
2. Remove cases from pillows and place
   the pillows on a chair or bedside table.
3. Loosen the top and the bottom linen
   from the mattress, moving around the
   bed from head to foot on one side and
   from foot to head on the opposite side.
4. Remove items to be reused (spread,
   blankets, sheets), fold them in quarters,
   and place them across the back of a
   chair.
5. Remove the remaining linen and place
   it in a laundry hamper.
6. If the mattress is to be turned, do so at
   this point by grasping it, pulling it
   toward you, and turning it.
7. Move the mattress to the head of the
   bed.

Closed (Unoccupied) Beds

1. Wash your hands.
2. Gather the linen to be used and place it
   in order, so that the first item to be
   used will be on top, the second item
   next, and so on.
   a. Mattress pad
   b. Bottom sheet (some facilities will
      have fitted bottom sheets)
   c. 1 rubber or plastic drawsheet (may
      be optional)
   d. 1 cloth drawsheet (a top sheet folded
      in half may be used in some settings)
   e. 1 top sheet
   f. 1 blanket
   g. 1 spread
   h. 1 pillowcase for each pillow on the
      bed.

If linen is stacked in this order, the stack need merely be turned over for it to be in the correct order.

3. Place a mattress pad on the mattress, securing it smoothly.

4. Place a bottom sheet on the bed, center fold at the center of the bed, lower hem even with the edge of the mattress at the foot of the bed, and the seam toward the mattress. Spread the sheet, tucking it under at the head of the bed.

5. Miter the corner where the sheet has been tucked under. (This will not be necessary if you use fitted bottom sheets.)
   a. Pick up the side edge of the sheet, holding it straight up and down with the edge of the mattress.
   b. Lay the upper part of the sheet on the bed as shown in Figure 6.2, part B.

c. Tuck the part of sheet that is hanging below the mattress smoothly under the mattress.

d. Hold the sheet in place beside the mattress with one hand. Lift the corner of the sheet laying on the bed with the other hand, bring it down over the side of the mattress, and tuck the hanging portion under the side of the mattress.

6. Tuck the remainder of the sheet under the side of the mattress all the way to the foot of the bed.

7. If a rubber or plastic drawsheet is to be used, place it over the middle part of the bed, center fold at the center. Unfold the drawsheet toward the far side of the bed, tucking the near edge smoothly under the mattress.

8. Place the cloth drawsheet over the rubber drawsheet, and place it on the

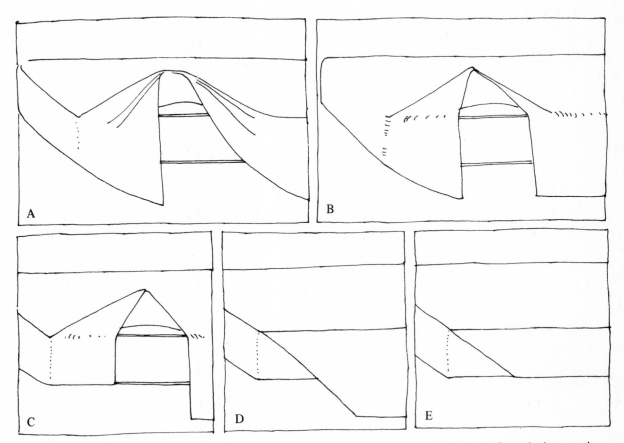

FIGURE 6.2 MITERING A CORNER *A and B:* Pull sheet up at corner and fold back; *C:* tuck sheet under at corner; *D and E:* fold rest of sheet down and tuck under.

bed as in step 7, making sure that the rubber or plastic drawsheet is completely covered.

You may be taught to make the entire side of the bed (both bottom and top linen) before moving to the other side. If so, omit steps 9–12 and finish the first side, beginning with step 13 below.

9. Go to the other side of the bed. Tuck the bottom sheet under the head of the mattress and make a mitered corner.

10. Tuck the bottom sheet along the side of the bed, pulling and straightening, moving toward the foot of the bed.

11. Pull the rubber drawsheet toward you from the center. Tuck it under the mattress with palms down, as snugly as possible. Grasp the top corner of the drawsheet, pull it diagonally, and tuck it under the mattress snugly. Repeat this activity with the lower corner of the drawsheet.

12. Repeat step 11 with a cloth drawsheet. Some people prefer to tuck rubber and cloth drawsheets together.

13. Place the top sheet on the bed, center fold at the center of the bed, seam side up. Align the top edge of the sheet even with the top edge of the mattress. Unfold it toward the far side of the bed.

14. Make a toe pleat (optional—follow the procedure at your clinical facility) by folding a 2-inch pleat across the sheet about 6 to 8 inches from the foot of the bed. Then tuck the end of the sheet under the mattress.

15. Place the blanket on the bed, center fold at the center of the bed, so that the top edge of the blanket is about 6 inches from the top of the mattress. Unfold the blanket toward the far side of the bed. Tuck it under the foot of the mattress, making a toe pleat if used. In warm weather, or at the patient's request, a blanket may not be used.

16. Place the bedspread on the bed, center fold at the center of the bed. The top edge of the spread should be about 6 inches from the top of the mattress. Unfold the remainder of the spread toward the far side of the bed. Tuck it under at the foot of the mattress, making a toe pleat if used. Some prefer to tuck all three—top sheet, blanket, and spread—together.

17. Miter the corner of the top linen at the foot of the bed. Do not tuck in the upper portion; allow it to hang down smoothly and freely.

18. Move to the other side of the bed. Straighten and tuck the top sheet, blanket, and spread at the foot of the bed. Miter the corner.

19. Fold the top sheet back over the top edge of the blanket and the spread. In the event there is more spread than blanket at the top of the bed, fold the excess spread back over the blanket to form an even line. Then fold the top sheet over as described. In some facilities the upper edge of the spread is left even with the upper edge of the mattress to designate a closed bed.

20. Put a pillowcase on the pillow. One way to do this is as follows:
    a. Grasp the pillowcase at the center of the closed end of the case. (See Figure 6.3.)
    b. Gather the case up over that hand and grasp the zipper, or open end of the pillow cover, with the same hand, pulling the case down over the pillow with the other hand.
    c. Straighten and smooth the case over the pillow and place it at the head of the bed with the open end away from the door (for neater appearance).
    d. Keep the pillow and case away from your uniform as you apply the case.

21. Replace the call light in the patient's reach and leave the bed in high or low position, depending on your facility's policy.

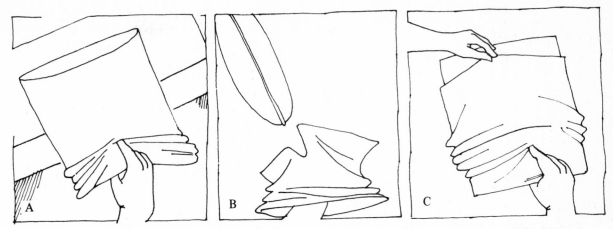

FIGURE 6.3 PUTTING A CASE ON A PILLOW *A:* Hold pillowcase at closed end, from outside; *B:* gather pillowcase over your hand, inside out; *C:* holding pillow with same hand, pull case back over pillow, right side out.

Open Beds

Open beds are usually made when patients are either up for a brief period in the room or perhaps out of the unit for x-ray or lab procedures. If beds are left open, it is easier to assist patients back to bed when they are ready.

Opening a bed is usually done by grasping the upper edge of the top linen with both hands, bringing it all the way to the foot of the bed, then folding it back toward the center of the bed. This is known as *fan-folding*.

Post-op, or Surgical, Beds

The post-op bed is also called the *anesthetic* or *surgical bed*. Make the base of the bed as any unoccupied bed, applying a mattress pad, bottom sheet, rubber or plastic draw-sheet, and cloth drawsheet. In some settings a bath blanket is placed over the base of the bed for extra warmth. Fold the top linen out of the way, so that the patient can be transferred from a stretcher to the bed with a minimum of motion and discomfort, and then covered with the top linen, which is easily within reach. (See Figure 6.4.) The

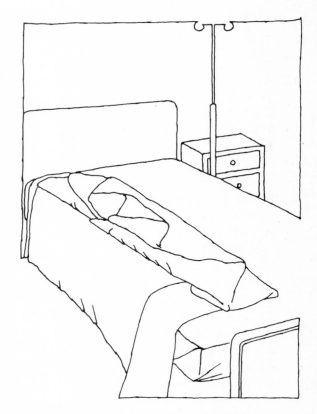

FIGURE 6.4 POST-OPERATIVE BED Top sheet, blanket, and spread are fan-folded for convenient transfer of patient from stretcher to bed.

top linen may be handled in a variety of ways, but in most cases the top sheet, blanket, and spread are placed as usual but are not tucked in at the bottom. Instead, fold these covers back toward the head of the bed to make a cuff, and then fan-fold them to the far side of the bed or, as required in some facilities, to the foot. Place the pillows on a table or chair or on top of the fan-folded top covers, and leave the bed in the high position to receive the patient. Place emesis basin, tissues, and IV standard, which are usually among the necessary post-op items, by the bed. Check your facility's procedures for other specific items that may be necessary.

Occupied Beds

There are many instances when a bed must be wholly or partially made with a patient in it. In most cases this is because the patient is too ill or disabled to get out of bed.

Practice making an occupied bed, keeping the safety and comfort of the patient foremost in your mind, and taking care to avoid bumping the bed or exposing the patient. The order of activities remains the same; the procedure differs only because a patient is in the bed.

1. Wash your hands and explain what you plan to do. The cooperation of the patient will be a great help to you. Provide for the privacy of the patient.
2. Gather linen as in step 2, Closed Beds, page 64. You will need a hamper or laundry bag for soiled linen.
3. Remove the call light (and other equipment), spread, and blanket from the bed. If the spread and the blanket are to be reused, fold them as in step 4, Stripping the Bed, page 64.
4. Before removing the top sheet, place a bath blanket over it. Ask the patient to hold the top edge of the bath blanket while you pull the sheet out from under it. Discard the top sheet. In some facilities the top sheet is saved and used as a bottom sheet; follow the procedure

used in your facility. If the mattress must be moved toward the head of the bed, you will probably need the assistance of another person.
5. Move the patient to the far side of the bed, making sure that the pillow is moved with him or her. If possible, the patient should be on his or her side, facing away from you. The side rail on the far side of the bed should be up.
6. Loosen the foundation (bottom linen) of the bed on the near side, leaving the mattress pad in place unless it is wet or soiled.
7. Fan-fold each piece toward the center of the bed, with the last fold toward the opposite side of the bed and tucked under the patient's back and buttocks.
8. Straighten the mattress pad.
9. Put the bottom sheet on the bed as in step 4, Closed Beds, page 65.
10. Tuck the sheet under at the top, miter the top corner, and tuck it in along the side of the mattress to the foot of the bed.
11. Fan-fold the other half of the sheet toward the center of the bed as you did the soiled linen, tucking it *under* the soiled bottom sheet.
12. If a rubber or plastic drawsheet is in use, unfold it at this point, pull it over the folded bottom sheets, and tuck it in snugly and smoothly.
13. Place the cloth drawsheet on the bed as in steps 7 and 8, Closed Beds, page 65. Tuck the near side under the mattress. Fan-fold the other half toward the center of the bed, tucking it under the patient's back and buttocks.

    You may be taught to make the entire side of the bed (both bottom and top linen) before moving to the other side. If so, omit steps 14–20 and finish the first side, beginning with step 21 below.
14. Help the patient roll over the folded linen and onto the clean linen. Adjust the pillow under his or her head. Put up the side rail.

15. Move to the other side of the bed. Lower the side rail.

16. Loosen the foundation of the bed. Remove the soiled linen (bottom sheet and cloth drawsheet) and place it in a laundry hamper or bag.

17. Straighten the mattress pad. Straighten, pull, and tuck the bottom sheet as in step 10, Closed Beds, page 66.

18. Pull and tuck the rubber drawsheet as in step 11, Closed Beds, page 66.

19. Pull and tuck the cloth drawsheet snugly and smoothly.

20. Now move the patient to the center of the bed in a position of comfort.

21. Place the top sheet on the bed over the bath blanket. Remove the bath blanket, instructing the patient to hold the sheet as you pull the blanket from the top to the bottom.

22. Add the blanket and the spread and proceed as in steps 13–19, Closed Beds, page 66. Instead of making a toe pleat, you may have the patient point his or her toes up, which allows room for the toes after the bed has been made.

23. Remove the pillow and put on a clean pillowcase as in step 20, Closed Beds, page 66. Replace the pillow under the patient's head.

24. Reattach the call light and any other equipment you removed.

25. Place the bed in the low position, adjusting the side rails according to your facility's policies and the individual situation.

Accessories for the Bed

Among the devices often added to the bed are the bedboard, the footboard, and the cradle, or Anderson frame. These devices may be ordered by a physician, but in many facilities they are added at the nurse's discretion.

BEDBOARDS

A bedboard is used when the patient needs an especially firm bed; it is placed directly under the mattress. Bedboards are often used for orthopedic patients or for those who have a history of back problems. Some patients are simply more comfortable sleeping on a firm surface.

FOOTBOARDS

A footboard may be placed at the foot of the bed for a variety of reasons, most commonly to keep the patient from sliding to the foot of the bed and/or to give him or her a firm surface to exercise against. Some physicians routinely order a footboard for their patients. Linen is tucked in around the footboard and is held up off the patient's

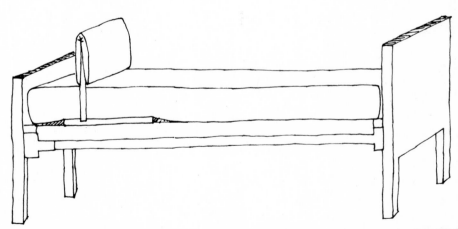

FIGURE 6.5   FOOTBOARD   The bottom part, or shelf, slides under the mattress at the foot of the bed like a bookend. Footboards are usually padded.

feet, though this is not the primary function of the device.

All footboards are not alike. Some are merely boards that fit at the foot of the mattress. Some require that a box or "block" be added, so that the feet of a shorter patient can reach the board. Other footboards fit under the mattress and slide up to the appropriate point on the bed (Figure 6.5). Footboards that allow the patient's feet to rest flat against them help to prevent foot-drop.

CRADLES

A cradle, or Anderson frame, is a device designed specifically to keep linen up off the feet and lower legs of patients when necessary, as in cases of edema, leg ulcers, and burns. Arrange the top linen over the device and pin it in place. Some facilities do not allow pinning because it can tear the linen. In these situations, linen must simply be tucked as securely as possible around the frame.

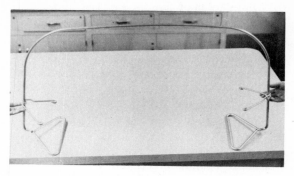

FIGURE 6.6 CRADLE The triangles at the base of the cradle slide under the mattress; the V-shaped parts just above fit over the top of the mattress. *Courtesy Ivan Ellis*

There are several varieties of cradles, including a simple rod that arches over the bed, which is held in place by the mattress (see Figure 6.6), and a latticework affair, which is also arch-shaped and which sometimes includes a socket for light treatments. If your facility has no cradle, you can make one by simply cutting one side out of a strong cardboard box.

PERFORMANCE CHECKLIST

	Unsatisfactory	Needs more practice	Satisfactory	Comments
Asepsis				
1. Wash hands before beginning bedmaking activity.				
2. Handle linen carefully.				
3. Hold linen away from uniform.				
4. Wash hands after bed is made.				
Body mechanics				
1. Raise bed to appropriate height.				
2. Avoid bending back.				
3. Face in direction you are moving.				
4. Conserve steps.				
Stripping the bed				
1. Gather equipment needed.				
2. Remove linen, folding that to be reused.				
3. Move mattress to head of bed.				
Closed beds				
1. Gather linen in the order to be used.				
2. Place bottom linen on bed using center fold as guide; lower hem of bottom sheet should be even with mattress at foot.				
3. Miter top corners of bottom sheet.				
4. Place top linen on bed, using center fold as guide. a. Make toe pleat if appropriate to facility.				
b. Miter lower corners of top linen.				
5. Apply pillowcase, taking care to keep pillow and case away from uniform.				
6. Replace call light and other items attached to bed.				
7. Leave bed in position indicated by facility policy.				

	Unsatisfactory	Needs more practice	Satisfactory	Comments
Open beds				
1. Use Performance Checklist for closed beds.				
2. Fan-fold linen to foot of bed after bed is made.				
Post-op beds				
1. Use first three steps of Performance Checklist for closed beds.				
2. Place top linen on bed, using center fold as guide, but do not tuck at bottom.				
3. Fold back top linen toward head of bed to make cuff.				
4. Fan-fold top linen to far side or foot of bed.				
5. Place pillow on chair or atop fan-folded linens.				
6. Leave bed in high position.				
7. Arrange appropriate items (emesis basin, tissues, IV standard) at bedside.				
Occupied beds				
1. Explain to patient what is to be done. Provide for privacy.				
2. Gather linen in the order to be used.				
3. Raise bed to convenient working level.				
4. Strip bed of all top linen except sheet.				
5. Position bath blanket and remove top sheet.				
6. Move patient to far side of bed, making sure side rail is up.				
7. Loosen bottom linen and fan-fold it toward center of bed.				
8. Place and tuck clean bottom linen on bed, mitering sheet at top corner.				
9. Fan-fold other half of clean bottom linen and tuck under patient.				
10. Help patient roll over folded linen. Raise side rail on that side of bed.				
11. Loosen soiled linen, remove from bed, and place in laundry hamper.				

	Unsatisfactory	Needs more practice	Satisfactory	Comments
12. Pull bottom linen through, straighten, and tuck, mitering sheet at top corner.				
13. Assist patient to position of comfort.				
14. Apply top linen, removing bath blanket and mitering lower corner of top linen.				
15. Change pillowcase.				
16. Reattach call light and arrange unit.				
17. Place bed in low position.				

QUIZ

Multiple-Choice Questions

_____ 1. Mr. Green is to be up in a chair each morning for 30 minutes. Given this information, what type of bed would be most appropriate for you to make for him?

    a. Closed bed   c. Occupied bed
    b. Open bed   d. Post-op bed

_____ 2. Mrs. Pine is going to x-ray for some special tests. She will arrive back on the floor via stretcher. Under these circumstances, what type of bed would be most appropriate for you to make?

    a. Closed bed   c. Occupied bed
    b. Open bed   d. Post-op bed

_____ 3. A patient who has severe edema of the lower legs should be provided with which accessory device?

    a. Cradle   c. Footboard
    b. Bedboard   d. Mattress pad

_____ 4. Patients who are confined to bed should be provided with which accessory device to help footdrop?

    a. Cradle   c. Footboard
    b. Bedboard   d. Mattress pad

_____ 5. Which of the following beds is left in the high position on completion?
(1) closed bed; (2) open bed; (3) occupied bed; (4) post-op bed

    a. 1 only   c. 2 and 3
    b. 4 only   d. 1 and 4

Short-Answer Question

6. Number the following pieces of linen in the order they would be used in the usual unoccupied hospital bed.

_____ Blanket   _____ Mattress pad

_____ Pillowcase   _____ Cloth drawsheet

_____ Top sheet   _____ Spread

_____ Bottom sheet   _____ Rubber drawsheet

Module 7 Assisting with Elimination and Perineal Care

MAIN OBJECTIVES

To assist patients with the use of bedpans or urinals in a hygienic manner, taking into account psychological factors.

To provide perineal care according to individual needs.

RATIONALE

Many patients are unable to use the bathroom for purposes of elimination. They may have an order for complete bed rest or for appliances (traction, casts) that impose immobility. Certain patients who have had recent surgery may be unable to use the bathroom for a day or so. Others who are generally weak may not be able to ambulate to the bathroom part or all of the time. Also because of their condition, some patients cannot clean themselves properly after eliminating and need the nurse's assistance.

It is one of the nurse's fundamental tasks to help patients with either a bedpan or urinal and to give perineal care skillfully, being aware of the psychological implications of this care.

PREREQUISITES

Successful completion of the following modules:

VOLUME 1
Assessment
Charting
Medical Asepsis

77

SPECIFIC LEARNING OBJECTIVES

	Know Facts and Principles	Apply Facts and Principles	Demonstrate Ability	Evaluate Performance
Assisting with Elimination				
1. Equipment	Describe equipment needed	Given a patient situation, gather appropriate equipment	When caring for patient, select correct equipment	Evaluate own performance with instructor
2. Assisting with bedpan or urinal	State three principles for carrying out procedures	Given a patient situation, explain and discuss medical asepsis, psychological needs, and normal conditions of elimination	In the clinical setting, carry out medical asepsis, provide psychological comfort, and approximate normal conditions of elimination	Evaluate own performance with instructor
3. Procedure				
a. Positioning	Describe positions used for individual patients	Given a patient situation, plan particular procedure correctly	In the clinical setting, individualize procedure to particular patient and carry out plan	Evaluate with instructor using Performance Checklist
b. Privacy	State measures to ensure privacy	Given a patient situation, plan privacy measures	In the clinical setting, provide privacy for patient	
c. Providing bedpan or urinal	Describe several techniques employed in giving bedpan or urinal	Given a patient situation, plan appropriate technique for giving bedpan or urinal	In the clinical setting, individualize technique for giving bedpan or urinal	Evaluate own performance with instructor
d. Cleaning patient after use	Recognize need for cleanliness	Demonstrate correct cleaning of patient	In the clinical setting, provide cleanliness for patient after use of bedpan or urinal	
4. Charting	State what should be recorded	Given a hypothetical situation, record as if on chart	Record complete observations in correct format	Evaluate recording with instructor

Giving Perineal Care

1. *Equipment*	Describe various equipment	Given a patient situation, simulate correct method for postpartum patient, and patient with a catheter	In the clinical setting, give perineal care to postpartum patient, nonsurgical patient, and catheterized patient, adapting equipment and procedure correctly	Evaluate with instructor using Performance Checklist
2. *Psychological comfort*	Explain why giving psychological support is important	Given a patient situation, discern possible causes of psychological discomfort	In the clinical setting, provide psychological support to patient	
3. *Procedure* a. *Postpartum patient* b. *Nonsurgical patient* c. *Patient with catheter*	Describe appropriate adaptations in procedure related to particular patient condition	Given a patient situation, adapt procedure appropriately for a particular patient	In the clinical setting, carry out procedure for postpartum patient, nonsurgical patient, and catheterized patient, safely and correctly	Evaluate own performance with instructor
4. *Charting information*	List what should be recorded	Given a patient situation, record as if on chart	Record observations correctly	Evaluate own performance with instructor

LEARNING ACTIVITIES

1. Review the Specific Learning Objectives.
2. Read the chapter on elimination in Ellis and Nowlis, *Nursing: A Human Needs Approach,* or a comparable chapter in another textbook.
3. Look up the module vocabulary terms in the glossary.
4. Read through the module.
5. In the practice setting:
   a. Become familiar with the various pieces of available equipment (different types of bedpans, urinals, perineal packs).
   b. Select a partner and perform the following:
      (1) Pretend you are a patient. Have your partner place you on the bedpan following procedures.
      (2) For three minutes remain on the bedpan in a flat position, then another three minutes in a sitting position.
      (3) Have your partner remove the bedpan as though you were incapacitated.
      (4) Describe any discomfort you experienced.
      (5) Reverse the roles, repeating (1), (2), (3), and (4).
   c. Using a mannequin, go through the specific procedure for giving perineal care to each of the following:
      (1) A postpartum or perineal surgical patient
      (2) A nonsurgical patient
      (3) A patient with a catheter
6. In the clinical area, with your instructor's supervision:
   a. Place a patient on a bedpan using both methods.
   b. Give a urinal to a male patient.
   c. Administer perineal care to a postpartum patient, a nonsurgical patient, and a catheterized patient.
7. Using the Performance Checklist, evaluate yourself with the help of your instructor.

VOCABULARY

ADL
bedpan
catheter
defecation
foreskin
fracture pan
genital area
guaiac
Hematest
labia
lumbosacral
penis
perineum
renal calculi
smegma
sutures
urethral meatus
urinal
urination
void
vulva

ASSISTING WITH ELIMINATION AND PERINEAL CARE

Helping a patient to use a bedpan is a basic task, which you should perform with a minimum of embarrassment for the patient and maximal skill. It becomes necessary when a patient cannot use the usual bathroom facilities either for medical reasons or because of immobility.

Principles

Keep several principles in mind. First, observe medical asepsis throughout for your own protection as well as the patient's. When performing these procedures, your hands may come in contact with mucous membrane, which is receptive to infection. It is even more important to protect the patient from the dangers of cross-contamination (contamination from other patients). For practical as well as aesthetic reasons, you must use good aseptic technique.

Second, the procedure can be embarrassing to you and to the patient. It is important to recognize these feelings in yourself and to know that, with experience, assisting with intimate procedures will become less personal and more routine to you. To lessen a patient's embarrassment or discomfort, maintain a straightforward attitude and protect the patient's privacy, keeping exposure to a minimum.

Lastly, when you help a patient with any substitution or adaptation of the usual activities of daily living (ADL), it is important—in terms of efficiency and patient comfort—that you approximate the normal as closely as possible. For a female patient the normal position for urination or defecation is a sitting one; a male commonly stands to urinate and sits to defecate. Therefore, having a patient assume these positions when using a bedpan or urinal is very helpful and may, in some cases, be a strong factor in whether the patient will be able to eliminate. A male patient, for example, will usually be more successful if he is allowed to stand to

urinate. If the patient is unable to stand alone, have him lean on the edge of the bed for stability with his feet on the floor. Other normal behaviors that should be encouraged are giving a patient privacy, allowing a patient to use tissue by himself or herself, and allowing a patient to wash his or her hands afterward. If a patient is unable to perform these activities, you should perform them for the patient.

Types of Bedpans

Bedpans are made of either metal (Figure 7.1) or plastic and come in two sizes, the smaller for pediatric patients. In most facilities, each patient has a personal bedpan, which is kept in a storage unit in the patient's room. Generally, it is stored with a bedpan cover over it. The cover may consist of a square of heavy fabric or paper in the form of a large envelope into which the bedpan can easily be slipped. The paper-type cover is disposable. A cover should be used for aesthetic reasons, to conceal the sight of the contents and to decrease odor after the patient has used the bedpan.

A *fracture pan* is a type of bedpan that was originally designed to be used by patients in casts, who could not use a pan with a high lip. It is now used for any patient who is unable to be placed on the higher bedpan. Fracture pans also come in two sizes, in plastic or metal, and with a handle for easier placement (Figure 7.2).

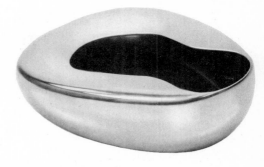

FIGURE 7.1 BEDPAN
Courtesy American Hospital Supply Corp., McGaw Park, Illinois

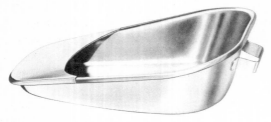

FIGURE 7.2   FRACTURE PAN
Courtesy American Hospital Supply Corp., McGaw Park, Illinois

A *urinal* is used by the male patient for urination. It is made of plastic or metal with a bottlelike configuration. A flat side allows it to rest without tipping. Urinals are available with or without attached tops or lids (Figure 7.3). Female urinals are also available.

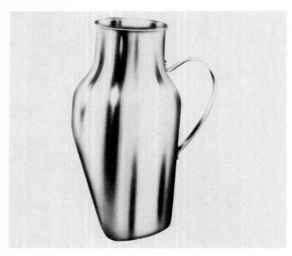

FIGURE 7.3   URINAL FOR MALE USE
Courtesy American Hospital Supply Corp., McGaw Park, Illinois

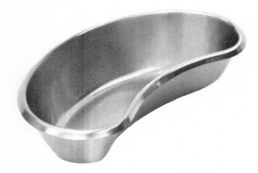

FIGURE 7.4   EMESIS BASIN FOR USE WITH IMMOBILE FEMALE PATIENT
Courtesy American Hospital Supply Corp., McGaw Park, Illinois

An *emesis basin* (Figure 7.4) can be used for the rare female patient who, because of extreme pain or for a medical reason, should not be raised to bedpan height except for defecation. After placing a pad or Chux under the patient, hold the emesis basin lengthwise between the legs, firmly against the perineum. Instruct the patient to void. At first a patient may be hesitant, fearing she will soil the bed. Encourage the patient to void freely. Usually the urine flows into the pan with only a drop or so on the pad, and the patient will be very grateful for this easy, more comfortable way to urinate.

Comfort Considerations

Although often unavoidable, using a bedpan or urinal is not a pleasant experience. A thin, fragile patient may even feel pain from the pressure of the hard surfaces. Fold a soft rag or small towel over the edges of the pan to lessen this discomfort. Another source of discomfort arises from metal pans, which feel cold to patients. Warm metal pans by holding them under running warm water and then drying them. These simple measures can make the experience less disagreeable.

The Procedure for Assisting with a Bedpan

1. Wash your hands. Use the principles of medical asepsis throughout. (Washing your hands before you undertake any procedure should become automatic, to protect both patients and yourself.)
2. Explain in general how you plan to proceed. (Of course, if a patient verbalizes the need to eliminate, do not go into detail.)
3. Provide privacy by closing the door and the bed curtains.
4. Raise the bed to the high position (for your convenience). For the patient's safety, put up the side rail on the opposite side of the bed from where you are standing.
5. Take the bedpan, cover, and toilet tissue out of the bedside storage unit. Set the cover and tissue aside. A fracture

pan can be used in the same way as a conventional bedpan.

6. There are several ways to put a patient on a bedpan, depending on the patient's condition and his or her ability to help you.

   a. With the patient in a recumbent position and your hand under the small (lumbosacral area) of the back, ask the patient to raise the buttocks by pushing up with the feet as you push the pan into position under the patient.

   b. A patient in the sitting position, who is able to, will prefer to simply lift himself or herself up by pushing down with the hands and feet as you place the pan into position.

   c. A more immobilized patient must be rolled onto the pan. For this maneuver, again elicit the patient's cooperation. Ask the patient to grasp the side rail on the opposite side of the bed (across from where you are standing) as you roll the patient away from you in one plane. Place the pan against the patient, in position. (You may want to pad the pan with a towel.) Now, hold the pan firmly in place as you roll the patient back. Finally, check the position of the pan. If the patient must remain flat, you may want to place a small pillow above the bedpan under the patient's back, for support. *Note:* If the patient's bed has a trapeze, make use of this device for giving and removing the bedpan. Have the patient use the trapeze to lift the hips.

7. Raise the side rail nearest you.

8. Elevate the head of the bed to mid- or high-Fowler's position (see Module 12), as the patient grasps the rails.

9. Place the toilet tissue and the call bell within the patient's reach.

10. Leave the patient. Because our culture emphasizes privacy during elimination, it is very difficult for some patients to eliminate with a nurse in attendance. If possible, it is best to leave the patient for a period of time; if this is not possible, you might step just outside the bed curtains.

11. When the patient signals, return promptly. It can be very irritating and uncomfortable for a patient to sit for unnecessarily extended periods of time on a bedpan because a nurse is inattentive. If a patient does not signal you in a reasonable amount of time, return to the patient to check that he or she is all right.

12. If necessary, clean the genital area with toilet tissue. Most alert patients will be able to clean themselves adequately. Some who are incapacitated may need further assistance. With fresh tissue always clean from the anterior (urinary) region to the posterior (rectal) region. Cleaning in this direction minimizes the chance of contaminating the urinary tract with fecal microorganisms.

13. Remove the bedpan, reversing the method that you used when you placed the patient on the bedpan. If you used the rolling technique, hold onto the pan firmly or get help, so that the contents do not spill.

14. Place a cover on the pan.

15. Carry the pan to the bathroom and, if ordered, measure the urine. If a patient is on intake and output, a measuring container is usually kept in the bathroom. You must estimate as accurately as possible, taking into account the amount of toilet tissue used. (See Module 11, Intake and Output.)

16. Collect a specimen of urine or feces, if ordered. (See Module 18, Collecting Specimens.)

17. Even when precise measurements or specimens are not ordered, note the amount, color, consistency, and odor, as well as the presence of blood, mucus, or foreign material. A patient who is being observed for renal calculi (kidney stones) may have an order to have all

urine strained. If you even suspect that a patient's urine or feces contain blood, in most facilities you can guaiac or Hematest a specimen on your own to verify your suspicion. (See Module 27, Common Laboratory Tests.)

18. Empty the contents into the toilet and flush.

19. Thoroughly clean the pan with cold water. State health regulations require that a container of disinfectant solution and a long-handled brush be kept in the bathroom for cleaning bedpans. Wash and rinse the pan thoroughly. Use paper towels for drying. Then, return the pan to the patient's storage unit.

20. Give the patient a basin of warm water, a washcloth, soap, and a towel, or a packaged moist towelette.

21. Allow the patient to wash his or her hands and perineal area, if desired. A nurse usually remembers to wash his or her own hands after assisting a patient with a bedpan but sometimes forgets that the patient would also like to wash. At home, patients normally wash their hands after elimination; therefore, this is no less important after using a bedpan.

22. Adjust the bed back to the low position and lower the rail on the stand side, if appropriate. Make the patient comfortable.

23. Dispose of the washing equipment.

24. Wash your hands.

25. Record any pertinent data. For example:

> 8 a.m. Moderate am't soft, very dark brown stool. Guaiac negative. 450 ml clear straw-colored odor-free urine.   G. Jones, SN

The Procedure for Assisting with a Urinal

The steps used to assist a male patient in using the urinal are essentially the same as those used to assist with a bedpan (see the Performance Checklist), except for a few adaptations.

Never place a urinal for long periods of time between a patient's legs in an effort to control incontinence. This can irritate and erode the skin of the penis. If a patient is unable to use the urinal himself, place the head of the penis into the opening and tell the patient he can now urinate without soiling the bed linen.

Giving Perineal Care

In the clinical setting, this procedure is sometimes called *pericare*.

1. Wash your hands.

2. Explain what you are about to do. Use words the patient understands: "washing your genital area" or "washing between your legs." Again, the patient may be embarrassed, so proceed in a professional manner.

3. The selection of equipment will vary with the type of patient to whom you are administering care.
   a. Postpartum or surgical patient
      (1) Bedpan
      (2) Chux
      (3) Pitcher
      (4) Tap water or antiseptic
      (5) Cotton balls or gauze squares
      (6) Clean pad or dressing
   b. Nonsurgical patient
      (1) Chux
      (2) Washcloth and towel
      (3) Basin of warm water
      (4) Mild soap or cleansing agent
   c. Patient with catheter, in addition to b, above
      (1) Catheter care kit (Figure 7.5)
         or
      (1) Swabs
      (2) Antiseptic or iodine solution

4. Provide privacy by shutting the door and closing the bed curtains.

5. Place the patient in the dorsal recumbent position and drape with a bath blanket as you would to catheterize a patient. (See Module 39, Catheterization.)

6. Proceed as follows:
   a. *Postpartum or surgical patient* Remove dressing or pads. After placing

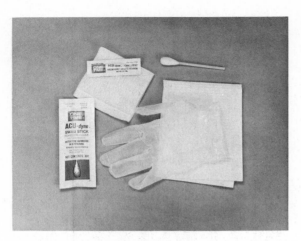

FIGURE 7.5   CATHETER CARE KIT
*Courtesy American Hospital Supply Corp.
McGaw Park, Illinois*

a Chux under the patient, position the bedpan following the procedure in step 6, page 83. Pour tepid tap water or the solution used in your facility over the perineum. Rinse with clear water. Wipe from anterior to posterior, which lessens the possibility of contamination of the urinary tract from the anal area, with cotton balls or gauze. Always clean gently, to prevent pain and avoid pressure on sutures (stitches). Use extra gauze squares or cotton balls if needed, but use each only one time and then discard. Replace pad or dressing, using sterile materials. Remove the bedpan, make any necessary observations, and discard the contents. This procedure can also be done with the patient sitting on a toilet.

b. *Nonsurgical patient*   After placing a Chux or pad under the patient, wash the perineum using warm water and mild soap. Gently separate the labia of the female patient as you clean, in order to remove secretions and *smegma* (an odorous collection of desquamated epithelial cells and mucus). Clean the male patient

beginning with the penile head, moving downward along the shaft. Retract the foreskin of the uncircumcised male gently to avoid causing irritation or pain, so that the underlying tissue can be cleaned. All patients should be rinsed, to remove soap residue, and dried thoroughly. Replace the foreskin over the head of the penis. Remove the damp pads and make the patient comfortable. Dispose of the equipment, wash your hands, and record any pertinent observations. For example:

> 8 a.m. Pericare given. Vulva appears reddened. Small am't clear vaginal drainage.   J. Adams, SN

c. *Patient with a catheter*   After cleaning the perineal area with soap and water as described in b, use the catheter care kit to provide additional protection against ascending infection. The kit usually contains an antiseptic solution (such as water-soluble iodine), an antiseptic ointment, applicator swabs, and a sterile glove. Open the kit using sterile technique (see Module 36). When you open the packages of ointment and swabs, be careful not to touch the applicator tips. Squeeze some ointment onto one applicator and some solution onto others. Put a sterile glove on your nondominant hand. If infection is suspected, you may use two gloves.

For a female patient, using your nondominant hand, spread the labia apart. Clean with swabs, using each swab once in a downward stroke. Clean first on one side of the catheter and then on the other. Retract the catheter slightly. Use a third swab to clean the catheter itself, starting at the meatus and cleaning along 6 inches of the catheter. Use the applicator swab with ointment to place ointment around the base of the catheter and along approximately 1 inch of it.

For a male patient, using your gloved nondominant hand, hold the penis at a right angle to the patient's body. Use swabs to clean the penis, starting from the meatus in a circular pattern. Retract the catheter slightly and use one swab to clean it. Apply the ointment to the urethral meatus and along 1 inch of the catheter.

PERFORMANCE CHECKLIST

Assisting with a bedpan	Unsatisfactory	Needs more practice	Satisfactory	Comments
1. Wash your hands.				
2. Explain what you are going to do.				
3. Provide privacy.				
4. Raise bed to high position with far side rail up.				
5. Obtain bedpan, cover, and toilet tissue.				
6. With as much assistance from patient as possible, position bedpan.				
7. Raise other side rail.				
8. Instruct patient to grasp side rail as you elevate head of bed.				
9. Make sure toilet tissue and call bell are in patient's reach.				
10. Leave patient if possible.				
11. Return to patient.				
12. If necessary, clean genital area with toilet tissue.				
13. Remove pan, reversing method used to position it. Hold pan securely if roll technique is used.				
14. Place cover on bedpan.				
15. Carry to bathroom and measure urine if necessary.				
16. Collect specimen of urine or feces if ordered.				
17. Observe contents.				
18. Empty contents into toilet.				
19. Thoroughly clean pan and return to storage unit.				
20. Give patient handwashing materials.				
21. Allow patient to wash hands. Genital area may also be washed (see Perineal Care).				
22. Adjust bed to low position and make patient comfortable.				
23. Dispose of equipment.				
24. Wash your hands.				
25. Record any pertinent observations.				

Assisting with a urinal	Unsatisfactory	Needs more practice	Satisfactory	Comments
1. Wash your hands.				
2. Explain what you are going to do.				
3. Provide privacy.				
4. Obtain urinal and cover.				
5. Assist patient to desired position.				
6. Give patient urinal, holding in place if necessary.				
7. Place call bell within reach.				
8. Leave patient if possible.				
9. Return to patient.				
10. Remove urinal.				
11. Place cover on urinal.				
12. Carry to toilet and measure contents if ordered.				
13. Collect specimen if ordered.				
14. Observe contents.				
15. Empty contents into toilet.				
16. Clean urinal and return to storage unit.				
17. Give patient handwashing materials.				
18. Allow patient to wash hands. Genital area may also be washed (see Perineal Care).				
19. Make patient comfortable.				
20. Dispose of equipment.				
21. Wash your hands.				
22. Record any pertinent observations.				
Perineal care				
1. Wash your hands.				
2. Explain what you are going to do.				
3. Obtain appropriate equipment.				
4. Provide privacy.				
5. Position and drape patient.				

6. Proceed as follows:
  a. Postpartum or surgical patient
    (1) Remove dressings or pads.				

(2) Position bedpan.				

	Unsatisfactory	Needs more practice	Satisfactory	Comments
(3) Pour tap water or prescribed solution on perineum.				
(4) Follow with rinse if solution used.				
(5) Wipe anterior to posterior with cotton balls or gauze squares, using each only once.				
(6) Use extra gauze squares and solution to clean more thoroughly if needed.				
(7) Discard.				
(8) Replace pad or dressing using sterile materials.				
(9) Remove bedpan, make necessary observations, and discard contents.				
b. Nonsurgical patient (1) Place pad or Chux under patient.				
(2) Moisten washcloth with warm water and apply mild soap or cleansing agent.				
(3) *Female* Wash perineal area from anterior to posterior; pay special attention to clitoral area and labial folds. *Male* Wash perineal area gently, beginning with head of penis and retracting foreskin; continue down shaft, around penis, and posteriorly to rectal area.				
(4) Rinse soap agents thoroughly from patient.				
(5) Dry area with soft towel. (Replace foreskin for male patient.)				
(6) Replace underpads.				
c. Patient with catheter (1) Perform routine perineal care.				
(2) Using swabs moistened with antiseptic solution, hold labia apart in female or penis erect in male, and clean catheter insertion area.				
(3) Retract catheter slightly and apply to catheter itself.				
(4) Do not rinse.				
(5) Apply ointment.				

	Unsatisfactory	Needs more practice	Satisfactory	Comments
7. Make patient comfortable.				
8. Dispose of equipment.				
9. Wash your hands.				
10. Record any pertinent observations.				

QUIZ

Short-Answer Questions

1. List three principles to be followed when assisting a patient with a bedpan or urinal.

   a. _____

   b. _____

   c. _____

2. Name four pieces of equipment that are used to help the bed patient to eliminate.

   a. _____

   b. _____

   c. _____

   d. _____

3. Which two comfort measures should you take for a thin elderly patient who must use a bedpan?

   a. _____

   b. _____

4. Describe two methods for placing a patient on a bedpan.

   a. _____

   b. _____

5. List five of the seven observations that you might make about a patient's urine or feces.

   a. _____

   b. _____

   c. _____

   d. _____

   e. _____

6. Identify three categories of patients who may need special pericare.

   a. _____

   b. _____

   c. _____

7. Describe the procedure for one of the three categories in question 6.

   _____

Module 8 Hygiene

MAIN OBJECTIVE

To provide patients with opportunities for hygiene according to their needs and with consideration of their conditions.

RATIONALE

Hospitalized patients have at least as many needs for hygiene measures in their daily lives as you do in yours. Indeed, they may have considerably more. Often, however, they cannot attend to those needs themselves without at least some help. It is the nurse's responsibility to provide patients with the opportunity for hygiene, with assistance as needed, taking into consideration their personal preferences and physical disabilities.

PREREQUISITES

Successful completion of the following modules:

VOLUME 1
Assessment
Charting
Medical Asepsis
Basic Body Mechanics
Bedmaking
Assisting with Elimination and Perineal Care

SPECIFIC LEARNING OBJECTIVES

	Know Facts and Principles	Apply Facts and Principles	Demonstrate Ability	Evaluate Performance

1. *Providing hygiene*
  a. *Baths*
  b. *Back rubs*
  c. *Oral care*
  d. *Hair care*
	Describe several aspects of hygiene, including baths, back rubs, oral care, and hair care	Given a patient situation, identify type of bath that should be given as well as appropriate type of oral and hair care.
		Explain rationale for types of baths, oral care, and hair care.		

2. *Procedures*	Describe procedures	Given a patient situation, state what should be done according to procedures	Demonstrate ability to perform several aspects of hygiene, including baths, back rubs, oral care, and hair care, according to patient's needs. Initiate performance of several aspects of hygiene independently, according to patient's needs.	Evaluate own performance with instructor using Performance Checklist
3. *Charting hygiene measures*	State items to be charted	Given a patient situation, chart appropriate information regarding hygiene	Chart hygiene procedures according to facility's procedure	Evaluate own performance with instructor

LEARNING ACTIVITIES

1. Review the Specific Learning Objectives.
2. Read the chapter on hygiene in Ellis and Nowlis, *Nursing: A Human Needs Approach,* or a comparable chapter in another textbook.
3. Look up the module vocabulary terms in the glossary.
4. Read through the module.
5. At home, give yourself a complete sponge bath using the technique for giving bedbaths. This can be done at the bathroom sink, but you should use the basin filled with water (not running water) to simulate a bedside situation. Pay special attention to the following:
   a. The temperature of water that feels comfortable to you
   b. Possible chilling due to exposure
   c. The amount of pressure or friction that is comfortable
   d. How easily soap can be rinsed off and how much soap should be used
   e. The effect of "trailing" ends of a washcloth
   f. The need for thorough drying
6. In the practice setting:
   a. Practice giving a complete bedbath, back rub, oral care, and hair care, using another student as your patient. Have the student comment on his or her comfort. Use the Performance Checklist to evaluate yourself. When you are satisfied with your performance, have your instructor evaluate you.
   b. Describe to your instructor what you would do differently to provide a partial bedbath or a self-bedbath with assistance.
   c. Describe the necessary safety measures for the patient receiving a shower or a tub bath.
   d. Practice denture care with dentures if provided in the practice setting. Use the Performance Checklist to evaluate yourself. When you are satisfied with your performance, have your instructor evaluate you.

7. In the clinical setting:
   a. Assist a patient with a tub bath or shower and morning care.
   b. Give a complete bedbath and morning care to a patient.

VOCABULARY

asepto syringe
aspirate
axilla
canthus
cariogenic
expectorate
Fowler's position
genital
semi-Fowler's position
sordes
supine
umbilicus

HYGIENE

Bathing the Patient

Apply the principles of asepsis and body
mechanics given in Module 6, Bedmaking,
to giving various types of bedbaths. Because a patient receiving a bedbath is very
likely to stay in bed while his or her bed
is being made, you may need to refer again
to the procedure for making an occupied
bed.

COMPLETE BEDBATH

1. Wash your hands.
2. Explain what you plan to do. Allow the
   patient to ask questions.
3. Provide for the patient's privacy.
4. Offer the patient an opportunity to use
   a bedpan or urinal. If you assist the
   patient in this activity, wash your hands
   afterward. Offer the patient an opportunity to wash his or her hands as well.
5. Gather the necessary equipment:
   a. Basin for water
   b. Soap (patient may have his or her
      own)
   c. Laundry hamper or bag
   d. Clean linen in the order of use (if
      you plan to make the bed as well)
   e. Bath blanket, towels, and wash-
      cloths as needed (Remember, you
      will want to leave a fresh towel and
      washcloth at the bedside for use at
      other times during the day.)
   f. Clean gown or pajamas
   g. Supplements to patient's personal
      toilet articles (Most patients will
      bring their own toothbrush and paste
      or powder, deodorant, comb, and
      the like; but in some situations this
      may not be true.)
6. Raise the bed to an appropriate working
   level.
7. Remove the top linen, placing a bath
   blanket over the patient before removing the top sheet. (See Occupied Beds,
   Step 4, page 68.)

8. Give oral care at this point if it has not
   already been done. (See Oral Care,
   pages 102–105.)
9. Obtain water for the bath. This may be
   done when you are rinsing the oral
   hygiene articles.
10. Position the patient for the bath. Usu-
    ally the supine position is used unless
    the patient cannot tolerate it. In some
    cases it may be necessary to use a semi-
    Fowler's, or even Fowler's position.
    Move the patient to your side of the
    bed to decrease the need for reaching.
11. Remove the patient's gown, leaving the
    bath blanket in place.
12. Spread a towel across the patient's
    chest, tucking it under the chin.
13. Make a mitt out of the washcloth.
    a. Tucking one edge of the washcloth
       under your thumb, wrap it in thirds
       around your hand, tucking the final
       edge under your thumb as well
       (Figure 8.1).
    b. Bring the far edge of the washcloth
       up and tuck it under the near edge.
       Using a mitt prevents loose, cool
       ends of the cloth from dragging
       across the patient.
    c. As long as the mitt does not come
       apart, it may be left on the hand.
14. Wash the patient's face. This is generally
    done *without* soap, but be certain to
    ask the patient for his or her preference.
    Many patients are able to do this por-
    tion of the bath themselves.
    a. Wash the eyes from the inner canthus
       to the outer canthus; rinse the cloth
       after washing each eye.
    b. Use gentle but firm strokes when
       you wash the face, so that the patient
       feels clean.
    c. Be sure to wash *behind* the ears as
       well as on the upper surfaces, using
       soap.
    d. You may want to use soap on the
       neck even if you didn't on the face.
       Wash just the front and the sides of
       the neck. The back part can be

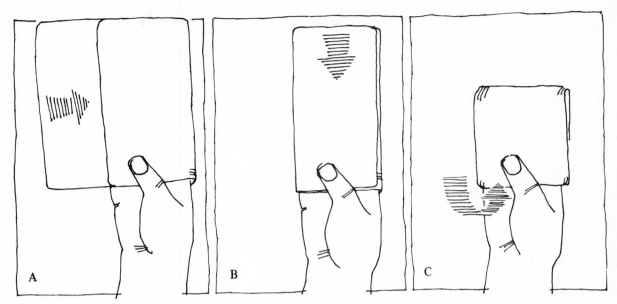

FIGURE 8.1   FOLDING A MITT FOR BATHING   *A:* Fold washcloth lengthwise in thirds around your hand; *B and C:* fold top end of cloth down and tuck under bottom end.

washed when the back is done. Rinse and dry the neck after washing.

15. Place the towel lengthwise under the far arm. If you have moved the patient toward the side of the bed on which you are working, it should not be too far to reach, especially if you place a towel across the patient's chest and have him or her place the arm on top of it (Figure 8.2). Do the far arm first to avoid leaning over and/or dripping dirty water on the part that is already washed. Using long firm strokes toward the center of the body (to increase venous return), wash the far hand, arm, and axilla in that order. Rinse and dry thoroughly.

Often the hands have been washed before the bath or are not very dirty. Some patients, however, really enjoy the opportunity to soak their hands in a basin. In any case, wash the hands thoroughly, being certain to dry well between the fingers. Use an orangewood stick to clean under the nails if needed.

16. Next place the towel under the near arm and wash the near hand, arm, and axilla in the same way.

17. Fold the bath blanket down to the waist. Place the towel over the bath blanket, so that it is close. It may also be used for warmth between washing and rinsing.

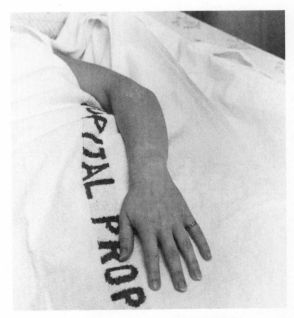

FIGURE 8.2   DRAPING FOR WASHING PATIENT'S ARM   Position patient's arm across body, with towel lengthwise underneath. *Courtesy Ivan Ellis*

Wash the chest, being certain to wash, rinse, and dry thoroughly under the breasts of a female patient. Leave the chest covered with the towel while rinsing the mitt. Rinse and dry the chest.

18. Fold the bath blanket down to the pubic bone, leaving the towel over the chest. Wash, rinse, and dry the lower abdomen, paying particular attention to the umbilicus. Remove the towel and replace the bath blanket over the chest and arms.

19. Remove the bath blanket from the far leg only, tucking it under the near leg and up around the hip to avoid exposure and/or draft. Place the towel lengthwise under the far leg (Figure 8.3).

20. Bending the leg at the knee, slide the basin onto the bed and place the patient's foot in it. Place the foot carefully in the basin, so as not to spill the water. In some facilities the basins used for bathing may be too small to carry out this procedure for patients with large feet.

21. Wash the leg, using long firm strokes toward the center of the body (to increase venous return). Rinse and dry.

22. Wash and rinse the foot, being careful to do each toe separately. Remove the basin from the bed. Dry the foot, giving special attention to the areas between the toes.

23. Wash the near leg and foot in the same way (steps 18–21).

24. Change the bath water.

25. Turn the patient on his or her side, facing away from you. Very few patients will be comfortable lying on the abdomen, although this may be done. Drape the patient as shown in Figure 8.4, the bath blanket drawn down to the hips and a towel tucked lengthwise behind and beside the back.

26. Wash, rinse, and dry the back, using long firm strokes. Remember to include the back of the neck.

27. Wash, rinse, and dry the buttocks.

28. A back rub may be given at this point if the purpose is to stimulate and/or invigorate the patient. If, however, you wish to make the back rub a more relaxing experience for the patient, you can wait until after the bath is completed.

29. Wash the genital area.

   a. In many cases, a patient will be able to wash himself or herself. In this case, your responsibility is to see to it that everything needed is within reach. You may want to stay within hearing distance or instruct the patient to call you with the call light. Be sure the patient understands what you expect him or her to do.

   b. If a patient is not able to wash his or her own genital area, you should do so, moving gently from front to back (clean to dirty), making certain to wash and dry carefully between opposing skin surfaces. (See Module

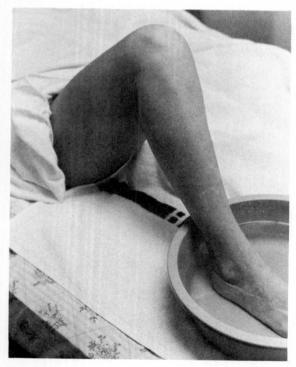

FIGURE 8.3 DRAPING FOR WASHING PATIENT'S LEG   Uncover only one leg at a time, keeping rest of patient's body covered.
Courtesy Ivan Ellis

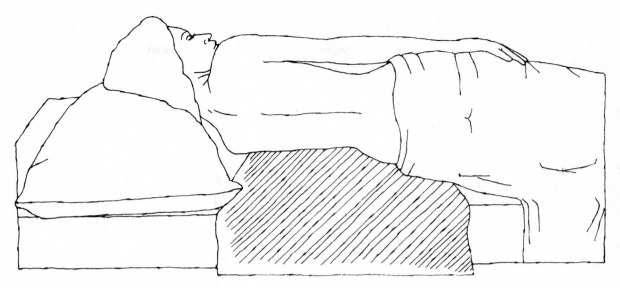

FIGURE 8.4   DRAPING FOR WASHING PATIENT'S BACK

7, Assisting with Elimination and Perineal Care.)

30. Help the patient put on a clean gown or pajamas.

31. Comb and/or brush and arrange the patient's hair. (See Hair Care, pages 105–106.)

32. File and/or cut the patient's fingernails and toenails. Since some facilities do not permit cutting nails, especially of diabetic patients, be sure you know the rules and follow them.

33. The male patient may shave at this point if he wants. You may have to assemble his shaving equipment, which will vary depending on the type of razor he prefers. If he is unable to shave himself, this task is also your responsibility. Most facilities have an electric razor you can use if the patient needs help. If your facility requires you to use a safety razor and you do not know how, ask for assistance.

34. Make the occupied bed. (See Occupied Beds, pages 68–69.) Be sure to return the bed to the low position at the completion of this procedure.

35. Set the patient's room in order; wash and return the bath basin to the patient's storage unit; and put away the patient's personal articles, leaving a washcloth and towel for use during the day. Be sure the patient has everything he or she will need throughout the day *within reach.*

36. Wash your hands.

37. Chart any pertinent observations and/or reactions of the patient.

PARTIAL BEDBATH

A partial bedbath is given for several reasons, including a patient's inability to tolerate a full bath and a lack of need or desire for a full daily bath. A partial bedbath usually includes the face, neck, hands, axillae, and perineum. The back may also be included if the patient can tolerate it. Perform a back rub for any patient on bed rest.

SELF-BEDBATH

This type of bath is given when a patient is, for some reason, unable to take a shower or a tub bath but is able to move about freely in bed. The self-bedbath is usually a complete bath. Your responsibility is to provide the basin of water, bath blanket, and other necessary articles and to be ready to assist at the call of the patient. Your assistance may be needed for the feet and legs, and is necessary for the back and buttocks. Do not omit the back rub simply because a patient is able to bathe unaided.

TUB BATH

Tub baths are generally used for cleaning purposes only, although at times therapeutic agents can be added. If your facility requires a physician's order for a tub bath, be sure you have the order before you offer the patient a bath.

1. Explain what you plan to do. Make sure your timetable is acceptable to the patient.
2. Prepare the tub area. It is frustrating for everyone involved to arrive at the tub room only to find it already in use.
3. After checking to make sure the tub is clean, fill the tub about half full with warm water (100–115° F).
4. Assist the patient to the tub room. Be certain to check which method of ambulation is appropriate. Bring all needed items (towel, deodorant, pajamas, and the like).
5. Hang a sign on the door indicating that the room is occupied.
6. Help the patient into the tub.
   a. If the patient is quite helpless, you may need a second person to assist while you wash. Other patients may be able to support themselves but will need your help with the bath. If there are no safety strips on the bottom of the tub, use an extra bath towel to prevent slipping.
   b. If the patient is quite independent, you may leave for a few minutes while the bath is being taken. The bed may be made at this time. Be certain, however, to tell the patient how to use the emergency call signal before you leave. If the patient seems weak, do *not* leave.
7. Return. Wash the patient's back.
8. Assist the patient out of the tub. *Get help* if you think you might need it. Both you and the patient are too valuable to injure.
9. Assist the patient with drying.
10. Help the patient to put on a clean gown or pajamas.

11. Assist the patient back to his or her room.
12. Return to the tub room.
    a. Clean the tub in the manner prescribed by your facility.
    b. Discard the used linen.
    c. Put the "unoccupied" sign on the door and/or notify the staff person next in line that the tub is ready for use.
13. Wash your hands.
14. Chart any pertinent observations and/or reactions of the patient.

SHOWER

A standing shower may be taken by a patient independently, or a shower may be given in a shower chair. In any case, patients usually prefer showers to bedbaths. If your facility requires a physician's order for a patient to have a shower, be sure you have the order before offering the patient a shower.

1. Explain your plan to the patient.
2. Prepare the shower area.
3. Assist the patient to the shower room or stall. If a chair shower is to be given, you can transport the patient in the shower chair. The safest way to do this is to pull the chair backward down the hall with at least one hand grasping the patient's shoulder.
4. Run the shower until the water is warm (100–115° F); then adjust it to the patient's preference. Place a paper shower mat or bath towel on the floor to prevent slipping.
5. Hang a sign on the door indicating that the room is occupied.
6. At this point, a patient who can take a shower independently may be left (with a call bell within reach), but leave for no more than ten minutes. A patient having a chair shower may need assistance throughout or only at the end of the shower. In any case, check frequently to be certain that the patient is all right.
7. Assist the patient with drying if necessary.

8. Help the patient put on a clean gown or pajamas.
9. Assist the patient back to his or her room.
10. Return to the shower room.
    a. Clean the stall and/or shower chair in the manner prescribed by your facility.
    b. Discard used linen.
    c. Put the "unoccupied" sign on the door.
11. Wash your hands.
12. Chart any pertinent observations and/or reactions of the patient.

Back Rub

Perhaps one of the most talked-about and least-performed aspects of nursing care is the back rub. A daub of lotion smeared over a patient's back in 30 seconds or less is *not* a back rub, but frequently that is all a patient gets.

All patients deserve a back rub at least twice a day (tradition dictates a back rub during or after the bath and at bedtime), but it is of particular importance for those confined to bed because it stimulates circulation and generally relaxes them. However, back rubs may certainly be done more frequently, as indicated by a patient's need and/or desire.

Use the lotion generally provided in the "hospitality kit" for rubbing the back. It is a nice touch to warm it slightly before use, by placing it under warm running water for a few moments. Once you begin a back rub, it is more pleasant and relaxing for the patient if at least one hand remains in contact with his or her back until you have finished (Figure 8.5). This is not difficult to do if the lotion is within easy reach.

Be aware of the patient's response to your touch and question the patient about areas that are especially tight or tense. Ask too which areas he or she would like you to give special attention. Also give special attention to any reddened areas. There are many acceptable ways to perform a back rub. We prefer the following method.

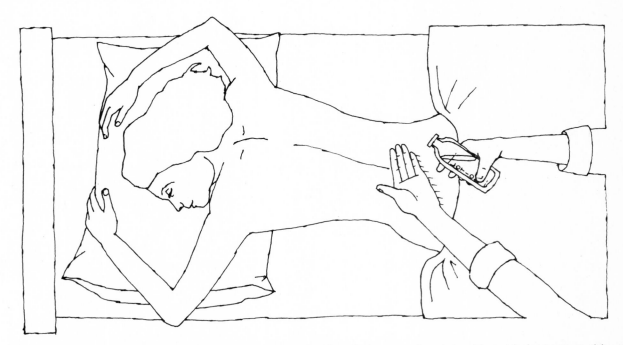

FIGURE 8.5 RETAINING TOUCH DURING BACK RUB   At least one hand should remain in contact with patient's back at all times, even when you are pouring lotion. (Let the back of your hand rest on the patient's back.)

1. Wash your hands.
2. Provide for privacy.
3. Secure lotion or another rubbing agent of the patient's preference.
4. Raise the bed to a comfortable working height for you.
5. Move the patient close to your side of the bed to decrease the distance you need to reach.
6. Position the patient on his or her abdomen if possible. If this is not possible because of the patient's condition or the presence of tubes, a side-lying position with the patient facing away from you is adequate, also. Pull the top covers down below the buttocks.
7. Pour a small amount of lotion in your hand and rub your palms together, to get the lotion on both hands.
8. With your feet apart (the outside one ahead of the inside one so that you can rock back and forth), place your hands at the sacral area, one on either side of the spinal column.
9. Rub toward the neckline, using long, firm, smooth strokes.
10. Pause at the neckline and, using your thumbs, rub up into the hairline, while using your fingers to massage the sides of the neck.
11. With a kneading motion, rub out along the shoulders.
12. Continue the kneading motion and move down one side of the trunk with both hands until you are again at the sacral area.
13. Then, placing your hands side by side with the palms down, rub in a figure-8 pattern over the buttocks and sacral area (Figure 8.6). Move the figure 8 back and forth to include the entire buttocks area, an area that is often neglected.
14. Next, again using the kneading motion, move up the opposite side toward the shoulder.
15. Ask the patient if there are any areas that he or she would especially like rubbed.
16. Complete the back rub using long firm

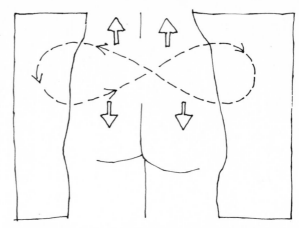

FIGURE 8.6   FIGURE-8 TECHNIQUE IN BACK RUB

strokes up and down the back (shoulders to sacrum and back to shoulders).
17. Replace the top covers, reposition the patient, and lower the bed.
18. Return the lotion to the bedside stand.
19. Wash your hands.
20. Chart any significant observations (condition of the skin, reddened areas, morale, any concerns of the patient). This is often a comfortable time for the patient to talk with you.

Oral Care

Oral care is a too-often neglected or inadequately done aspect of hygiene. Ideally the patient should be offered the opportunity for oral care before breakfast, after all meals, and at bedtime. Not all patients will want oral care this frequently, but it should still be offered. Oral care is especially important for patients receiving oxygen and for patients who have nasogastric tubes in place, as well as for those on NPO (nothing by mouth). Many will be able to take care of this aspect of their hygiene independently, provided the equipment is conveniently placed.

If a patient can perform his or her own oral care but is confined to bed, you should provide the necessary articles: toothbrush, toothpaste and/or powder (usually brought to the facility by the patient), cup of water, emesis basin, and face towel. Some patients also use dental floss.

TOOTHBRUSHING

Brushing is correctly done using a small soft brush. Many dentists recommend a four-row, level, straight-handled brush. Hold the brush at a 45° angle, making a small, vibrating, circular motion with the bristles at the junction of the teeth and gums. Use the same action on the front and the back of the teeth.

Use a back-and-forth brushing motion over the biting surfaces of the teeth. Brush the tongue last and then rinse the mouth. It is wise to rinse after eating if brushing cannot be done. Mouthwashes can be used if desired, but remember that their antiseptic value is questionable.

FLOSSING

Flossing should be done once daily to remove placque (organisms trapped in a mucus base), which if not removed causes tooth and gum disease. Placque forms in 24 hours, after which it can only be removed by

a visit to the dentist's office. Floss is correctly held as demonstrated in Figure 8.7; however, remember that control of the floss is more important than how it is held.

Flossing is carried out both between the teeth and between the gums and each individual tooth, taking care not to injure the delicate mucous membranes. The mouth should be rinsed after flossing.

Patients who can sit in Fowler's or even semi-Fowler's position can often do most of their oral care independently. If they cannot, use the following procedure.

1. Wash your hands.
2. Assemble the equipment. Raise the bed to a comfortable working height.
3. Place a towel under the chin, tucking it behind the patient's shoulders.
4. Moisten the toothbrush with water from a glass and spread a small amount of toothpaste on it. If no cleansing agent is available, plain water is satis-

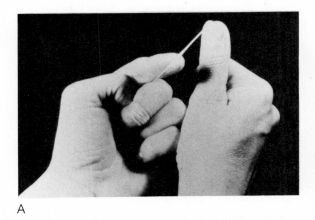

A

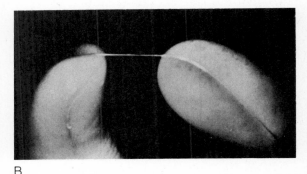

B

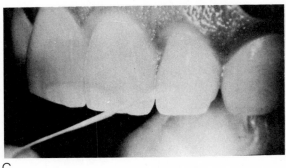

C

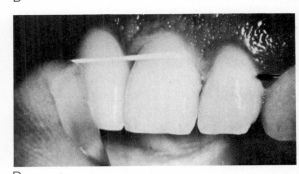

D

FIGURE 8.7   FLOSSING THE TEETH
Courtesy Ivan Ellis

factory in terms of dental care. Baking soda is a substitute that also freshens the breath.

5. Brush the teeth according to the procedure above, allowing the patient to expectorate into the emesis basin.
6. Allow the patient to rinse his or her mouth with water, followed by a mouthwash if desired.
7. Wipe the patient's mouth.
8. Rinse and return equipment to its appropriate place.
9. Wash your hands. Return the bed to the low position.

Unconscious patients are completely dependent on you for their oral care. Because these persons may be "mouth breathers" and are not taking food or fluids by mouth, sordes accumulates rapidly. A suitable procedure for the oral care of unconscious patients is as follows.

1. Wash your hands.
2. Assemble the equipment. Many facilities have mouth care kits prepared, which include tongue blades, applicators, mouthwash, and the like. Suction should be available. Raise the bed to a comfortable working height.
3. Place the patient in semi-Fowler's position, if possible, with his or her head turned to the side toward you. If the patient's head cannot be raised, leave him or her flat and turn the head to the side toward you.
4. Place a towel under the patient's chin, tucking it in beneath the shoulders.
5. Place a padded tongue blade (made by wrapping 4 x 4s around a tongue blade and taping them securely) in the patient's mouth.
6. Using oversized cotton-tipped applicators, or gauze or a washcloth wrapped around your index finger, clean all surfaces of the mouth, including the palate, inner cheeks, and tongue. A variety of cleansing agents can be used. A mixture of hydrogen peroxide and water, half and half, is probably as good as anything, and it is not cariogenic, as

are buttermilk and milk of magnesia. Commercial agents often contain lemon, which can etch the teeth, and glycerin, which actually adsorbs moisture from the tissue. Therefore the use of such agents is not wise, particularly for unconscious patients or patients who are receiving nothing by mouth. If a large accumulation of sordes is present, it may be necessary to remove it in stages, so as not to damage the tissue.

7. Brush the teeth (see Toothbrushing, page 103–104).
8. Rinse the patient's mouth with small amounts of water, either allowing it to drain into the emesis basin by gravity or using an asepto syringe to aspirate it.
9. Wipe the patient's mouth.
10. Lubricate the lips as needed. Use a water-soluble agent to prevent the aspiration of any oils.
11. Rinse and replace the equipment.
12. Wash your hands. Return the bed to the low position.

CARE OF DENTURES

Patients often want to care for their dentures themselves. If so, your responsibility, once again, will be to provide them with the necessary articles. A patient may have brought a denture brush and cleansing agent to the hospital, but, if not, a regular toothbrush and paste or powder will suffice. Provide the patient with a partially filled bath basin over which to wash the dentures, so that if they fall they will not break. The patient will also need a glass of water for rinsing.

If you care for the dentures yourself, keep the following facts in mind.

1. Handle dentures with care. If dropped, they often break. For this reason they are usually cleaned over a sink that is partially filled with water, to break the fall in case they are dropped.
2. To assist a patient with removal, apply downward pressure with the index fingers from above the dentures. It may help if the patient inflates his or her

cheeks to break the suction. If no assistance is needed, it works well to have the patient remove his or her own dentures and place them in a denture cup for you.

3. Take the dentures to the sink in the denture cup. Use a denture brush if the patient has one. Note that the longer side of the brush is used for the tooth surface and that the smaller part is used for brushing the inner surface. Be certain to do the brushing over a basin of water. Some people like to pad the basin with a towel instead of putting water in it. Both measures are taken to prevent breakage in case the dentures are dropped.

4. Have the patient rinse out his or her mouth before reinserting the dentures. Some like to use a soft toothbrush to brush the gums and tongue.

5. Then rinse the dentures and return to the patient, fitting the upper dentures in first. Dry the patient's mouth.

6. If dentures are to be stored (for an unconscious patient or at night if necessary), they should be stored in a covered container, carefully labeled, and preferably placed in a drawer or other area where they would not be likely to be brushed off onto the floor. Whether or not they should be stored in water depends on the material of which they are made. Check with the patient or the patient's family.

Hair Care

A patient's hair should be combed and brushed on a daily basis. Generally this is done along with other hygiene activities and at other times throughout the day as necessary. This aspect of care is especially important to the patient, since morale is often directly related to appearance.

Hair care is usually done at the completion of the bath. Whenever it is done, these are some important points to remember.

1. Explain what you plan to do. If the patient can participate, encourage him or her to do so. If assistance is needed, you should be prepared to give it.

2. Wash your hands.

3. Assemble the equipment. The patient will probably have brought his or her own comb, brush, and other preferred hair care items to the facility. A mirror may be available as a part of the over-bed table.

4. Place a face or bath towel over the pillow to keep it clean.

5. The patient who can attend to the combing and brushing of his or her own hair should be placed in Fowler's position with the hair care items on the overbed table. Assist the patient as necessary.

6. The helpless and/or unconscious patient may be flat or in a semi-Fowler's position.

7. Turn the patient's head away from you and bring the hair back toward you. Brush hair with minimal tangles in two or three large sections. Matted hair may have to be separated into small sections and treated with cream rinse or alcohol to remove the snarls.

8. Hold a section of hair 2 to 3 inches from the end. Comb the end until it is free of tangles. Gradually move toward the scalp, combing 2 to 3 inches at a time until the hair is tangle-free. You should be very gentle to avoid causing pain.

9. Turn the patient's head in the opposite direction and repeat steps 7 and 8.

10. Arrange the hair as neatly and simply as possible. Braiding may be the most appropriate style for long hair. (The family can bring in barrettes and ribbons to make your job easier.) Use cream or spray as necessary and as preferred by the patient.

11. Remove the towel and place it in a laundry hamper or bag.

12. Clean the comb and brush and return them, along with the other toilet articles, to the bedside stand.

13. Wash your hands.

14. Chart any pertinent observations and/or reactions of the patient.

SHAMPOOS

Many patients whose illnesses keep them in the hospital only a few days do not want or need shampoos during that time. Other patients, however, may *need* shampoos, not only to remove oil and dirt and to increase circulation to the scalp, but to improve appearance and morale as well. Before giving a shampoo, check to see if a physician's order is needed.

Generally, a shampoo is not given at the same time as the bath because it is a tiring procedure. The obvious exception is when a patient can shower. The equipment and general procedure you will use for those patients who need a shampoo and cannot shower will vary with the facility. In some places, the patient is taken on a stretcher to an area away from his or her room where there is a sink at the right height with room for the stretcher too. In most facilities, however, the patient remains in bed and the shampoo is given using pitchers of warm water and a trough arrangement to guide the water into a receptacle on the floor or chair beside the bed.

Use this general procedure for giving a shampoo.

1. Explain what you plan to do. Often the patient will have requested a shampoo.
2. Wash your hands.
3. Assemble the equipment, including bath blanket, two towels, shampoo, commercial rinse or vinegar, plastic square to protect the bed, pitcher, trough (if available in the facility, or you can make one from a plastic or rubber sheet with rolled towels under the edges), and a basin to collect water. (See Figure 8.8.)
4. Remove the top linens and position a bath blanket. (See Occupied Beds, step 4, page 68.)
5. Place the plastic square under the patient's head and shoulders.
6. Place a towel around the patient's

shoulders and neck, with the ends of the towel coming together in front.
7. Place or arrange a trough under the patient's head with one end extending to the receptacle for water.
8. Wet the hair, taking care to keep water out of the patient's eyes. Some patients like to hold a folded washcloth over their eyes.
9. Shampoo and rinse two times, using only a small amount of shampoo and rinsing thoroughly. Use cream rinse or half-and-half vinegar and water rinse as desired by the patient. Rinse again.
10. Dry the patient's hair, ears, and neck with a towel. If an electric hair dryer is available, you may find it helpful, particularly if a patient has long hair.
11. Comb and/or brush and arrange the hair, allowing the patient to assist if able. If hair-setting materials are available, a female patient may wish to set, or have you set, her hair, in which case you would comb it at a later time.
12. Remove the plastic square, towels, trough, pitcher, and basin.
13. Replace the top bed linen, removing the bath blanket after the top sheet is in place.
14. Allow the patient to rest.
15. Wash your hands.
16. In addition to the procedure itself, record the patient's response and any pertinent observations.

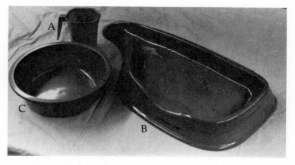

FIGURE 8.8 EQUIPMENT FOR SHAMPOOING PATIENT'S HAIR IN BED Water is poured from the pitcher *(A)* over the patient's hair, drains down through the trough *(B)* beneath the patient's head, and falls into the basin *(C)* below.
Courtesy Ivan Ellis

PERFORMANCE CHECKLIST

Complete bedbath	Unsatisfactory	Needs more practice	Satisfactory	Comments
1. Wash your hands.				
2. Explain procedure to patient.				
3. Provide for privacy.				
4. Gather equipment (see Complete Bedbath, step 5, page 96).				
5. Raise bed to working level.				
6. Remove top linen and place bath blanket.				
7. Obtain water.				
8. Position patient (see Complete Bedbath, step 10, page 96).				
9. Remove patient's gown.				
10. Spread towel across patient's chest; make mitt; and bathe patient's eyes, face, ears, and neck.				
11. Spread towel under far arm and then near arm, bathing, rinsing, and drying hands, arms, and axillae.				
12. Spread towel across patient's chest and wash, rinse, and dry chest to waist.				
13. Wash, rinse, and dry abdomen.				
14. Place towel under far leg and then under near leg, washing patient's feet and legs and taking care not to expose him or her.				
15. Change water.				
16. Assist patient to turn, and wash, rinse, and dry back and buttocks.				
17. Wash genital area or give patient an opportunity to do so.				
18. Help patient put on clean gown.				
19. Assist patient with hair and nail care.				
20. Tidy up area.				
21. Wash your hands.				
22. Chart.				

	Unsatisfactory	Needs more practice	Satisfactory	Comments
Tub bath				
1. Explain procedure.				
2. Prepare tub area.				
3. Fill tub about half full with warm water (100–115° F).				
4. Assist patient to tub room.				
5. Hang "occupied" sign on door.				
6. Assist patient into tub.				
7. Assist with bath as necessary, especially back.				
8. Assist patient out of tub, securing help if needed.				
9. Assist patient with drying.				
10. Help patient put on clean gown or pajamas.				
11. Assist patient back to room.				
12. Ready tub room for next occupant.				
13. Wash your hands.				
14. Chart.				
Shower				
1. Explain procedure.				
2. Prepare shower area.				
3. Assist patient to shower room or stall.				
4. Adjust shower to 100–115° F.				
5. Hang "occupied" sign on door.				
6. Assist patient with shower as indicated.				
7. Assist patient with drying.				
8. Help patient put on clean gown or pajamas.				
9. Assist patient back to room.				
10. Ready shower room or stall for next occupant.				
11. Wash your hands.				
12. Chart.				

	Unsatisfactory	Needs more practice	Satisfactory	Comments
Back rub				
1. Wash your hands.				
2. Provide for privacy.				
3. Secure lotion.				
4. Raise bed.				
5. Move patient to your side of bed.				
6. Position patient.				
7. Rub patient with lotion, starting at sacral area and moving toward neckline using long firm strokes.				
8. Massage into hairline.				
9. Knead along shoulders.				
10. Knead down one side to sacral area.				
11. Rub in figure-8 pattern over buttocks and sacral area.				
12. Knead up opposite side toward shoulders.				
13. Seek response from patient.				
14. Complete back rub moving from shoulders to sacrum and back to shoulders.				
15. Replace covers, reposition patient, and return lotion.				
16. Wash your hands.				
17. Chart.				
Oral care (The student serving as patient should provide his or her own toothbrush and cleansing agent.)				
1. Wash your hands.				
2. Gather equipment.				
3. Place towel under chin.				
4. Moisten toothbrush and apply cleansing agent.				
5. Brush teeth of patient according to Toothbrushing, page 103.				
6. Allow patient to rinse with water.				
7. Wipe patient's mouth.				
8. Rinse and return equipment.				
9. Wash your hands.				
10. Chart.				

	Unsatisfactory	Needs more practice	Satisfactory	Comments
Care of dentures				
1. Wash your hands.				
2. Gather equipment, including basin of water.				
3. Assist patient with removal of dentures.				
4. Brush all surfaces of dentures.				
5. Have patient rinse his or her mouth.				
6. Rinse dentures and return to patient, upper dentures first, or store dentures appropriately.				
7. Assist patient to dry his or her mouth.				
8. Wash your hands.				
Hair care				
1. Explain procedure to patient.				
2. Wash your hands.				
3. Gather equipment (see Hair Care, step 3, page 105).				
4. Place towel over pillow.				
5. Turn patient's head away and comb hair, starting close to ends and keeping hand between scalp and hair ends.				
6. Turn patient's head in opposite direction and repeat step 5.				
7. Arrange hair.				
8. Remove towel.				
9. Return equipment to bedside stand.				
10. Clean the equipment.				
11. Wash your hands.				
12. Chart.				
Charting				
1. Procedure.				
2. Patient's response.				
3. Observations made.				

QUIZ

Multiple-Choice Questions

_____C_____ 1. The temperature of the water for bathing and shampooing has been described as "warm." This means

    a. 75–90° F.
    b. 90–105° F.
    c. 100–115° F.
    d. 110–125° F.

_____B_____ 2. The preferred position for bathing the patient in bed is

    a. prone.
    b. supine.
    c. semi-Fowler's.
    d. Fowler's.

_____D_____ 3. The partial bedbath usually includes which of the following areas of the body? (1) face and neck; (2) hands; (3) axillae; (4) perineum

    a. 1 and 2
    b. 1 and 2
    c. 2, 3, and 4
    d. All of these

True-False Questions

_____F_____ 4. A patient's face should be washed with soap and water.

_____F_____ 5. When washing the arms, long firm strokes toward the center of the body are used to decrease venous return.

_____T_____ 6. The back of the neck is washed separately from the front of the neck.

_____F_____ 7. You should always cut and file the toenails and fingernails of the patient.

_____T_____ 8. A patient should be offered the opportunity for oral care before breakfast, after all meals, and at bedtime.

_____F_____ 9. The unconscious patient does not need oral care.

_____T_____ 10. Toothbrushing is correctly done using a small soft brush.

_____T_____ 11. Dentures should be brushed over a basin of water.

_____F_____ 12. The hair of the hospitalized patient should be washed and combed and/or brushed on a daily basis.

Module 9 Basic Infant Care

MAIN OBJECTIVE

To provide basic daily care for infants and to implement safety measures in all aspects of care.

RATIONALE

Included in the care of hospitalized infants are feeding, bathing, and diapering. Special efforts are needed to maintain safety for infants both in general care and throughout all procedures. To provide this safety, the nurse must carry out special measures and use equipment, such as restraints, correctly.

PREREQUISITES

Successful completion of the following modules:

VOLUME 1
Assessment
Charting
Medical Asepsis
Basic Body Mechanics
Hygiene

SPECIFIC LEARNING OBJECTIVES

	Know Facts and Principles	Apply Facts and Principles	Demonstrate Ability	Evaluate Performance
1. *Diapering*				
a. Types	Identify types of diapers in common use			
b. Folding cloth diapers	Know methods of folding cloth diapers and advantages of each method	Determine appropriate way to fold diaper for particular situation	Fold diaper in both triangle and fan-folded shapes	Evaluate own performance using Performance Checklist
c. Cleaning	State rationale for frequent diaper changes. Know purpose of cleaning perineal area and buttocks with each diaper change.	Decide when to change infant's diaper based on rationale. Given a situation, select appropriate materials for cleaning infant during diapering.		
d. Fastening diapers	List two ways diapers are fastened	Given a situation, determine appropriate way to fasten diaper	Fasten diaper, handling safety pins correctly	
e. Skin problems	Describe symptoms of diaper rash and scald	Given a description of infant, identify whether diaper rash or scald is present	In the clinical setting, identify diaper rash and/or scald	
f. Diapering procedure	List steps of procedure		Change infant's diaper correctly and safely	Evaluate diapering by checking for fit and comfort. Evaluate own performance using Performance Checklist.

2. *Bathing*	Discuss special considerations for bathing infant	Given a situation, describe correct procedure for bathing infant	Bathe infant correctly and safely	Evaluate own performance with instructor
3. *Bottle feeding*	Describe two positions for bottle feeding	Plan appropriate feeding position for particular infant	Bottle-feed infant	Evaluate by measuring infant's intake
a. *Temperature*	State usual temperature for bottle. State method for testing temperature.	Given a situation, decide whether to warm formula	Correctly distinguish safe temperature for bottle feeding	Evaluate own performance with instructor
b. *Burping*	Describe two positions for burping		Burp infant after feeding	Evaluate by checking whether infant has burped
4. *Feeding solids*	Describe two positions for feeding solids to infant	Plan appropriate position for particular infant	Feed solids to infant correctly	Evaluate by recording infant intake
a. *Temperature*	State proper temperature for solid foods	Identify safe method for warming infant's food	Demonstrate method to determine temperature of food	Evaluate own performance with instructor

SPECIFIC LEARNING OBJECTIVES (*cont.*)

	Know Facts and Principles	Apply Facts and Principles	Demonstrate Ability	Evaluate Performance
5. *Safety Measures*				
a. *Tying a clove hitch*	State purpose of clove-hitch restraint	Identify situation in which clove-hitch restraint needed	Correctly and safely tie clove-hitch restraint	Evaluate own performance using Performance Checklist
b. *Using crib restraints*	State purpose of crib restraints	Identify situations in which crib restraints needed	Correctly and safely apply crib restraints	Evaluate own performance using Performance Checklist
c. *Elbow restraints*	State purpose of elbow restraints	Identify situations in which elbow restraints needed	Correctly and safely apply elbow restraints	Evaluate own performance using Performance Checklist
d. *Mummying*	State purpose of mummying	Identify situations in which mummying needed	Correctly and safely apply mummy restraint to infant	Evaluate own performance using Performance Checklist
		Given a situation, identify correct type of restraint to be used		Evaluate choice with instructor

LEARNING ACTIVITIES

1. Review the Specific Learning Objectives.
2. Look up the module vocabulary terms in the glossary.
3. Read through the module.
4. In the practice setting:
   a. Diapering
      (1) Inspect both cloth and disposable diapers.
      (2) Practice folding diapers using both the fan-folded and triangle-folded methods. Fold them to provide extra thickness in the front (used for males and females lying on the abdomen). Then refold to provide extra thickness in the back (used for females lying on the back).
      (3) Diaper an infant mannequin using the Performance Checklist as a guide. Practice opening and closing safety pins with one hand while keeping other on the "infant."
      (4) Arrange for your instructor to check you when you feel competent.
   b. Bathing
      (1) Bathe an infant mannequin using the procedures as described.
   c. Bottle feeding
      (1) Practice holding an infant mannequin for bottle feeding.
      (2) Practice both methods of holding an infant mannequin for burping.
      (3) Have your instructor check your performance.
   d. Feeding solids
      (1) Practice feeding an infant mannequin solids while holding it on your lap.
   e. Safety measures
      (1) Practice tying a clove-hitch knot. Have your instructor check the knot.
      (2) Improvise an arm or use a mannequin's arm and tie it to a stationary object (the bed frame, armboard) using a clove-hitch knot.
      (3) Inspect elbow restraints if they are available.
      (4) Practice mummying an infant mannequin using the two methods outlined in the module.
      (5) Have your instructor check your performance.

VOCABULARY

burp
circumcise
clove hitch
colic
cradle cap
fontanel
foreskin
macerate
macular
smegma

BASIC INFANT CARE

Diapering

TYPES OF DIAPERS

Many hospitals use disposable diapers (Figure 9.1). These have the advantage of decreasing laundry and ensuring that no cross-contamination occurs. Most have a waterproof cover that protects the linen from urine and stool. Disposable diapers come in a variety of sizes based on weight, making proper fit possible. Some infants do develop skin sensitivity to paper products, however.

Cloth diapers can be softer and less irritating for some infants. Plastic pants are optional, and should be omitted for an infant, for example, a newborn, whose skin is sensitive to urine accumulation. Cloth diapers generally come in one size but can be folded to accommodate different-size infants. Also, several diapers can be folded together to provide an absorbent diaper for overnight use on older infants or toddlers. Some cloth diapers are available in prefolded shapes.

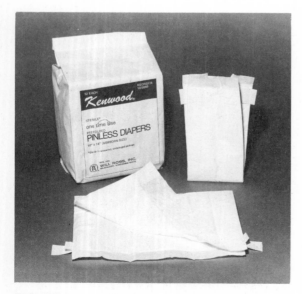

FIGURE 9.1   DISPOSABLE DIAPER
Courtesy Searle Medical Products USA Inc.

FOLDING CLOTH DIAPERS

There are a variety of methods for folding diapers. We explain two common ones in this module. The purpose of any type of fold is to provide a diaper that:

a. is the correct size for the infant.
b. fastens safely and securely.
c. is the thickest where greatest absorbency is needed.
d. is comfortable for the infant to wear.
e. retains both urine and stool in the diaper.

No one folding method is ideal, and you may devise your own adaptations for specific situations.

Triangle folding provides the greatest mobility for an infant's legs. A diaper can be folded with its maximum thickness in the front for boys or for girls who sleep on the abdomen, and with maximum thickness in the back for girls who sleep on the back. Alter the size by changing the size of the initial square into which the diaper is folded and by changing the width to which the triangle is folded.

To fold, follow the diagrams in Figure 9.2.

1. Fold the diaper into a square (A). The size may be altered at this point.
2. Holding one corner of the square firmly in place, fold the two adjacent corners toward the middle of the diaper, forming an elongated diamond shape (B). The final width of the diaper can be altered by changing the amount the two corners overlap.
3. Fold the corner you have been holding down over the other two, creating a long triangle.
4. Now, fold the last corner, which is the smallest angle of the triangle, toward the center (C). The length of the diaper may be altered by changing the amount that is folded up.

Fan-folding provides the greatest width between the legs and is often better at containing loose stools than is a triangle-folded diaper. The size can be changed very simply. Alter the width by changing the width of the

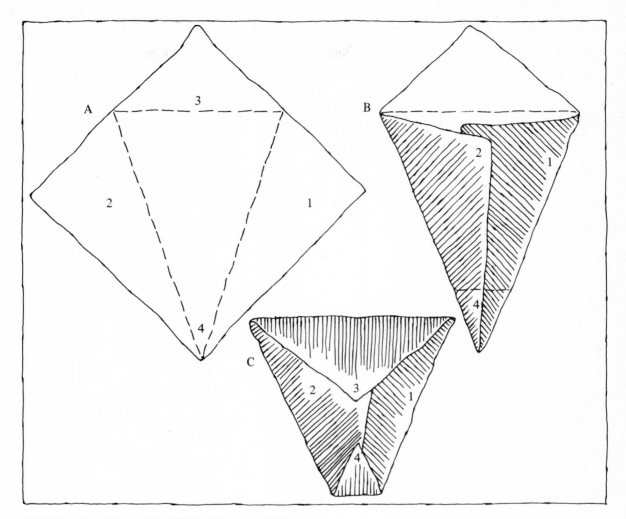

FIGURE 9.2   TRIANGLE-FOLDING A DIAPER

initial fold, alter the length by simply fold-ing over the front or the back until the diaper is the desired length.

To fold, follow the diagrams in Figure 9.3.

1. Pick up an oblong diaper by two ad-jacent corners on the short side (A).
2. Lay enough of the diaper on the table to provide the desired width.
3. Make recurrent folds over the center of the diaper, so that the diaper has many layers in the center (B).
4. Fold one front end over to create the correct length for the infant. Use the folded end in either the front or back as needed.

CLEANING AT DIAPER CHANGES

Facilities usually establish a routine for this procedure. Several ways are presented here.

1. The simplest method is to wash with a mild soap and water, and then to rinse thoroughly. Keep a washcloth and towel at the side of the crib for this purpose.
2. Use cotton balls saturated in baby oil or baby lotion. This method does not require rinsing because the baby oil does not irritate the skin.
3. Use disposable wipes that contain baby oil or lotion for cleaning. Again, rinsing is not needed because there is no ir-ritating substance present.

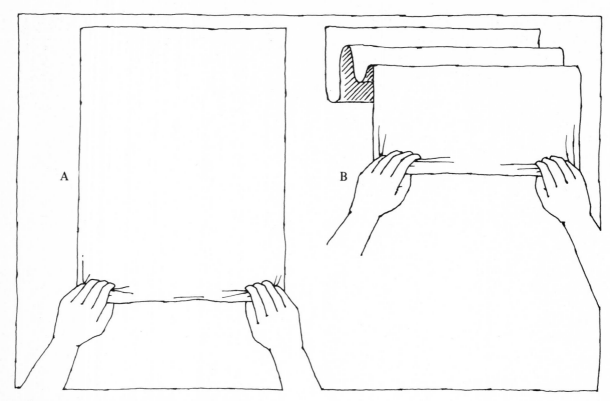

FIGURE 9.3   FAN-FOLDING A DIAPER

FASTENING DIAPERS

Some disposable diapers come with attached tapes for fastening. These are both convenient and safe. Use safety pins to fasten all other diapers. Remember that opened safety pins are *always* a hazard. Fasten pins in the closed position as soon as they are removed and place them out of reach. Then, even if you have misjudged the infant's reach, he or she will pick up a closed, not an open, pin.

When you are ready to fasten a diaper, place the pin so that the open end points to the infant's side. If the pin later opens, it will be less likely to cause injury. Also, always place your hand between the infant and the diaper you are pinning. Then, if you push the pin completely through the diaper, you will stick your own hand and *not* the infant. If a safety pin does not slide easily into the diaper, stick the point into a bar of soap to lubricate it, so that it enters easily.

SKIN PROBLEMS

Diaper rash is a skin reaction that appears as a macular to solid redness in the perineal area. It may be caused by

a. prolonged contact with urine.
b. the irritation of ammonia formed as the urine decomposes.
c. maceration from wetness.
d. irritation from residual detergents or cleansing agents in a diaper.
e. irritation from the harsh surface of a diaper.

Scald occurs rapidly and appears as a totally reddened area much like a burn. It happens when the stool or urine contains harsh ingredients, which cause a chemical-type burn of the skin.

The best method to prevent diaper rash and/or scald is to change diapers frequently, to clean the skin with each change to remove residual urine or feces, and wash diapers correctly (with mild soap and

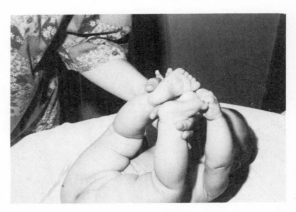

thorough rinsing). If diaper rash persists, consult a physician. Infants are prone to candida (a fungal infection), which can have an appearance similar to diaper rash.

If an infant is having frequent, loose, or diarrheal stools, a heavy non–water soluble ointment (petroleum jelly, A & D ointment) may be applied at the time of the diaper change to protect the skin from contact with the stool. You must check your facility's policy regarding whether an ointment may be used.

Powders also can be used to help the skin remain dry. Do not let powder get into the air, where the infant might inhale it, because it acts as an irritant to the respiratory tract. Place a small amount on your hand, and then smooth it over the infant's skin. Use only a thin coating; large amounts tend to gather in clumps that can irritate the skin. Some infants are sensitive to the perfume in baby powder, and this can cause skin irritation also. Because of the potential problems associated with its use, some facilities do not use baby powder at all. Cornstarch is an inexpensive substitute for it and does not tend to cause irritation.

DIAPERING PROCEDURE

1. Wash your hands so that you do not introduce microorganisms to the infant.
2. Obtain a clean diaper and cleansing equipment.
3. Fold the diaper if necessary.
4. Place the infant on his or her back in the crib or on a clean surface. Make sure the infant is safe from falling. *Never* leave an infant when he or she is out of the crib.
5. Unfasten the soiled diaper, close the safety pins as you remove them, and set them aside out of the infant's reach.
6. Remove the soiled diaper, using the clean portion of the diaper to wipe away stool. Wipe from front to back. Do not leave the infant.
7. Clean the diaper area thoroughly. Take extra care to clean in all folds, around the scrotum on a boy and between the

FIGURE 9.4   LIFTING AN INFANT BY THE ANKLES TO PLACE A DIAPER
Courtesy Ivan Ellis

labia on a girl. For a girl, be sure you clean from anterior region to posterior region, so you do not contaminate the urinary meatus with bacteria from the rectal area. If there was a large amount of stool or urine, the infant may need more extensive bathing. Change all wet or soiled clothing. Be careful about leaning over a male infant—urine can be sprayed a long distance.

8. Lift the infant's buttocks by grasping both ankles with one hand and place a clean diaper under the infant (Figure 9.4).
9. Pull the front of the diaper up between the infant's legs, so that it fits snugly around the abdomen. Fasten with pins or tapes. (See Figure 9.5.)

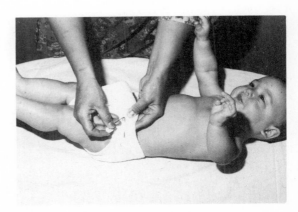

FIGURE 9.5   DIAPER IN PLACE
Courtesy Ivan Ellis

10. Be sure that the infant is secure and protected from falling.
11. Dispose of the soiled diaper.
12. Wash your hands.
13. Chart the appearance of the stool and check voiding. All stools and voidings are usually recorded for infants.

Bathing

An infant is given a bedbath in much the same manner as an adult. Keeping the infant warm and safe are primary elements. Among the special considerations for bathing an infant are the following:

Safety   Everything must be in reach before beginning; one hand must remain in contact with the infant.

Holding the infant   Any way of holding an infant must provide support for the head and neck and keep the infant close to your body to lessen the chance of injury or dropping. The *football hold* does all of these things. In the football hold the infant is held with the head in the palm of the hand, the back on the forearm, and the feet between the arm and your side (Figure 9.6). If the infant can sit in a basin with support, keep one of your arms behind the infant, holding onto the infant's far arm. This leaves your other arm free, yet keeps the infant secure. With an older infant who can sit unaided, you should still keep one hand on the infant

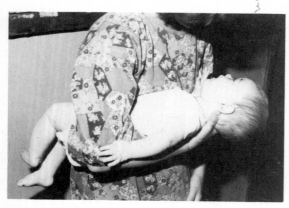

FIGURE 9.6   THE FOOTBALL HOLD
Courtesy Ivan Ellis

at all times. Remember, a tub is slippery and infants move very quickly. Do not immerse an infant with an umbilical cord.

Shampooing   This is usually done each time an infant is bathed to prevent a scale accumulation called *cradle cap*. Hold the infant football-style, with the head over the basin, so the scalp can be gently scrubbed and thoroughly rinsed with strokes going away from the infant's face.

Eye care   Without soap, clean each eye from inner to outer canthus, using a clean area of the washcloth for each eye.

Folds   Infants have many creases and folds. Take care to wash and dry carefully in all of them.

Perineal care   For the female infant, be sure to clean between the labia and in all folds from front to back. For the uncircumcised male infant, retract the foreskin to clean and then replace it.

BATHING PROCEDURE

1. Wash your hands.
2. Gather the necessary equipment. You will need a basin, mild soap, a washcloth, a towel, clean clothing for the infant, and possibly clean linen.
3. Fill the basin with warm water. Check the temperature by using a sensitive part of your arm, such as the elbow. It should be comfortably warm, never hot. If a bath thermometer is available, use water at 100° F to 105° F.
4. Place the basin on a firm surface. On a towel in the crib may be the safest place.
5. Wash and dry the infant's face. Be very careful with the soap.
6. Hold the infant securely in a football hold, with the head over the basin. (See Figure 9.6.)
7. Shampoo the scalp. Use your fingertips, not your fingernails, and massage firmly. If any scales are present, remove them from the hair with a fine comb. Do not hesitate to wash over the fontanels (soft spots). In some facilities, the scalp (including the area behind the ears) is

wiped with a small amount of baby oil on a cotton ball to help prevent scales.

8. Rub the head dry with a towel.

9. Undress the infant. Keep the infant dressed during the shampoo to prevent chilling.

10. Hold the infant securely as you place him or her into the water. Use a towel in the basin to decrease slipping.

11. Keep one hand securely on the infant while bathing with the other (Figure 9.7).

12. Wash and rinse the shoulders, arms, and chest, and then move on down the body.

13. Lift the infant out of the water and lay him or her on the towel.

14. Wrap the infant while you dry, to prevent chilling.

15. Diaper and redress the infant.

16. If the crib must be made, place the infant at one end while you make up the other.

17. Put side rails up before you leave the infant. Refasten the crib net if necessary.

18. Empty and clean the basin.

19. Dispose of soiled linen.

20. Wash your hands.

21. Chart observations made during the bath and enter bath on the checklist or flow sheet.

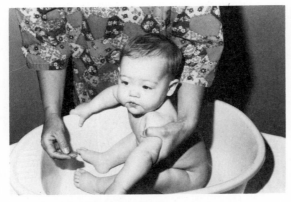

FIGURE 9.7   BATHING AN INFANT IN A BASIN
Courtesy Ivan Ellis

Bottle Feeding

1. Check the order for formula. Today, prefilled disposable bottles are commonly used in hospitals. These are convenient and offer a stable, standard product. Most have a nipple already attached, and specialized formulas are also available. Always check to be sure which formula has been ordered.

   A variety of specialized nipples are made for infants with feeding problems. These may be substituted for the regular nipple.

2. Wash your hands.

3. Be sure to correctly identify the formula before you begin. Obtain a bib.

4. Warm the formula if necessary. Studies have shown that formula temperature does not cause gas or colic. However, an infant with decreased energy levels will have to use energy to restore body heat if given cold formula. Also, chilled food takes longer to digest. Therefore, the feeding should be at room temperature or slightly warmer. If the feeding is warmer than room temperature, use it as soon as it is warmed, so that it is not a source of bacterial growth. Most hospitals routinely use formula at room temperature.

5. Test for temperature. This is commonly done by shaking a few drops of formula onto the inner aspect of the arm. The formula should feel only lukewarm—not hot.

6. Check the infant's identification.

7. Try to sit in a comfortable position, in a pleasant area, while you feed an infant. Atmosphere is transmitted to infants and affects their feeding and digestion.

8. Ideally, hold the infant in your arms while you bottle-feed. In the instances when an infant cannot be removed from the crib or isolette (due to equipment, traction, need for oxygen), substitute hand touch and support for whole-body contact. Tuck a bib or clean cloth under the infant's chin to wipe up dribbles and spills.

9. Hold the infant with the head slightly elevated to facilitate swallowing. Hold the bottle so that the nipple is filled with fluid, not air (Figure 9.8). Although the sucking infant commonly does swallow air, you should minimize it. Excessive swallowed air causes distention, discomfort, and possibly regurgitation.

10. If the infant eats quickly, remove the bottle for an occasional rest.

11. After the feeding is completed, burp the infant to help him or her expel swallowed air. Two positions are most commonly used: the *over-the-shoulder* and the *on the lap* (Figures 9.9 and 9.10) positions. A small infant should be burped after each ounce as well as at the end of the feeding. Place the bottle on a clean safe surface while you burp the infant; do not place it on the floor.

12. By *gently* patting or rubbing the infant's back you encourage the relaxation of the cardiac sphincter and the release of retained air. Place the bib or cloth where it will protect your clothing while you burp the baby.

13. Change the infant's diaper if necessary. Small infants commonly move their bowels while eating due to the gastrocolic reflex.

14. Return the infant to the crib.

15. Position the infant on the abdomen, with the head to the side, or on the side, so that if the infant spits up he or she

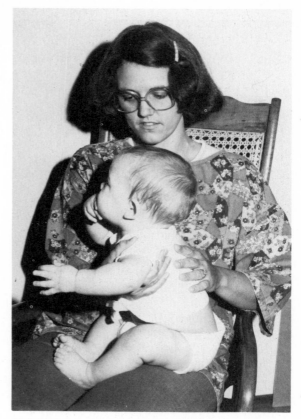

FIGURE 9.9   HOLDING AN INFANT ON THE LAP FOR BURPING
Courtesy Ivan Ellis

will not aspirate. An infant positioned on the right side is most likely to burp out air without bringing formula with it because the sphincter is on the left side of the stomach.

16. Chart the kind and amount of formula taken.

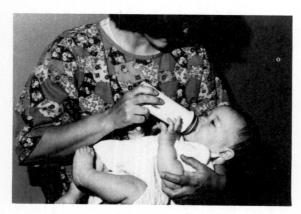

FIGURE 9.8   BOTTLE-FEEDING AN INFANT
Courtesy Ivan Ellis

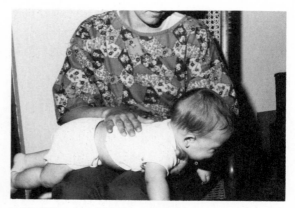

FIGURE 9.10   LYING AN INFANT ON THE LAP FOR BURPING
Courtesy Ivan Ellis

Feeding Solids to an Infant

Always wash your hands before you begin. Obtain the proper food and a small spoon. Position the infant comfortably, either on your lap (Figure 9.11) or in a highchair (Figure 9.12). Use a bib to protect the infant's clothing.

Check the food to be sure it is a comfortable temperature. Hot food can burn an infant's tender mouth and chilled food takes longer to digest, so slightly warm or room-temperature food is usually used. Remember that infants have not established the strong likes and dislikes of adults and will usually eat what they are fed. They do, however, respond to nonverbal cues of aversion from the person who is feeding them. Also, feeding plainer foods (cereals, vegetables) before feeding fruits usually results in better acceptance of the plainer foods. This is because once infants have tasted the naturally sweet fruit they will prefer to continue eating it.

Give small bites and place them well into the mouth. Scrape the food that is pushed back out of the mouth into the spoon and refeed. Hungry infants will often eat rapidly and complain loudly if food appears too slowly.

Infants frequently put their hands into their mouths, smearing the food. You can minimize this by providing something for the infant to hold, by fending off the hands

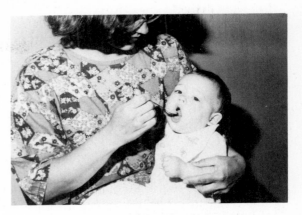

FIGURE 9.12   FEEDING AN INFANT ON THE LAP
Courtesy Ivan Ellis

with your free hand, or by actually holding the arms. (Note Figures 9.11 and 9.12.)

When you have finished, wash the infant. Diapering also may be needed because the stimulus of food often causes the bowels to move.

Safety Precautions

There are many different kinds of restraints available for infants. *Crib nets* are used to keep an active infant or toddler in the crib while still allowing some freedom of movement. Clear Plexiglas *domes* (Figure 9.13) also are used for the same purpose.

Chest restraints can be used to secure an infant to a highchair. On occasion, they may be used to keep an infant restrained in a crib. (See Module 13, Applying Restraints.)

Sandbags provide a useful way to immobilize an infant. A sandbag is heavy enough so that an infant cannot push it out of the way, but make sure that the sandbag does not cause pressure on the infant's tender skin.

A soft *fabric tie* can be used to immobilize an extremity. Use a clove-hitch tie (Figure 9.14) which ensures that the loop will not tighten and restrict circulation if the infant struggles. Whenever you use a tie for a restraint, watch the infant closely to make sure that he or she does not become entangled in it. Always attach the end of a tie to a stable part of the crib (bed), like the frame, and

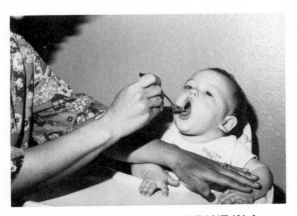

FIGURE 9.11   FEEDING AN INFANT IN A HIGHCHAIR
Courtesy Ivan Ellis

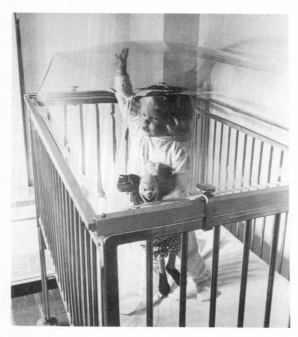

FIGURE 9.13   PLEXIGLAS CRIB DOME
Courtesy American Hospital Supply Corp. and Bafti-Dom Crib Top

not to a movable part, like the side rail. This prevents injury when the movable part is moved.

Elbow restraints are used to immobilize the elbow joint and to prevent an infant or young child from touching his or her own face and head. To be effective, elbow restraints must be incorporated in a jacket or applied over a long-sleeved shirt and pinned at the wrist. This prevents the infant from pulling the arms up and out of the restraint. (See Module 13, Applying Restraints.) Commercial elbow restraints are commonly available, but substitutes can be constructed from tongue blades, tape, and cardboard.

MUMMYING

One method to safely immobilize an infant during a procedure such as venipuncture is to wrap the infant tightly in a manner called *mummying* or *swaddling.* A secure restraint allows the procedure to be done more quickly and protects the infant from the harm that might occur if he or she were to move during the procedure. You can alter the swaddling to provide access to whatever part of the body is needed. To expose only the neck and head, follow the diagrams in Figure 9.15.

1. Wash your hands.
2. Obtain a clean small sheet and fold it into a triangle.
3. Place the sheet under the infant with a long straight edge lying across under the

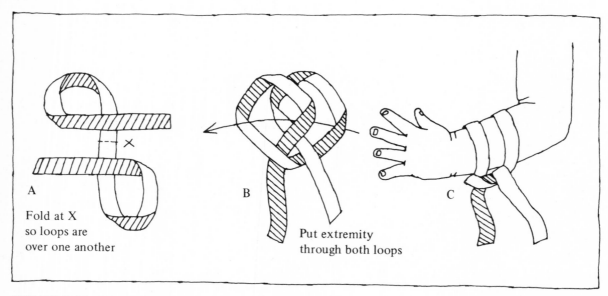

A
Fold at X
so loops are
over one another

B
Put extremity
through both loops

C

FIGURE 9.14   CLOVE HITCH

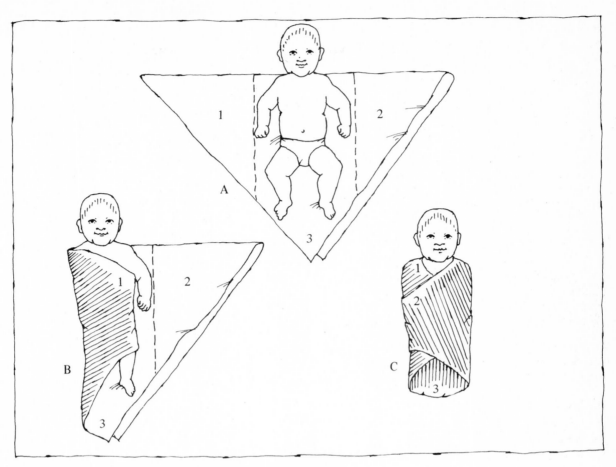

FIGURE 9.15   MUMMY RESTRAINT: CHEST COVERED

shoulders and the opposite point under the feet (A).

4. Fold one side corner over the infant's arm and across the chest. Tuck this side under the infant's back (B). This securely anchors the arm back.
5. Fold the bottom point up over the feet.
6. Then wrap the other side corner over the top of and around the infant. Note that one person can then hold the infant, yet all extremities are restrained.
7. Pin or simply hold in place.

A mummy wrap can also be done to allow the chest and abdomen to be uncovered, as shown in Figure 9.16.

1. Wash your hands.
2. Start with a triangle-folded sheet.
3. Place the sheet under the infant as before (A).

4. Wrap one corner over the infant's arm and under the infant's back.
5. Repeat with the other arm (B). The ends of the sheet will emerge on either side of the infant's legs and hips.
6. Wrap first one end and then the other tightly around the infant's legs (C).
7. Fold the bottom point up over the feet.
8. Pin or tuck the bottom edge over the infant's arms (D).

WRAPPING FOR CIRCUMCISION

To immobilize an infant during circumcision, usually a *circumcision board* is used. The infant is wrapped securely, in the correct position, against the board, which prevents the infant's movement during the procedure. The exact manner of wrapping using the board is determined both by the device itself and by the specific procedure in your

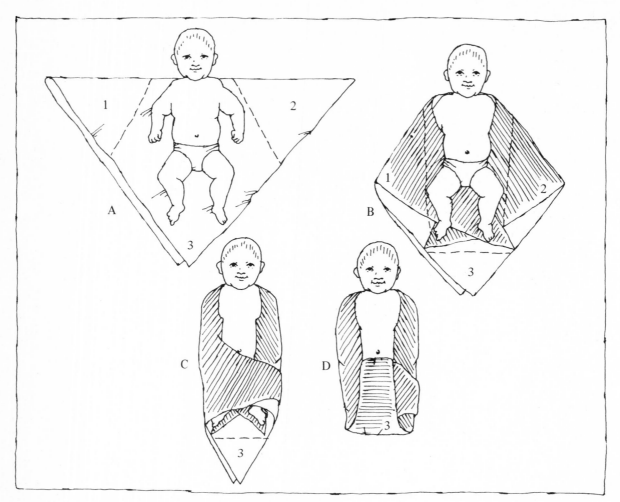

FIGURE 9.16 MUMMY RESTRAINT: CHEST EXPOSED

hospital. If the facility has no specific
procedure, modify the swaddling procedures
given above for use with the available device.

PERFORMANCE CHECKLIST

	Unsatisfactory	Needs more practice	Satisfactory	Comments
Diapering				
1. Triangle folding				
a. Fold into square.				
b. Hold one corner and fold adjacent corners into center forming diamond shape.				
c. Fold corner down creating long triangle.				
2. Fan-folding				
a. Pick up diaper by adjacent corners.				
b. Lay first layer on table to provide desired width.				
c. Make recurrent folds over center.				
d. Fold front end over to desired length.				
Diapering procedure				
1. Wash your hands.				
2. Obtain clean diaper and cleansing equipment.				
3. Fold diaper if necessary.				
4. Place infant on clean safe surface.				
5. Remove any pins, close, and place out of reach.				
6. Remove soiled diaper, wiping away stool, and set aside.				
7. Clean according to facility's policy or follow cleaning procedure in step 7, page 121.				
8. Lift infant's buttocks by grasping both ankles, and slide clean diaper underneath.				
9. Pull diaper between legs and fasten safely and securely.				
10. Leave infant in safe place.				
11. Dispose of soiled diaper according to facility's policy.				
12. Wash your hands.				
13. Chart.				
Bathing				
1. Wash your hands.				
2. Gather equipment.				

	Unsatisfactory	Needs more practice	Satisfactory	Comments
3. Fill basin and check water temperature.				
4. Place basin on safe surface.				
5. Wash and dry infant's eyes and face.				
6. Hold infant football-style over basin.				
7. Shampoo scalp.				
8. Rub head dry.				
9. Undress infant.				
10. Sit infant in water.				
11. Hold with one hand while bathing with other.				
12. Starting with shoulders and moving down body, bathe infant.				
13. Lift infant out of water and lay on towel.				
14. Wrap infant in towel and dry.				
15. Diaper and redress infant.				
16. Make crib.				
17. Put side rail and crib net (or top) in place.				
18. Empty and clean basin.				
19. Dispose of soiled linen.				
20. Wash your hands.				
21. Chart.				

Bottle feeding

	Unsatisfactory	Needs more practice	Satisfactory	Comments
1. Check order for formula.				
2. Wash your hands.				
3. Obtain correct formula and bib.				
4. Warm formula if necessary.				
5. Test temperature of formula.				
6. Check infant's identification.				
7. Pick up infant and sit down comfortably.				
8. Hold infant in correct position and tuck bib under chin.				
9. Offer bottle, tilted so nipple remains full of formula.				
10. Remove bottle for occasional rest as needed.				

	Unsatisfactory	Needs more practice	Satisfactory	Comments
11. When infant stops feeding, position for burping.				
12. Rub infant's back or pat gently until he or she burps.				
13. Change infant's diaper if necessary.				
14. Return infant to crib.				
15. Position on abdomen or right side.				
16. Chart formula taken.				
Feeding solids				
1. Wash your hands.				
2. Obtain correct food, spoon, and bib.				
3. Position infant.				
4. Put bib on infant.				
5. Check temperature of food.				
6. Give small bites.				
7. Refeed as needed.				
8. Wash infant as needed.				
9. Diaper if necessary.				
Mummying				
1. Head and neck exposed a. Wash your hands.				
b. Get and fold clean sheet				
c. Place sheet under infant.				
d. Fold one corner over arm, across chest, and under back.				
e. Fold bottom up.				
f. Fold second corner over top of infant and around body firmly.				
g. Pin or hold in place.				
2. Chest and abdomen exposed a. Wash your hands.				
b. Obtain triangle-folded clean sheet.				
c. Place sheet under infant.				
d. Wrap one corner over arm and under back.				

	Unsatisfactory	Needs more practice	Satisfactory	Comments
e. Repeat for other side.				
f. Wrap ends securely around legs.				
g. Fold bottom point up over feet.				
h. Pin or tuck bottom edge over arm.				

QUIZ

Short-Answer Questions

1. What is an advantage of a triangle-folded cloth diaper? _____
   _____

2. Why is the perineal area cleaned at the time of a diaper change? _____
   _____

3. What should be done with safety pins while changing a baby's diaper?
   _____

4. Differentiate between diaper rash and scald. _____
   _____

5. How would you test a bottle feeding for proper temperature? _____
   _____

6. Why is a clove hitch used to tie an arm restraint? _____
   _____

7. List three safety measures that must be followed when bathing an infant.
   a. _____
   b. _____
   c. _____

Module 10 Admission and Discharge

MAIN OBJECTIVE

To admit and discharge patients, taking into consideration both general nursing concerns and individual patients' needs.

RATIONALE

Entering a health care facility is a major crisis in the lives of most persons. Individuals have many needs and concerns that must be identified and for which action must be taken. In addition, each health care facility must maintain certain routine procedures and gather the specific information about incoming patients that will facilitate the performance of its functions. Identifying both these aspects and meeting both sets of needs are challenging tasks for the nurse.

The same two aspects are present when persons are ready to leave a health care facility. Again, the nurse must strive to create an optimum balance in trying to meet these two sets of needs.

PREREQUISITES

1. Successful completion of the following modules:

   VOLUME 1
   Assessment
   Charting
   Medical Asepsis

2. Modules 15 and 16, Transfer and Ambulation, may be essential for admitting some incapacitated patients.
3. Modules 18, 20, and 21, Collecting Specimens, Temperature, Pulse, and Respiration and Blood Pressure, may be necessary in a facility that requires the admitting person to collect such data.

SPECIFIC LEARNING OBJECTIVES

Admission

	Know Facts and Principles	Apply Facts and Principles	Demonstrate Ability	Evaluate Performance
1. *Introduction and orientation* a. *Staff* b. *Environment* c. *Expectations and role*	State rationale for introducing patient to staff and environment. State rationale for orienting patient to expectations and role and discussing patient's expectations.	List information specific patient would need on admission	When admitting a patient, introduce staff present and environment, and discuss expectations for patient's behavior	Elicit patient's evaluation of adequacy of introductions and orientation
2. *Immediate needs* a. *Physical* b. *Emotional*	Discuss various physical needs patient may have on admission. Discuss various emotional needs patient may have on admission.	Given a patient situation, identify physical needs that take priority. Given a patient situation, identify emotional needs that take priority.	When admitting a patient, take action to meet immediate needs, both physical and emotional	Check patient for evidence of comfort and relaxation
3. *Baseline assessment* a. *Observation* b. *Physical examination* c. *Interview and history taking*	List initial observations that must be made. List information that should be obtained.	Given data on a new patient, identify observations needed for patient. Given data on a new patient, outline interview to be done.	When admitting a patient, make appropriate observations. Obtain needed information through interview.	Use Performance Checklist in Module 1, Assessment, to evaluate completeness of assessment
4. *Care of personal property*	Discuss nurse's responsibility toward patient's property	State usual disposition of personal effects in own facility	Arrange for safekeeping of patient's property	
5. *Record keeping*		List records required in own facility	Record observations, interview, disposition of personal property	Evaluate own performance using list of forms in Performance Checklist

Discharge

1. Planning for continuity of care	State rationale for continuity of care. List resources for continuing care.	Given a situation, identify which resources would be needed for continued care	For a patient in the clinical area, plan appropriately for care after discharge from unit	
2. Patient teaching	List common learning needs for patients being discharged	Given a situation, identify learning needs	Teach patient in clinical area before discharge within limits of own ability	
3. Final assessment	Explain why final assessment is needed	Given a situation, list appropriate final assessment information for patient	Make complete final assessment of patient	Evaluate own performance using Performance Checklist in Module 1, Assessment
4. Care of personal property	List places personal effects may be kept	List forms for own facility that must be completed at discharge regarding patient's belongings	Retrieve all of patient's personal effects and see that they accompany patient	Use Performance Checklist to see that all items are completed
5. Business functions	Discuss usual business functions for which nurse is responsible	List business functions required in facility	When discharging patient, see that financial arrangements are completed. Obtain medications and supplies if needed.	
6. Record keeping	Discuss usual records to be filled out	List discharge records required in facility	Record data on entire discharge procedure	Evaluate own performance using list of forms in Performance Checklist

LEARNING ACTIVITIES

1. Review the Specific Learning Objectives.
2. Read the section on threats to the patient's mental health (in the chapter on mental health) in Ellis and Nowlis, *Nursing: A Human Needs Approach,* or comparable material in another textbook.
3. Look up the module vocabulary terms in the glossary.
4. Check the procedure book at your facility in relation to forms and processes required for admission and discharge.
5. Assist a staff member or more experienced student with the admission of a patient. Discuss the procedure:
   a. Were all steps included?
   b. Did more than one person participate in the process?
6. With the supervision of your instructor, admit a patient. Evaluate your own performance using the Performance Checklist. Consult with your instructor regarding your performance.
7. Repeat steps 5 and 6 for the discharge of a patient.

VOCABULARY

assessment
chart
nursing history
referral
urinalysis

ADMISSION AND DISCHARGE

Admission

When admitting a person to a health care facility, you have many responsibilities. They can be grouped under the following headings.

1. Immediate needs of the person
   a. Physical
   b. Emotional
2. Introduction and orientation
3. Baseline assessment
   a. Observations and physical examination
   b. Interview and history taking
4. Care of belongings
5. Record keeping

These activities will not always be done in the same order. For example, an item from baseline assessment may most conveniently be done at the same time that you begin record keeping. The needs of the individual patient and your own convenience will guide you.

IMMEDIATE NEEDS

A brief general assessment of a new patient to ascertain his or her immediate needs is essential. This should be your first concern. A person does not enter the hospital unless he or she has a health care problem. This problem may not be causing any immediate distress or it may be acute. A well-founded criticism of some health care workers is that they are so concerned about routines and forms that the patients' primary problems remain uncared for.

Immediate needs can be either physical or emotional. If a patient is in acute pain, contact the physician immediately regarding orders for medication and care; meanwhile, institute nursing measures to relieve pain. If a patient is upset or distraught, spend a short time listening and talking to the patient; this can facilitate his or her transition to the hospital environment. If a patient feels that those around are concerned about his or her immediate needs and are taking action to

meet them, a relationship of trust may well have begun.

INTRODUCTIONS AND ORIENTATION

When you deem it appropriate, it is your responsibility to introduce the patient to persons in the environment. This may be the very first thing you do, but it can wait until some immediate need has been met. Here you must use your judgment.

Your greeting should convey interest in and concern for the patient. A person just entering a hospital is really not concerned about your problems of staffing or time except as they directly affect his or her own care. If it is necessary for a patient to wait, an explanation is appreciated.

Although you should not expect a patient to remember the names of all staff members initially, introducing yourself and others by both name and position helps the patient to orient himself or herself to what is happening. Other patients who are in the same room should also be introduced.

Explain what will occur during the admitting process. This relieves the patient's anxiety created by fear of the unknown.

A thorough patient orientation to the unit includes how all items for the patient's use work, which areas are for personal belongings, and the location of the bathroom. Especially important are directions on how to call a nurse.

Explain anything you expect a patient to do, in detail. From exactly what to wear under the hospital gown to what activity is ordered, a patient will be better able to participate in his or her own care if what is expected is clear.

BASELINE ASSESSMENT

The information to be gathered in baseline assessment varies from one facility to another. It almost always includes temperature, pulse, and respiration (TPR); blood pressure (BP); height; and weight. In some facilities, a complete physical examination is done by the nurse. In others, the nurse may do a thorough nursing assessment that does not encompass the traditional physical examination.

A nursing history is usually taken. Even if a formalized nursing history is not used, information in relation to allergies, current medications, and the patient's perception of his or her entering problem (often called the *chief complaint*) is gathered. An interview is used to gather subjective information regarding the patient. (See Figure 10.1.)

These baseline data are necessary in order to evaluate future observations and other data gathered.

PERSONAL PROPERTY

One of the more difficult problems in an institution, large or small, is keeping track of a patient's personal property. The loss of valued items is upsetting to patients and can be costly to an institution.

Most facilities have a routine for checking and noting all personal items brought or worn to the facility by a patient. Those items that are not needed can be sent home with family members. This is perhaps the best safeguard. Large sums of money and valuable items are usually kept in a safe in the business office with proper documents attesting to their location and their value. The amount of money that a patient should keep at the bedside depends on the policy of the facility and the patient's personal wishes and needs.

Items that are kept with the patient are less likely to get lost if they are marked with the patient's name, but this is not always possible. Arrange to keep these possessions together in a place that is accessible to the patient. A printed list of clothing and personal effects that you can quickly check off is often used to make an exact inventory. (See Figure 10.2 for an example of a clothing and personal effects list.)

RECORD KEEPING

Charting all parts of the admission process is essential for legal records. The baseline assessment serves as a reference throughout the period of care; and frequently the record

of care of personal effects must be consulted. In addition, you may be responsible for a variety of other records (notification of the dietary department, starting a Kardex card and medication record, filling out census forms). You will have to consult the procedure book at each facility to determine which forms are your responsibility. (See Figure 10.3.)

Discharge/Transfer

Whether you are planning for a patient's discharge to home, to another facility, or simply to another unit, your responsibilities are similar. They include the following.

1. Planning for continuity of care
2. Patient teaching
3. Final assessment
4. Care of personal property
5. Business functions
6. Record keeping

ORDER FOR DISCHARGE

Often you will know that a patient is leaving before an official discharge or transfer order is written. In that case, planning can begin earlier. However, no official documents or processes should be started until the order is written.

CONTINUITY OF CARE

Your nursing responsibility for a patient does not end when he or she leaves the area in which you work. You have a responsibility to see that plans are made for continuing care as needed. If the patient is going home, this planning can be done with the patient and the family. You may have to consult the official discharge planner of your facility if home nursing care or an extended-care facility is needed. If a patient is moving to another unit, you must consider how best to communicate the needs of the patient to the next nursing unit.

PATIENT TEACHING

Wherever the patient is going, explain what will happen, where he or she is going, and

INITIAL PATIENT INTERVIEW — 3 SOUTH

Reason for hospitalization

Symptoms

HISTORY

Infections

Diabetes
   how long

Heart

Hypertension

Peripheral
   Vascular disease

Respiratory

Other problems or illnesses

Previous use of steroids

G.U.

G.B.

G.I.
   constipation
   diarrhea

Special diet
   food allergies

Tobacco   amt.
Alcohol   amt.

Prior hospitalizations

Current meds.

PHYSICAL
CIRCULATORY
Pulse AP _____ R _____
Rhythm_____
Pedal pulse_____
Edema _____
Homan's sign _____
Calf tenderness _____

RESPIRATORY
Lung sounds _____
Dyspnea _____
Cough _____
Sputum _____

DERMATOLOGY
Color _____
Condition _____
Lacerations _____
Bruises _____
Decubiti _____

C.N.S.
Level of
   consciousness _____
Pain _____
   location _____
   type _____
   precipitated _____
   by _____

G.I.
Bowel sounds _____
Distention _____
Abd. Soft _____
      Firm _____
Palpitation _____
   tenderness _____

G.U.
Any problems vd. _____
Frequency _____
Pain _____
Incontinence _____
Catheter_____
   date inserted _____

MUSC. — SKEL.
Fractures _____
Deformities _____
Arthritis _____
Ambulatory _____
   Needs assist. _____

PSY. — SOC.
Anxiety _____
Introduce to
   roommates
   and unit _____
Pre-op
   teaching _____

DISCHARGE PLANNING
Home responsibilities?
Do you live alone?
Someone to help after discharge?
Admitted from SNF or protected care?

Sign _____

FIGURE 10.1   A SAMPLE NURSING HISTORY
Courtesy Ballard Hospital, Seattle, Washington

NORTHGATE GENERAL HOSPITAL				Patient's Clothes List		Admission Data

AMT.	CLOTHING	AMT.	CLOTHING	AMT.	MISCELLANEOUS	AMT.	DENTURES	ADM. TIME
	BATHROBE		NIGHTGOWN		CANE		UPPERS	B.P.
	BED JACKET		PAJAMAS		CONTACT LENS		LOWERS	T. P. R.
	BELT		PANTI HOSE		ELECTRIC RAZOR		PARTIAL	WT. HT.
	BLOUSE		SCARF		GLASSES			TRANSFUSIONS
	BRA		SHIRT		HEARING AID			ALLERGIES
	COAT		SHOES (PAIR)		LUGGAGE		VALUABLES	
	DRESS		SKIRT		RADIO		BANK BOOK	
	GARTER BELT		SLACKS		T.V.		RING	
	GIRDLE		SLIP				WALLET	
	GLOVES (PAIR)		SLIPPERS (PAIR)				WATCH	MEDICINES MED. DR.
	HANDKERCHIEF		SOCKS (PAIR)				PURSE	
	HAT		SUIT					
	HOSE		SWEATER				VALUABLES ENVELOPE NUMBER	
	JACKET		UNDERSHIRT					
	NECKTIE		UNDERWEAR					

ANY VALUABLES OR FUNDS NOT DEPOSITED WITH THE HOSPITAL ARE RETAINED AT MY OWN RISK AND ANY VALUABLES, ELECTRICAL APPLIANCES, RADIOS, T.V., ETC., BROUGHT TO ME WHILE A PATIENT WILL BE MY OWN RESPONSIBILITY.

DIET

DINNER DRINK

SNACK

1. SIGNATURE OF PATIENT _____

2. CHECKED IN BY (NURSE-AIDE) _____ DATE _____

3. SIGNATURE OF PERSON RECEIVING ITEMS ABOVE _____

4. SIGNATURE OF PERSON RECEIVING VALUABLES ENVELOPE _____

5. CHECKED OUT BY (NURSE-AIDE) _____ DATE _____

PLEASE COMPLETE IN INK ONLY

DISCHARGED _____

FIGURE 10.2 PERSONAL PROPERTY LIST
Courtesy Northgate Hospital, Seattle, Washington

PATIENT RECORD

DATE	HOUR	ASSESSMENT

ADMITTED PER _wheelchair_   GLASSES _yes_   CONTACTS _no_

DR. _Brown_   NOTIFIED TIME _4⁰⁰ pm_   DENTURES (NATURAL)

T.P.R. _98⁴-96-22_   B.P. _164/98_   (ARTIFICIAL) ↑ ↓

WEIGHT _160 lbs._   ADMISSION BATH _none given_   HEARING AID _no_

LAB WORK DONE: BLOOD ✓   URINE ✓   TRANSFUSIONS (YES) _2_ (NO)

MEDICINES (BRING TO DESK) _Aldoril_   (WHERE) _Army_ (WHEN) _1943_

ALLERGIES _none_   PREGNANCIES _none_

Psy-Soc 61-y.o. black male admitted to 462-B. States he feels
"uptight" about coming to the hospital. States chief complaints
are dizzyness and S.O.B. See Initial Patient Interview for
complete systems review. ————————————— R. Johnson, R.N.

Patient Assessment	Circulatory (Circ.) Genitourinary (G.U.)	Central Nervous System (C.N.S.) Musculoskeletal (Musc.-Skel.)	Dermatology (Derm.) Psycho-Social (Psy.-Soc.)	Gastrointestional (G.I.) Respiratory (Resp.)

BALLARD COMMUNITY HOSPITAL
SEATTLE, WASHINGTON

FIGURE 10.3   A SAMPLE ADMISSION RECORDING FROM A PATIENT'S CHART
Courtesy Ballard Community Hospital, Seattle, Washington

Original Copy Goes To Receiving Facility.
Carbon Copy Retained In Patient Record.

Patient's Last Name	First Name	MI	Name and Address of Facility Transferring:

From:

Address, City, State, Zip Code	Phone

To:

Date of Birth	Age	Sex	Marital Status	Church
			S M W D Sep.	

Adm. Date:_____Discharge Date:_____

Relative or Guardian (specify relationship) name, address	Phone

Previous Hospitalization and/or Nursing Home Stay (within last 90 days):

Attending Physician:

Health Insurance Info.:   Soc. Sec. No._____

Consulting Physician(s):

Medicare_____Medicaid_____

Physician after transfer:

Other_____

MEDICAL SUMMARY   (To be completed by Physician)

Admitting Diagnosis:

History and Physical (photo copy to be included). Any significant changes from initial H & P. ☐ yes ☐ no   If yes, changes are:

Discharge Diagnosis:
  Primary:

  Secondary:

Course of Treatment (include Medical/Surgical Procedures Done and Date):

ALLERGIES. ☐ yes ☐ no   Type:_____

Does ☐ Patient ☐ Family know diagnosis: ☐ yes ☐ no

PHYSICIAN ORDERS

DIET ☐ Regular ☐ Sodium Restriction,_____gm. ☐ Diabetic,_____calories ☐ Low Residue ☐ Bland

☐ Mechanical ☐ Soft ☐ Tube,_____ cc per_____hr ☐ Other_____

DRUGS   (If PRN, state reason for giving and max. amt. to be given. List discontinuation date, if any, on all medications ordered)
Note: Any brand or form of drug identical in form and content may be dispensed unless checked here: ☐

ACTIVITY ORDERS   (List activity level, restrictions and/or precautions, etc.)
Note: if ordering restraints indicate reason for use.

SPECIAL TREATMENTS   (Including Physical Therapy, Speech, O.T., etc.)
Specify frequency.

REHABILITATION POTENTIAL   (Describe the highest level of independent functioning the patient can be expected to achieve.)

Certification: ☐ I certify that post hospital skilled nursing care is medically necessary on a continuing basis for any of the conditions for which he/she received care during this hospitalization.   ☐ I certify that my above orders regarding home health services (skilled nursing care, therapy, or others as defined) are medically necessary because my patient is confined to home. These services are related to the condition(s) for which he/she received inpatient hospital or ECF care.

Signature of Physician_____ M.D.   Phone:_____ Date:_____
This form has been approved by the Seattle Area Hospital Council and the Washington State Health Facilities.

PATIENT TRANSFER FORM

FIGURE 10.4 DISCHARGE/TRANSFER SUMMARY
Developed by the Seattle Area Hospital Council

PATIENT CARE PLAN   ATTACH Kardex or Patient Care Plan

ACTIVITIES OF DAILY LIVING

Self Care Status (√ level)	Indep.	Assist.	Unable	Additional Comments
Baths Self				
Dresses Self				
Feeds Self				
Oral Hygiene				
Shaves Self				
Transfers Self				
Ambulates				

Sleep Habits:_____

√ If Uses: ☐ walker   ☐ crutches   ☐ cane   ☐ wheelchair

☐ toilet   ☐ commode   ☐ bedpan   ☐ urinal

PHYSICAL TRAITS (Check if Applicable)

Impairments: ☐ speech   ☐ hearing   ☐ visual   ☐ sensation   ☐ other

Disabilities: ☐ amputation   ☐ paralysis_____
                                      (Describe)

☐ contractures_____   ☐ foot drop R___L___
                    (Describe)

Prosthesis: ☐ dentures - partial___ upper___ lower___

☐ eyes R___ L___   ☐ glasses   ☐ contact lens

☐ hearing aid   ☐ limb RA___ LA___ LL___ RL___

DIETARY INFORMATION   (Describe appetite, special needs, likes/dislikes, if on tube feeding, the time of last feeding, etc.)

BEHAVIOR/MENTAL STATUS

☐ Alert   ☐ Oriented   ☐ Confused   ☐ Forgetful   ☐ Wanders

☐ Noisy   ☐ Depressed   ☐ Combative   ☐ Withdrawn   ☐ Other

Comments:

SOCIAL-EMOTIONAL   (List according to number) 1. attitude toward illness or disease. 2. adjustment/coping ability. 3. emotional support from family/friends. 4. feeling about transfer. 5. financial. 6. other.

Prior to Present Pt. Lived:
☐ alone
☐ with family
☐ with friends
☐ nursing home
☐ boarding home
☐ other

Signature_____   Date_____

PATIENT CARE INFORMATION

Patient Abilities (√ level)	Usually	Occ.	Rarely
Able to communicate			
Motivated to do self care			
Follows direction			
Bladder control (Date cath. inserted_____)			
(Date cath. last changed_____)			
Bowel control (Date of last BM_____)			
(Date of last Enema_____)			

Last 8° I_____ O_____   Bladder/Bowel Program ☐ yes ☐ no

Vital Signs (last): T____ P____ R____ BP____ Wt.___ _Ht._____

SKIN CONDITION
(Show by code) 1. Potential decubiti, 2. Existing decubiti, 3. Draining wounds, 4. Tubes, 5. Other

CURRENT MEDICATIONS

Time of last medication(s) on day of transfer_____

_____

_____

Effective PRN meds (state reason for and freq. given)_____

_____

_____

Antibiotics received during present stay: ☐ yes ☐ no Type_____

ADDITIONAL NURSING INFORMATION
ATTACH ADDITIONAL PAGE IF NECESSARY. Describe special treatment(s) or condition(s), details of care, safety measures, teaching done and/or needed as well as level of pt. understanding, and other pertinent information.

VALUABLES ACCOMPANYING PT.
(Money, Prosthesis, Jewelry)

Signature_____ Date____
(Responsible or transporting party)

Copies sent:
☐ H & P   ☐ Discharge Summary
☐ X-ray   ☐ Lab   ☐ Path Report
☐ Other_____

Nurses Signature_____   Unit_____ Date_____

FIGURE 10.4   DISCHARGE/TRANSFER SUMMARY (continued)

when this will happen. The patient may need information about his or her medications, treatments, activity, diet, and continued health supervision. Ideally, teaching will have begun earlier so that the patient is not overwhelmed with stimuli and information at the time of discharge. However, occasionally this is not done in advance, and essential teaching must be done on the day of discharge. Often the family is included in the teaching, also.

In the event that data indicate that the patient is not ready for discharge (for example, an elevated temperature), report the information to the physician immediately for his or her evaluation.

FINAL ASSESSMENT

Before a patient leaves your unit, you must prepare a final assessment of his or her total status. Include physical status, emotional status, and the patient's ability to continue or participate in his or her own care.

PERSONAL PROPERTY

Be sure that all personal belongings accompany the patient. Especially critical are dentures, glasses, and special appliances, such as crutches. If a list of personal effects was made on admission, this will help, but remember that items brought in after admission may not be on the list. Check your list with the patient. Do not forget that there may be items in the safe or in the medicine room.

BUSINESS MATTERS

Before a patient leaves a hospital, it is customary for either the patient or the family to consult with the business office regarding financial matters. This may have been taken care of on admission through identification of an insurance company or a third-party payer. Be sure you know the usual routine in your facility. You may have to get drugs from the pharmacy or supplies from elsewhere for the patient to take home. Planning for these items should be done when you consider continuity of care and patient teaching.

RECORD KEEPING

Again, forms will vary according to facility. Record your final assessment, patient teaching, plans for continuity of care, disposition of personal items, and completion of business functions. Some facilities use a form in the chart that should help to remind you of all these points. (See Figure 10.4.)

DELEGATION OF TASKS

If a nursing assistant, a volunteer, or anyone else is able to assist with a patient's admission or discharge, you must carefully evaluate which tasks require greater skill and judgment. For example, decision making and assessment are nursing functions that do not lend themselves to delegation to nonnursing personnel. A routine task, however, such as orientation to the physical unit, can be delegated.

PERFORMANCE CHECKLIST

Admission	Unsatisfactory	Needs more practice	Satisfactory	Comments
1. Check for orders.				
2. Meet immediate needs. a. Physical				
b. Emotional				
3. Make introductions and orient patient. a. Greet patient (done first).				
b. Introduce self.				
c. Explain admission routine.				
d. Orient patient to individual unit: bed, bathroom, call light, supplies, and belongings.				
e. Orient patient to entire unit: location of nurses' station and day room or lounge.				
f. Explain expected behavior.				
g. Introduce other staff and roommates.				
4. Perform baseline assessment. a. Observation and physical examination (1) TPR				
(2) BP				
(3) Weight and height				
(4) Total assessment				
b. Interview and history (1) Medications				
(2) Allergies				
(3) Entering complaints and concerns				
5. Take care of personal property. a. Items to be kept at bedside				
b. Items to be put in safe or medicine room				
c. Items to be sent home				
6. Keeping records. a. All data recorded				
b. Special forms for facility completed (add your own list of forms)				

Discharge/Transfer	Unsatisfactory	Needs more practice	Satisfactory	Comments
1. Check for orders.				
2. Plan for continuing care. a. Referrals as needed				
b. Information for new persons involved in care				
c. Contacting family or significant others if needed				
d. Transportation				
3. Teaching patient. a. What to expect				
b. Medications				
c. Treatments				
d. Activity				
e. Diet				
f. Needs for continued health supervision				
4. Perform final assessment. a. Physical status				
b. Emotional status				
c. Ability to continue own care				
5. Check and return personal property. a. Personal items on unit				
b. Items from safe or medicine room				
6. Perform business functions. a. Financial matters				
b. Obtaining supplies				
7. Keep records. a. Discharge note				
b. Special forms for facility (add your own list of forms)				

QUIZ

Multiple-Choice Questions

_____ 1. The first thing you should do when admitting a patient is

a. orient the patient to the unit.
b. ascertain and meet the patient's immediate needs.
c. take TPR and BP.
d. make a baseline assessment.

_____ 2. When orienting a patient to the environment, which of the following is not necessary?

a. The location of the utility room and kitchenette
b. How to call a nurse
c. The location of the bathroom
d. How to operate the bed

_____ 3. If a patient is very distraught on admission, you should

a. hurry as quickly as possible.
b. go slowly to provide calm as you follow the usual routine.
c. temporarily omit routine items.
d. continue with the regular admission procedure as usual.

_____ 4. If a volunteer is available to assist with admission, which task would be most appropriate to delegate to him or her?

a. Baseline assessment
b. Ascertaining immediate needs
c. Orientation to the unit
d. Charting data

_____ 5. Which of the following should you consider if you are transferring a patient to another unit? (1) continuing care; (2) patient teaching; (3) care of belongings; (4) final assessment

a. 1, 2, and 4
b. 2, 3, and 4
c. 1 and 2 only
d. All of these

_____ 6. A patient has a very valuable jeweled ring. You would suggest

a. that the patient wear it.
b. that the patient hide it well in his or her suitcase.
c. keeping it at the nursing station.
d. putting it in the office safe.

————— 7. Which of the following are usually nursing responsibilities related to *discharge*? (1) planning for transportation; (2) teaching the patient about medications; (3) making a final assessment; (4) making sure that the patient's personal property is sent along

   a. 1, 2, and 3
   b. 2, 3, and 4
   c. 1, 3, and 4
   d. All of these

————— 8. If a patient is being *transferred to another unit,* which of the tasks listed in question 7 are usually needed?

   a. 2 and 3
   b. 1 and 4
   c. 1, 3, and 4
   d. All of these

————— 9. Which of the following patients is most likely to need a referral to provide continuing care after discharge? (1) one who had a routine appendectomy; (2) one who had a stroke and has right-sided paralysis; (3) one who had acute pneumonia; (4) one with a new colostomy

   a. 1 and 3
   b. 2 and 4
   c. 3 and 4
   d. All of these

Module 11 Intake and Output

MAIN OBJECTIVE

To be able to measure correctly and keep accurate records of patients' fluid intake and output.

RATIONALE

Many illnesses cause changes in the body's ability to maintain fluid balance. Intake can be decreased due to anorexia, nausea, vomiting, and many other conditions. Output can be altered by various disease processes in the body, especially kidney and heart problems. There are a number of drugs in current use that alter urinary elimination. These and many other conditions make a careful measurement of both intake and output essential to total patient assessment. A record of this measurement is maintained for all health team members' use.

PREREQUISITES

Successful completion of the following modules:

VOLUME 1
Assessment
Charting
Medical Asepsis

SPECIFIC LEARNING OBJECTIVES

	Know Facts and Principles	Apply Facts and Principles	Demonstrate Ability	Evaluate Performance
1. *What is measured*	State what items must be measured for intake and output	Given a sample patient diet, identify items to be measured. Given a patient situation, identify intake, other than dietary, that must be measured. Given a patient situation, identify which excretions must be measured for output.	Measure intake accurately. Measure output accurately.	With instructor, evaluate choices of what to measure
2. *Record-keeping forms*	List pertinent information that should be recorded at patient's bedside. List pertinent information that should be recorded on patient's chart.	Given a listing of information about patient's intake and output, record it on correct form in proper place	Record intake and output on proper forms	With instructor, evaluate use of forms
3. *Measurements used*	Identify when to add or subtract quantities to get correct totals	Given a patient situation with amounts of intake and output, figure correct totals	Total intake and output. Record totals on correct form.	Evaluate own performance using Performance Checklist

4. *Time periods for measurement*	Know variety of time periods that may be used for recording intake and output	Given patient's amounts of intake and output, compute total for 8-hour systems	Compute totals for 8- to 24-hour periods	Evaluate own performance using Performance Checklist
5. *Fluid balance*	Define fluid balance. Identify factors in addition to intake and output that must be considered regarding fluid balance.	Given a patient situation, identify factors that relate to fluid balance. State additional data that may be needed for accurate assessment of fluid balance.	Determine whether patient is in fluid balance. Report instances of fluid imbalance to appropriate person.	
6. *Patient's participation*	Identify ways of explaining to patient need for measurement of intake and output, and method to be used	Given a patient situation, devise plan for measuring intake and output that includes patient	In the clinical setting, successfully maintain intake and output record on patient from patient's list	Compare own results with those of staff person also assigned to care of patient

LEARNING ACTIVITIES

1. Review the Specific Learning Objectives.
2. Read the section on fluids (in the chapter on nutrition and fluids) in Ellis and Nowlis, *Nursing: A Human Needs Approach*, or comparable material in another textbook.
3. Look up the module vocabulary terms in the glossary.
4. Read through the module.
5. in the practice setting:
   a. Practice measuring, using containers showing metric measurement.

   Using the container measurements given on the sample form in Figure 11.1, compute the intake and output for the following patient:

FIGURE 11.1   INTAKE-OUTPUT WORKSHEET
Courtesy Ballard Community Hospital, Nursing Department, Seattle, Washington

Mr. Denner, on rising, brushed his teeth. After rinsing his mouth, he drank half a glass (small) of water. Breakfast arrived and was composed of:

Fruit juice, small glass
Cereal bowl of hot oatmeal with
   a pitcher of cream
Bacon and soft-boiled egg
Pot of coffee with small cream
Glass of milk

Shortly after breakfast, he felt nauseated and vomited 75 ml of semiliquid emesis. Throughout the morning, he voided two times: 50 ml and 225 ml.

By lunch, he was feeling much better and a light diet was ordered. When it arrived, he ate a small bowl of broth and half of a small bowl of gelatin.

He voided once more after lunch: 125 ml.

He was given oral medications twice, each time with 1 oz water.

At the end of the day shift, half of a 1,000-ml bottle of IV fluids had been absorbed.

Turn in the above computations. Have your instructor evaluate their accuracy.

6. In the clinical setting:
   a. Familiarize yourself with the various diets used in your facility.
   b. Check the form used by your facility for intake and output measurement.
   c. Keep an intake-output record on one of your assigned patients for one meal and for the time period you are on the unit. Have your instructor check your accuracy.
   d. For a patient in the clinical area who is on intake-output measurement, figure the last three 8-hour periods and total your figures for 24 hours.
   e. For the same patient, check the record and decide, based on recorded

data, whether this patient is in fluid balance. Present your data and your decision to your instructor for verification.

VOCABULARY

catheter
diaphoresis
diarrhea
diuresis
diuretic
infusion
minibottle
parenteral fluid
piggyback
preformed water
profuse
pureed
water balance

INTAKE AND OUTPUT

Initiating Measurement

A patient's fluid intake and fluid output (I and O) may be measured for a variety of reasons. For example, you may initiate measuring to verify whether a patient is taking adequate fluids or to verify a concern that the output is adequate for optimum kidney function. This specific information may be important to a complete and accurate assessment. Urinary output may also be measured to evaluate the effectiveness of a diuretic, which is a drug given to increase urinary output.

The physician may order that intake and output be measured for many of the same reasons as well as for diagnosis and treatment progress. Most post-op patients and patients with indwelling catheters are routinely on intake and output measurement. For some patients, whose water balance is crucial, daily weights are ordered as well.

Substances Measured

INTAKE

Measure all items that are naturally fluid at room temperature. This includes water, milk, juice, and all other beverages, as well as ice cream, gelatin, and soups. Do *not* measure pureed foods because they are simply solids that are prepared in a different form. Intravenous-infusion fluid, blood, and irrigating solutions that are not returned are included in intake.

OUTPUT

Urine is the major item that is measured for output. In the healthy person, this output should approximately equal fluid intake. However, fluids are also lost through the lungs with expired air, through the skin with perspiration, and in the feces. These items are not usually measured because they approximately equal the total of preformed water that is contained in solid foods and the water produced by the body's own metabolism. However, if these amounts become excessive (for example, in a case of diarrhea or of profuse diaphoresis), they must be measured or estimated, and added to the output record.

Vomitus, drainage from suction devices, wound drainage, and bleeding are abnormal losses of fluid. They should always be measured or estimated.

Units of Measurement

Intake and output are measured in metric liquid units called *milliliters* (ml).[1] Metric units are used as a standard because they lend themselves more easily to calculations that require the conversion of liquid and weight measures. Intravenous fluids have been standardized into metric measurements for this reason also.

Accurate intake and output records are greatly facilitated when a patient is involved in the process. If the patient understands what is to be done and the reasons for doing it, he or she may even remind personnel of the need for measuring intake and output. Also, he or she will be sure to save all urine for measurement and may even assist with recording intake.

Record Keeping

BEDSIDE RECORDS

First, a record must be kept at the patient's bedside, or in the patient's room, so that measurements can be recorded immediately. A form is often taped near the wash basin or on the door as a reminder to the health care team. Make a complete listing of the items measured and their quantities on this record. Many of these forms list the metric equivalents to the U.S. standard units of liquid measurement. (See Figure 11.1.)

PERMANENT RECORDS

There is a special record form on the patient's chart to make a permanent recording of the

---

[1]Traditionally the cubic centimeter (cc or cm^3) has been used as a milliliter equivalent.

patient's intake and output. (See Figure 11.2.) Do not record individual items on this form, but do record totals for each 8-hour or 24-hour period (according to the hospital's procedure) for each category. Thus the intake record might include a figure for oral intake, intravenous-fluid intake, miscellaneous intake, and a *total* intake figure. The output is recorded similarly, with totals for each category and then a comprehensive total for all outputs.

Parenteral fluids (those given by infusion) may be recorded on an independent record (Figure 11.3).

General Procedure

INTAKE

1. Initiate or continue the measurement of intake on either the order of the physician or your assessment.
2. Locate intake-output worksheet at the patient's bedside. Some facilities attach these sheets above the bathroom sink, others, to the door of the room. Familiarize yourself with the location at your facility.
3. Explain or reinforce the reasons for accurate intake measurement to the patient.
4. Encourage the patient to participate. Some patients feel more involved in their own care by helping you compute the values.
5. After a meal, record on the I and O sheet the amount of each fluid item taken.
6. Compute partial intake of any fluid item. This figure may have to be an estimate, except for a patient on very strict measurement for medical reasons.
7. Add free water, including any given with medications.
8. Add any nourishment given between meals.
9. Total your 8-hour measurements at the end of your shift for transfer to the permanent record.

OUTPUT

1. Follow steps 1–4 above.
2. With each voiding, use the measuring container to accurately measure the urine. Again, the patient may wish to do this for you and can be instructed to keep accurate account. Any fecal material would have to be removed from the container for accuracy. Toilet tissue displacement can be approximated and is usually not removed. It is sometimes easier to pour off the urine from the bedpan in order to measure it.
3. Record the output on the I and O sheet. Use proper column.
4. Add any other output, including liquid stools, emesis, drainage, and the like. The quantity of some of these items will have to be estimated; even so, they should be added.
5. Total your 8-hour measurements at the end of your shift, and transfer them to the permanent record.

TOTAL 24-HOUR RECORD

1. Wash your hands.
2. Enter the 8-hour intake figures in the proper column.
3. Enter the 8-hour output figures in the proper column.
4. Be sure to add the number of milliliters of intravenous fluid infused over the 24-hour period. Also add the milliliters of medication delivered by minibottle or piggyback methods.

FLUID BALANCE RECORD

| DATE | SHIFT | FLUID INTAKE | | | | FLUID OUTPUT | | | | |
		ORAL	PARENTERAL	BLOOD	8 HR. TOTALS	URINE	GASTRIC	DRAINAGE	OTHER	8 HR. TOTALS
	11-7									
	7-3									
	3-11									
	24 HR. TOTAL									
	11-7									
	7-3									
	3-11									
	24 HR. TOTAL									
	11-7									
	7-3									
	3-11									
	24 HR. TOTAL									
	11-7									
	7-3									
	3-11									
	24 HR. TOTAL									

BALLARD COMMUNITY HOSPITAL
Seattle, Washington

FLUID BALANCE RECORD

FIGURE 11.2 INTAKE-OUTPUT RECORD FOR PATIENT'S CHART
Courtesy Ballard Community Hospital, Nursing Department, Seattle, Washington

PARENTERAL FLUID SHEET

DATE	TIME	NO.	SOLUTION	ADDITIVES	Amount Start	Time De'd	Amount Remaining	Total Amt. Given	Signature & Remarks

BALLARD COMMUNITY HOSPITAL
Seattle, Washington

PARENTERAL FLUID SHEET

FIGURE 11.3   PARENTERAL-FLUID SHEET
Courtesy Ballard Community Hospital, Nursing Department, Seattle, Washington

PERFORMANCE CHECKLIST

Intake	Unsatisfactory	Needs more practice	Satisfactory	Comments
1. Initiate measuring intake of patient.				
2. Locate intake–output worksheet at bedside.				
3. Explain reason for intake measurement to patient.				
4. Encourage patient's participation.				
5. After meal, record amount of each fluid item taken.				
6. Compute correctly partial intake of any fluid item.				
7. Add intake of free water, including quantities given with medications.				
8. Add liquid nourishments provided.				
9. Total intake on worksheet at end of 8-hour work period.				

Output				
1. Initiate measuring output of patient.				
2. Utilize bedside intake–output worksheet.				
3. Explain reason for measurement of output to patient.				
4. Encourage patient's participation.				
5. With each voiding, use measuring container to accurately measure urine.				
6. Record on worksheet in proper column.				
7. Add other output (diarrheal stools, emesis, drainage, perspiration), if of significant quantity, deciding which items can be measured and which must be estimated.				
8. Total output on worksheet at end of 8-hour work period.				

Total 24-hour record	Unsatisfactory	Needs more practice	Satisfactory	Comments
1. Wash your hands.				
2. Locate 24-hour intake–output record in patient's chart.				
3. Enter 8-hour intake total in proper column.				
4. Enter 8-hour output total in proper column.				
5. By computing number of milliliters of intravenous fluids left in IV bottle (bag) at beginning of work period and number of milliliters infused during remainder of work period, record intravenous-fluid intake in designated column. Add this to intake total.				

QUIZ

Multiple-Choice Questions

_____ 1. Intake and output are measured in metric units because

    a. metric weights and measures lend themselves to easier conversion from one to another.
    b. metric measures are more accurate.
    c. intravenous fluids are measured in metric units.
    d. nursing is a science and scientific disciplines use metric measures.

_____ 2. The intake-output worksheet is used primarily to

    a. show the patient his or her fluid status.
    b. total fluid intake and output.
    c. record the various fluid items of intake and output at the bedside.
    d. provide a permanent record of intake and output.

_____ 3. The permanent record of intake and output is usually kept

    a. on the worksheet.
    b. in the nurse's notes.
    c. on a special form in the chart.
    d. on the graphic record with temperature and vital signs.

_____ 4. The following items should be included in the total measurement of intake: (1) dietary fluids; (2) irrigation fluids returned; (3) gelatin; (4) fluids at bedside; (5) cereal; (6) ice cream; (7) intravenous fluids; (8) pureed fruits and vegetables.

    a. 1, 4, 7, and 8
    b. 1, 3, 4, 6, and 7
    c. 1, 2, 4, 5, and 7
    d. All of these

_____ 5. The following items should be included in the total measurement of output: (1) urine; (2) normal stools; (3) diarrheal stools; (4) vomitus; (5) normal perspiration; (6) excessive perspiration; (7) wound drainage.

    a. 1, 3, 4, 6, and 7
    b. 1, 4, 5, 6, and 7
    c. 1, 3, and 4
    d. All of these

_____ 6. In checking an I and O sheet, Jane Smith, RN, noted a larger than usual 8-hour intake recorded for a certain elderly patient. She then checked the worksheet on which the exact items taken were recorded. The following were listed on the worksheet:

Breakfast	Snack	Lunch
cereal, 60 ml	pureed peaches, 100 ml	pureed peas, 60 ml
half and half, 50 ml		pureed meat, 50 ml
apple juice, 100 ml		applesauce, 100 ml
(water pitcher changed,		milk, 100 ml
100 ml)		

Jane Smith determined that an error had been made. The error resulted from

a. incorrect addition.
b. including the morning water pitcher amount which was actually taken during the previous 8-hour shift.
c. including amounts for things that should not have been measured.

_____ 7. A patient has taken the following amounts during the dayshift (7:00 a.m.–3:00 p.m.). This hospital records all intake and output for 24-hour periods only. At the end of your shift, you will record which of the following on the intake and output record?

Breakfast	Lunch	Snack	Water Pitcher
juice, 100 ml	milk, 240 ml	gelatin, 50 ml	500 ml
milk, 90 ml	pudding, 50 ml		
coffee, 150 ml			

a. 1080 ml
b. 1130 ml
c. 1180 ml
d. Nothing

_____ 8. Totals over 24-hour periods are helpful because

a. intake and output balance usually cannot be identified over shorter time periods.
b. they reduce the time needed for record-keeping.
c. physicians usually check them once every 24 hours.
d. a 24-hour total is most accurate.

_____ 9. The following items were eaten by Mr. Jones. What is his total intake for the day shift?

Water Pitcher, 7:00 a.m.
100 ml

Breakfast
coffee, 250 ml
juice, 90 ml

Snack
juice, 100 ml

Lunch
milk, 240 ml

Water Pitcher Change, 2:30 p.m.
300 ml

Dinner
coffee, 250 ml

Water Pitcher Change and Snack, 8:30 p.m.
broth, 150 ml
water, 350 ml

a. 980 ml
b. 1080 ml
c. 1230 ml
d. 1330 ml

_____ 10. If the hospital in question 9 records intake on the record every eight hours, the total recorded by the nurse working from 3:00 p.m. to 11:00 p.m. would be

a. 450 ml.
b. 750 ml.
c. 1400 ml.
d. zero.

_____ 11. Mr. Jones had an output of 400 ml for the two shifts. This might indicate

a. fluid imbalance.
b. water intoxication.
c. edema formation.
d. kidney malfunction.

_____ 12. Mr. Ford is to have all intake and output measured. He is 45 years old, a truckdriver, father of four children, and has been admitted with a problem of possible kidney infection. In planning for accurate measurement, you would

a. measure all urine yourself because this is a critical concern.
b. see that urine is measured by a staff person (aide, LPN, RN), to guarantee accuracy.
c. have Mr. Ford measure his own urine and record it.
d. ask Mr. Ford if he would prefer to measure his output himself or have a staff person do it.

Module 12 Moving the Patient in Bed and Positioning

MAIN OBJECTIVES

To move patients in bed while maintaining correct body mechanics for both patients and nurse.

To place patients in positions that are anatomically correct as well as comfortable.

To be able to place patients in the special positions required for examination and therapy.

RATIONALE

A very important function of the nurse is to be able to move and position patients properly. This ability requires a knowledge of anatomy and good body alignment. The nurse should learn a number of positions, so that patients can be repositioned approximately every two hours. A regime of good positioning prevents pressure sores (decubitus ulcers) and joint contractures. Muscle tone, respiration, and circulation are also improved with frequent movement.

Often, an examination or procedure requires a special position to improve visibility. It is usually the nurse's responsibility to assist patients into special positions and to arrange for maximum comfort in the situation.

PREREQUISITES

Successful completion of the following modules:

VOLUME 1
Assessment
Charting
Medical Asepsis
Basic Body Mechanics

SPECIFIC LEARNING OBJECTIVES

	Know Facts and Principles	Apply Facts and Principles	Demonstrate Ability	Evaluate Performance
Moving the patient in bed				
1. *General procedure*	Give assessment factors and safety precautions for both nurse and patient	State rationale for assessment and safety	Adapt procedure to individual patient	Evaluate own performance with instructor
2. *Moving patient closer to one side of bed*	Describe each move in detail	Choose best movement procedure for particular patient	In clinical area, perform each move with patient if possible	Using the Performance Checklist, evaluate moves performed with help of instructor
3. *Moving patient up in bed: one-person assist*				
4. *Moving patient up in bed: two- or three-person assist*				
5. *Turning patient in bed: back to side*				
6. *Turning patient in bed: back to abdomen*				
7. *Turning patient: logrolling*				
8. *Using turn sheet with any of above*				
Recording			Record plan for turning on care plan as well as on chart	

Positioning

1. *Reasons for frequent and proper positioning* — Give three reasons for frequent and proper positioning — State rationale underlying each reason — Make adaptations for individual patients

2. *Positioning aids* — List available aids that are used for positioning — From list, select appropriate aids for each body position — In clinical area, use aids correctly for patient situation — Evaluate own performance with help of instructor

3. *Supine position*
4. *Side-lying position*
5. *Prone position*
6. *Sitting position*
7. *Fowler's position*
8. *High-Fowler's position*
9. *Orthopneic position*
10. *Lithotomy position*
11. *Sim's position*
12. *Knee-chest position*
13. *Trendelenburg position*

(3–13) Describe each — Choose best position for particular patient — In clinical area, place at least one patient in each position if possible — Using the Performance Checklist, critically evaluate patient's body alignment and comfort

Recording — Record plan for turning and positioning on nursing care plan. Chart on record, using proper format.

LEARNING ACTIVITIES

1. Review the Specific Learning Objectives.
2. Read the section on the effects of immobility (in the chapter on activity and rest) in Ellis and Nowlis, *Nursing: A Human Needs Approach,* or comparable material in another textbook.
3. Look up the module vocabulary terms in the glossary.
4. Read through the module.
5. In the practice setting, select three other students and form a group of four.
   a. Changing so that each has the opportunity to play the role of the patient, perform each of the following procedures for moving the patient in bed. Use the Performance Checklist for guidance. Those not participating at a given time can observe and evaluate the performances of the others.
      (1) Move the "patient" closer to one side of the bed.
      (2) Move the "patient" up in bed: one-person assist.
      (3) Move the "patient" up in bed: two- or three-person assist.
      (4) Turn the "patient" in bed: back to side.
      (5) Turn the "patient" in bed: back to abdomen.
      (6) Turn the "patient" in bed: logrolling.
      (7) Perform two of the above using a pull sheet. Does this make the task easier? How?
   b. With the same group, change roles as you did before and position the "patient" in the following ways:
      (1) Supine position
      (2) Side-lying position
      (3) Prone position
      (4) Sitting position (in a chair)
      (5) Fowler's position
      (6) High-Fowler's position
      (7) Orthopneic position
      (8) Lithotomy position
      (9) Sim's position
      (10) Knee-chest position
      (11) Trendelenburg position
   c. Note the different positions you assume during a normal night's sleep. Is one particular position more comfortable for you than others? How often do you estimate you change your position during the night?
6. In the clinical setting:
   a. Consult with your instructor regarding the opportunity to move patients using a variety of techniques. Evaluate your performance with the instructor.
   b. Consult with your instructor regarding the opportunity to position patients in a variety of appropriate positions. Evaluate your performance with the instructor.

VOCABULARY

alignment
anatomical position
axilla
dorsiflexion
extension
external rotation
flaccid
flexion
footdrop
gravity
orthopneic
paralysis
plantar flexion
pronation
trapeze
trochanter

MOVING THE PATIENT IN BED

When you must move a patient in bed, correct body mechanics are essential for both you and the patient. Without correct body mechanics, you may injure your back. It is also possible to put excessive stress on a patient's joints or to cause severe discomfort with incorrect moving techniques.

General Procedure

1. Assess the patient's need to move, the patient's ability to move unaided, and the assistive devices available.

2. Plan the moving technique and obtain any needed supportive devices or assistance.
3. Wash your hands.
4. Raise the bed to the high position. This enables your own body mechanics to be correct and protects you from back injury.
5. Put the bed in the flat position, if possible. In this way you will not be working against the gravitational pull on the patient. If the patient is medically unable to lie flat, you will have to adjust to the altered position, possibly with the help of an assistant.

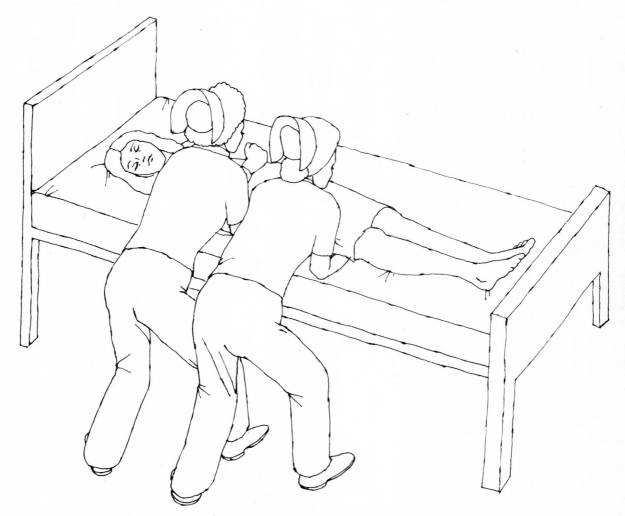

FIGURE 12.1 MOVING A PATIENT TO ONE SIDE OF A BED: TWO-PERSON ASSIST The nurses slide their arms under the patient (one at the shoulders, one at the hips) and pull toward themselves. Note the stance: back straight, hips and knees flexed, and right foot forward to give a broad base of support that can withstand a shift in weight as the patient is pulled toward the side of the bed.

6. Move the patient in one of the ways indicated in the following pages. In any move, remember to use smooth, coordinated movements.
7. Make sure all safety devices (side rails, pillows, protective restraints, call lights) are in place.
8. Wash your hands.
9. Record the patient's activity as required by your facility. Usually position changes from side to side or from back to abdomen are noted on a chart or flow sheet. Simply assisting a patient to move up in bed is not usually recorded.

You may note the techniques used for moving the patient on a nursing care plan for the use of other nursing care personnel. If the patient's ability to move is a significant part of the general assessment, you may have to write a progress note regarding the patient's activity.

MOVING A PATIENT CLOSER TO ONE SIDE OF THE BED

This activity is a needed part of many other moves; therefore, it is being presented separately. Most of the time, you will use this in conjunction with another type of movement.

1. Slide your hands and arms under the patient's head and shoulders, and pull them toward you. Be sure you bend from the hips and knees, keeping your back straight.
2. Move your hands and arms down under

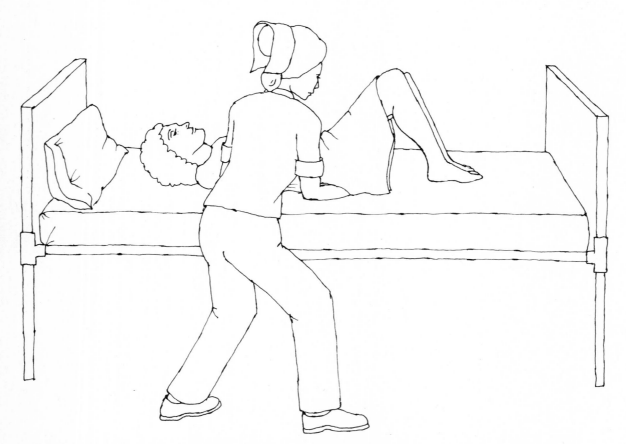

FIGURE 12.2 MOVING A PATIENT UP IN BED: ONE-PERSON ASSIST   The patient pushes with feet flat on the bed. The side rails and trapeze have been omitted to clarify the nurse's position. If they are not available, the patient pushes on the bed with the palms of the hands to further asisst in moving.

the patient's hips, and pull that section of the body toward you.

3. Slide your hands and arms under the patient's legs, and pull them toward you.

4. Repeat steps 1–3 in sequence until the patient is in the desired location on the bed.

If more than one person is available to assist, the same general technique is used except two sections of the body are moved at the same time. One nurse slides hands and arms under the patient's shoulders; the other nurse slides hands and arms under the patient's hips. To work together, one nurse must signal for the move by saying "One, two, three, *pull*!" (See Figure 12.1.)

MOVING A PATIENT UP IN BED: ONE-PERSON ASSIST

Follow the General Procedure above. For step 6, use the following technique for a patient who is able to cooperate and partially help. Independence should be encouraged, both to benefit the patient's physical progress and to support the patient's feelings of self-esteem and independence.

1. Have the patient bend the knees and place the soles of the feet firmly on the surface of the bed. The patient may need some assistance with this procedure.

2. Instruct the patient to grasp the overhead trapeze, if one is in place, or to grasp the side rails at shoulder level. Some patients may be able to grasp the headboard and pull themselves up.

3. Slide your hands and arms under the patient's hips, facing slightly toward the foot of the bed with your outside foot slightly ahead of your inside foot (Figure 12.2). Keep your back straight, bend at the hips and the knees, and keep your elbows bent so that you are using your strong leg muscles to pull.

4. Instruct the patient that you will both move at the same time, on the count

("One, two, three, *up!*"). All effort should be expended simultaneously.

5. Count, "One, two, three, *up!*" The patient should pull with the arms and push with the feet. From your position, you will *pull* the patient up in bed. In pulling, you use your strong flexor muscles in their most effective manner. Many persons do this same maneuver facing the head of the bed, pushing the patient up. This method has two drawbacks: first, you cannot move as much weight this way; second, you meet greater resistance from the bed surface in pushing along it than in pulling along it.

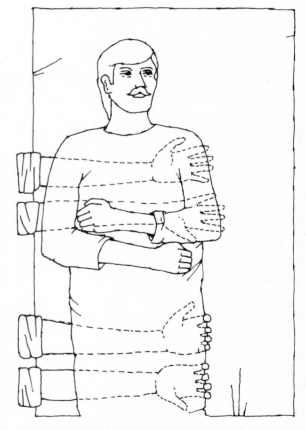

FIGURE 12.3 MOVING A PATIENT UP IN BED: TWO-PERSON ASSIST *Note:* The patient has been moved closer to one side of the bed. Both nurses slip their arms under the patient so that the patient can be pulled up in bed.

MOVING A PATIENT UP IN BED: TWO- OR THREE-PERSON ASSIST

When you must move a heavy patient or one who is unable to help, you will find it easier to use more than one person. In most cases, two persons are sufficient, however, for the exceptionally heavy patient, you may find that three persons are necessary. For step 6 in the General Procedure, page 172, proceed in the following manner.

1. Move the patient close to one side of the bed (Figure 12.3).
2. If the patient is able, have the patient bend the knees and plant the soles of the feet firmly on the bed. Even if the patient is unable to push with the feet and legs, this positioning of the knees and soles eliminates the need to drag the weight of the legs as well as the weight of the trunk.
3. The first nurse (nurse 1) slides his or her arms under the patient's head and shoulders. This nurse faces the foot of the bed.
4. The second nurse (nurse 2) slides his or her arms under the patient's hips from the same side of the bed. This nurse also faces the foot of the bed (Figure 12.4).
5. The nurse with the heaviest burden (usually nurse 2) counts, "One, two, three, *up!*" so that both pull the patient up in bed at the same time.

This procedure can be repeated several times until the patient is in the correct position.

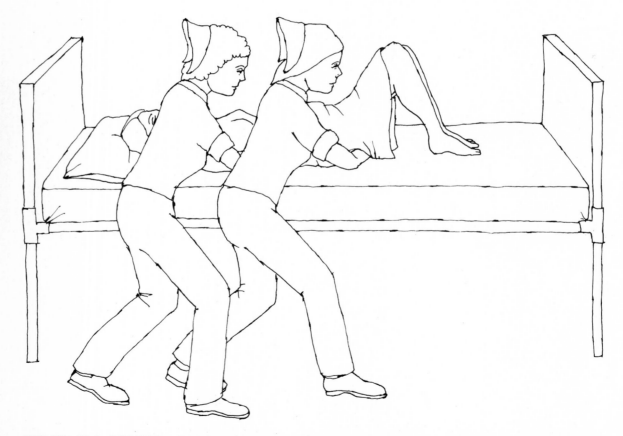

FIGURE 12.4   MOVING A PATIENT UP IN BED: TWO-PERSON ASSIST   *Note:* The nurses face toward the foot of the bed. The outside foot (right in this instance) is placed more toward the foot of the bed to provide a wide stance. The back is straight; knees and hips are slightly bent.

If a third person is necessary to move a patient, the three nurses should align themselves along the patient on the same side of the bed, distributing the weight among them. Since the patient is close to the side of the bed where the nurses are standing, it is possible for the nurses to maintain firm support with their legs, keeping their center of gravity over that base of support and working close to their bodies. This is an efficient way to use muscles. On occasion, it will be necessary to leave a patient in the middle of the bed. In that case, the lifters should position themselves on each side of the bed, paying close attention to their body mechanics. It is very easy to bend from the waist and put strain on the back.

Under no circumstances should a nurse pull a patient up in bed by grasping the patient under the axillae and pulling. This may work well for the nurse, but it is very uncomfortable for the patient and can cause a shoulder dislocation, especially for a person with extremely weak muscles or paralysis.

TURNING A PATIENT IN BED:
BACK TO SIDE

1. Move the patient so that the side the patient is to lie on is close to the center of the bed.
2. Raise the side rail on that side and move to the other side of the bed. You will be rolling the patient toward you.
3. Prepare the pillows needed for support. (See Side-Lying Position, page 181.)

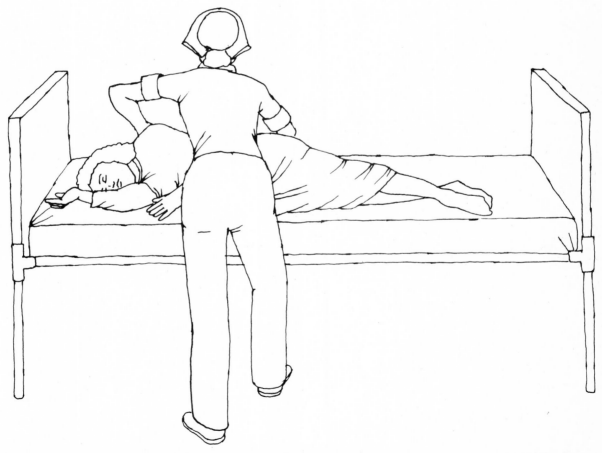

FIGURE 12.5 TURNING A PATIENT FROM BACK TO SIDE Use a wide base of support, with back straight and knees slightly bent. Then, use the entire weight of the body to rock backward, turning the heavy patient. (Side rails have been omitted for clarity.)

4. Two different ways are used to turn the lower body. The method you use will depend on your preference and the patient's ability.

   a. Cross the far ankle over the near ankle. Then grasp the patient with one hand behind the far hip.

   b. Raise the knee on the far leg. Then grasp the leg by reaching over the knee and holding the far side of the knee.

5. Move the near arm of the patient out away from the patient's body.

6. Place the patient's far arm across the chest.

7. Grasp the patient behind the far shoulder.

8. Roll the patient toward you (Figure 12.5).

9. Adjust the patient's position to the correct side-lying position.

TURNING A PATIENT IN BED: BACK TO ABDOMEN

1. Move the patient to the extreme edge of the bed.

2. Raise the side rail on that side and move to the other side of the bed.

3. Prepare the pillows needed for support. Frequently, heavy-breasted patients will need a pillow under the abdomen for comfort. A very thin patient might be more comfortable with a small pillow under the iliac crests.

4. Place the patient's near arm along the side of the body, so that the patient will roll over it, and the far arm up over the patient's head.

5. Turn the patient's face away from you, so that the patient will not roll onto his or her face during the turning procedure (Figure 12.6).

6. Roll the patient onto his or her side using the same technique noted in the last section.

7. Once the patient is on his or her side, check the arm and face carefully to see that they are correctly positioned.

8. Roll the patient over onto the abdomen.

9. Adjust the patient's position to a correct abdominal position.

TURNING A PATIENT: LOGROLLING

When a patient must maintain a straight alignment at all times, the patient is turned

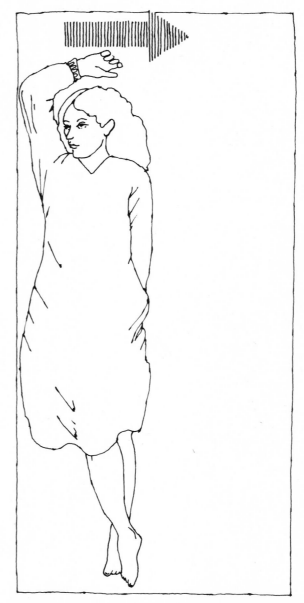

FIGURE 12.6   PATIENT READY TO BE TURNED FROM BACK TO ABDOMEN   The patient is at the the extreme edge of the bed. Face and arms are positioned for safety. The legs and far arm are positioned to facilitate rolling.

by a technique called *logrolling*. The technique requires at least two nurses, and, if the patient is very large, three nurses may be necessary.

1. Move the patient to one side of the bed as an entire unit. Each person assisting with the turn slides his or her arms under the patient. At a signal ("One, two, three, *move*!"), all pull the patient, making sure that the patient's body stays correctly aligned at all times.
2. Raise the side rail on that side of the bed.
3. All assistants move to the other side of the bed.
4. Arrange the pillows as will be needed for support after the patient has been turned. One is needed to support the head with the spine straight; another is needed between the legs (in fact, two may be needed here).
5. All assistants reach across the patient and grasp the far side of the patient's body.
6. At the signal ("One, two, three, *turn*!"), all turn the patient smoothly, keeping the patient's body perfectly straight (like a log). (See Figure 12.7.)

A turn sheet under the patient makes the turn smoother and easier. The assistants should proceed as outlined above, but instead of grasping the patient's body, they grasp the turn sheet on the far side of the patient and

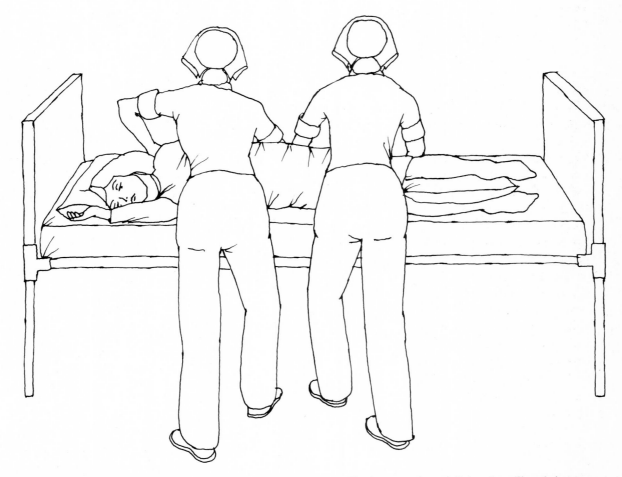

FIGURE 12.7 LOGROLLING Roll the patient as a unit. The legs remain parallel and a pillow is between them to keep the upper leg from dropping and causing a twisting action on the spine. Place a pillow under the head so that the head does not drop down. At least two nurses are essential for this procedure.

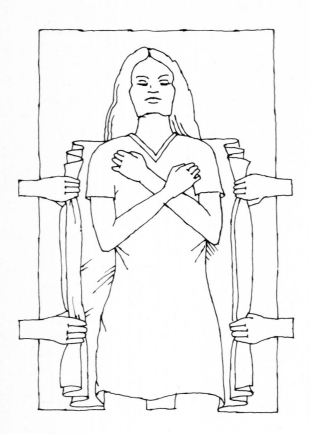

FIGURE 12.8 *(left)* TURN SHEET (PULL SHEET) IN PLACE The sheet extends from the shoulders to below the hips and is rolled or fan-folded at each side of the patient's body.

FIGURE 12.9 *(below)* MOVING A PATIENT UP IN BED USING A TURN SHEET Both nurses face the foot of the bed. Knees and hips are slightly bent and backs are straight. Feet are spread to form a wide base of support.

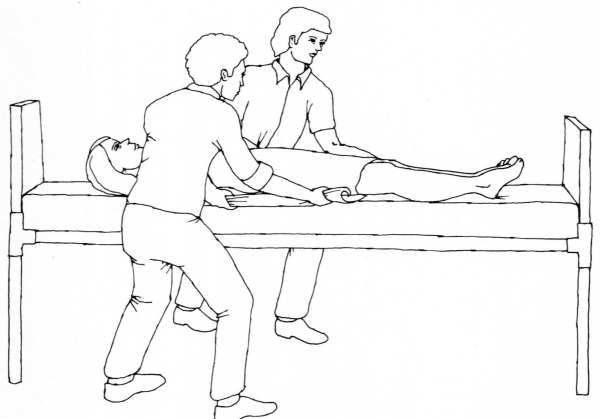

pull it toward them. The turn sheet supports the entire body and makes it easier to keep the patient straight. (See next section.)

USING A TURN SHEET OR PULL SHEET

A sheet can be used as an aid in turning and moving a patient in bed. Place the turn sheet, or pull sheet, under the patient's trunk, with the bottom edge below the patient's buttocks and the top edge at the top of the patient's shoulders. Do not tuck in the sides; fan-fold or roll them along the patient on each side. To move the patient up in bed or to turn the patient, grasp the fan-folded edges of the sheet instead of the patient's body. (See Figures 12.8 and 12.9.)

One advantage of using a turn or pull sheet is that the movement takes place between two layers of dry cloth, which produce less friction than does skin on cloth. Another advantage is that it is much easier to grasp a sheet firmly than it is to hold a patient's body. Your hands can slip off the patient if you do not grasp hard enough; and if you grasp too hard you can cause discomfort or even bruising. Do not lift the patient with the pull sheet; always slide the patient.

POSITIONING

Positioning a Patient in Bed

Positioning patients in bed in proper body alignment and changing their positions frequently are important nursing functions. Many alert patients automatically reposition themselves and readily move about in bed. They may not need special attention, but often need a reminder that comfort and good body alignment are sometimes not the

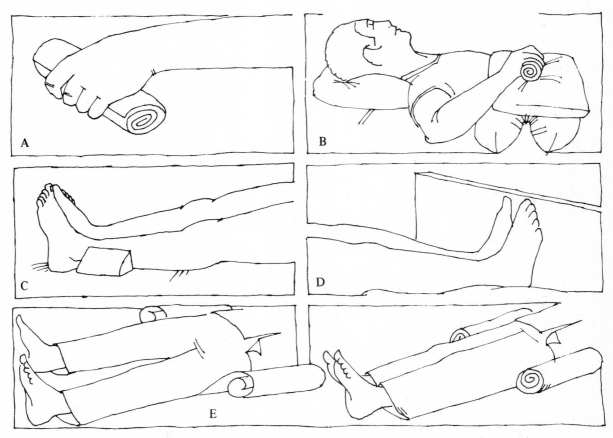

FIGURE 12.10 POSITIONING AIDS *A:* Washcloth in a handroll; *B:* pillows; *C:* sandbag; *D:* footboard; *E:* bath blanket in a trochanter roll.

same. For example, two large pillows under the head may be comfortable, but the neck, which is in constant flexion, can develop spasms and even contracture from this position. Patients' bodies must be repositioned during the night as well, keeping in mind the many turns and positions used by well persons during sleep. This is usually done every 2 hours. For some patients more frequent turning is needed to prevent skin breakdown. Without a 24-hour repositioning schedule, patients will develop pressure sores readily. It is helpful to give range-of-motion exercises (ROM) to patients at the time they are repositioned. (See Module 14.)

You can make positioning aids easily by using ordinary items found in your facility. Pillows, towels, washcloths, sandbags, footboards, and strong cardboard cartons can all be used to help maintain a patient's proper position. (See Figure 12.10.)

SUPINE POSITION

The patient should lie on his or her back, with the spine in straight alignment. Place a low pillow under the head to prevent neck extension. The arms may be at the patient's side with the hands pronated. The forearms can also be elevated on pillows. In either position, if the patient's hands are paralyzed, handrolls should be in place. Handrolls can be made of several washcloths (or other linen) that have been rolled and taped. Place the handroll in the palm of the patient's hand. The fingers and thumb should be flexed around it. The roll should be large enough so that the fingers are only slightly

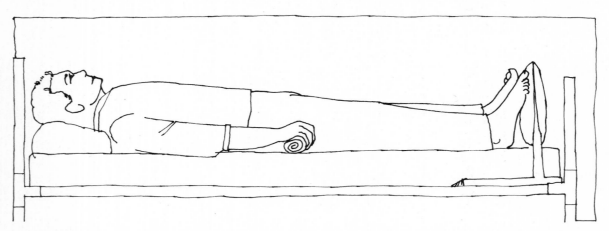

FIGURE 12.11   SUPINE POSITION   A small pillow and a footboard help put the patient in correct supine position. Handrolls are used for patients whose hands are paralyzed.

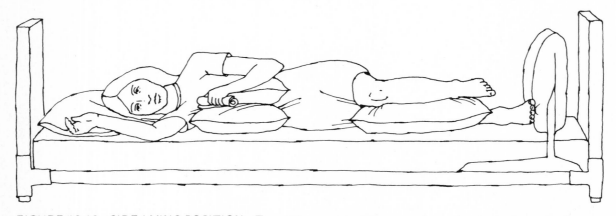

FIGURE 12.12   SIDE-LYING POSITION   Two pillows support the upper leg and arm; the lower leg lies straight.

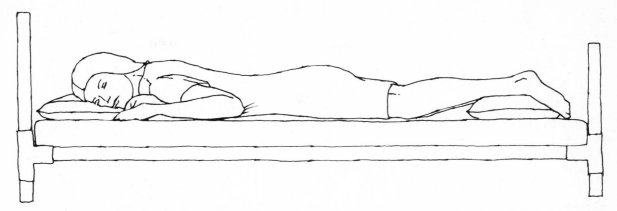

FIGURE 12.13 PRONE POSITION   A small pillow supports the patient's ankles. The patient's arms bend upward toward the shoulders. A small pillow may be used under the head.

flexed. A handroll may have to be secured to the hand with paper tape. (See Figure 12.11.)

When the body is lying flat on the bed, position the legs so that external rotation does not occur. A trochanter roll is effective in preventing external hip rotation. This roll can be made from a sheet, bath towel, or pad. Place one end flat under the patient's hip (*trochanter*) and roll the linen *under* to form a roll that stabilizes the leg and prevents it from turning outward. An ankle roll, which is made in the same way but is smaller than a trochanter roll, can accomplish the same purpose. If both legs are paralyzed, place a roll on either side at the hip or the ankle.

The foot should be supported so that the toes point upward in anatomical position and do not fall into plantar flexion. If plantar flexion were maintained for a long period of time, a permanent deformity, called *footdrop,* would occur. The foot would be unable to dorsiflex and would not be functional. A manufactured footboard, sandbags, or a strong cardboard carton can be used to maintain the feet at right angles to the legs.

SIDE-LYING POSITION

If done properly, the side-lying position can be particularly comfortable for the patient. (See Figure 12.12.) A patient who is paralyzed on one side can be placed on that side as well as on the unaffected side unless the

patient has discomfort. Give special attention to body alignment, however.

In this position, the patient is on his or her side with the head supported on a low pillow. Tuck a pillow *under* along the patient's back to both support the back and hold the position. Bring the underlying arm

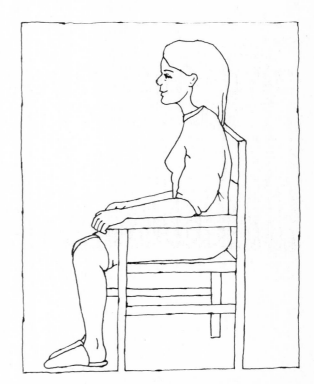

FIGURE 12.14 POSITIONING A PATIENT IN A CHAIR   The patient's buttocks should fit well back into the seat of the chair. The back is straight, the knees are bent, and the feet are flat on the floor. The elbows are supported by armrests.

forward and flex it onto the pillow used for the head. Bring the top arm forward, flex it, and rest it on a pillow in front of the body. Put handrolls in place if needed. The top leg should be flexed and brought slightly forward. A pillow, placed lengthwise under the top leg, keeps the legs separated and supports the top leg. Take care to support the feet to prevent plantar flexion and footdrop.

PRONE POSITION

The prone position (Figure 12.13) is used infrequently by nurses because many believe that respirations are compromised in this position. However, if it is done properly, a great number of patients can tolerate this position. Also, it can be used very effectively with a patient who has pressure sores, because it relieves the pressure on the buttocks and both hips as well.

With the patient on the abdomen, turn the head to one side. Do not use a pillow. Be sure that the spine is straight. Place a folded towel under each shoulder. With a female patient who has large breasts, put a flat pillow under her abdomen; this should add to her comfort and not defeat the principles of good alignment. The arms may be flat at the patient's side or flexed at the elbow with the hands near the patient's head. Place handrolls if needed. The feet should

either fall in the space between the mattress and the footboard or a roll should be placed under the ankles. This will keep the feet in proper alignment, preventing plantar flexion.

Positioning a Patient in a Chair

In a chair, a patient's feet should be flat against the floor with the knees and hips at right angles. The buttocks should rest firmly against the back of the chair, and the spine should be in straight alignment (Figure 12.14). Avoid placing pillows at the back because they may upset proper alignment. Support the patient's elbows with armrests. If needed, place handrolls in the patient's hands. A footrest of some type may be needed for shorter patients.

Therapeutic Positions

In addition to the horizontal resting position described above, a variety of special positions are used for therapeutic reasons. The reasons for use can be found in a medical-surgical text.

FOWLER'S POSITION

The patient is in the supine position with the head of the bed elevated 18 to 20 inches. (See Figure 12.15.)

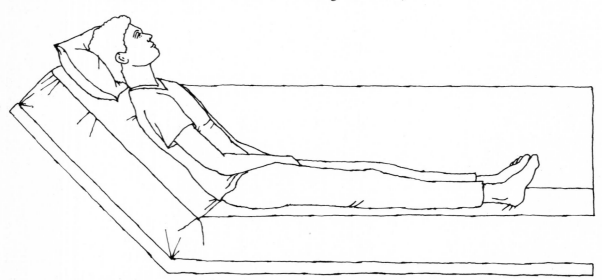

FIGURE 12.15 FOWLER'S POSITION   In the traditional Fowler's position, the knees were also elevated; today, this is seldom done because of potential pressure on the popliteal area.

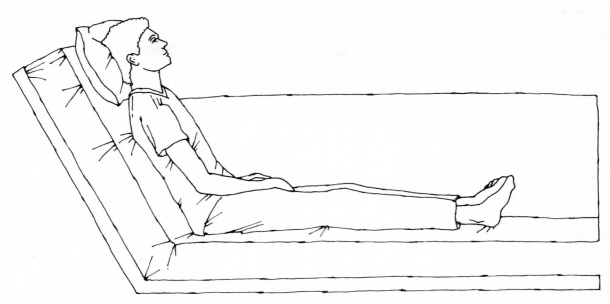

FIGURE 12.16   HIGH-FOWLER'S POSITION

HIGH-FOWLER'S POSITION

The patient is in the supine position with the head of the bed elevated to greater than a 45-degree angle. (See Figure 12.16.)

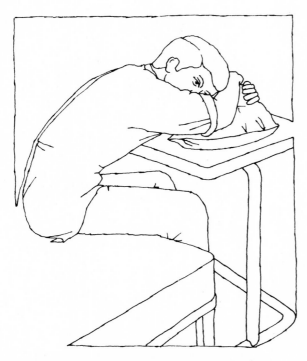

FIGURE 12.17   ORTHOPNEIC POSITION   A pillow is placed on the overbed table; the patient rests the elbows on the pillow.

ORTHOPNEIC POSITION

The patient sits up in or at the edge of the bed with an overbed table across his or her lap. The table is padded with a pillow and elevated to a comfortable height. The patient leans forward and rests head and arms on the table for support. (See Figure 12.17.)

LITHOTOMY POSITION

The patient is on his or her back. The legs are separated widely with the knees raised. When the patient is on the examining table, the feet are placed in stirrups. (See Figure 12.18.)

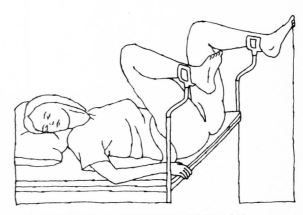

FIGURE 12.18   LITHOTOMY POSITION (Draping omitted for clarity.)

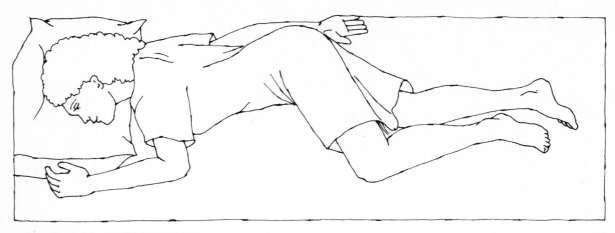

FIGURE 12.19   SIM'S POSITION

SIM'S POSITION

This is a side-lying position that uses only a single supporting pillow—that under the head. The patient is turned far enough onto the abdomen so that the lower arm is extended behind the patient's back and both knees are slightly flexed. (See Figure 12.19.)

KNEE-CHEST POSITION (GENUPECTORAL)

The patient kneels on the bed or table, and then leans forward with the hips in the air and the chest and arms on the bed. A pillow can be placed under the patient's head (Figure 12.20). There are special examination tables that are constructed to allow a patient to kneel on a platform and lean on the table.

TRENDELENBURG POSITION

In this position, the patient lies on the back. The head is lowered at a 45-degree angle below horizontal level. (See Figure 12.21.)

FIGURE 12.20   KNEE-CHEST POSITION
(Draping omitted for clarity.)

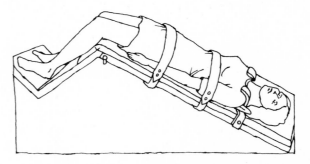

FIGURE 12.21   TRENDELENBURG POSITION
The knees are bent as would be common in the operating room.

PERFORMANCE CHECKLIST

	Unsatisfactory	Needs more practice	Satisfactory	Comments
Moving a patient in bed: General procedure				
1. Assess patient's need.				
2. Plan moving technique.				
3. Wash your hands.				
4. Place bed in high position.				
5. Place bed surface in flat position if possible.				
6. Move patient in method selected. (See following checklists.)				
7. Make sure safety devices are in place.				
8. Wash your hands.				
9. Record activity as required.				
Moving a patient closer to one side of a bed				
1. Slide your hands and arms under patient's head and shoulders, and pull toward you.				
2. Move your hands and arms under patient's hips, and pull toward you.				
3. Slide your hands and arms under patient's legs, and pull toward you.				
4. Repeat in sequence until patient is in correct position.				
Moving a patient up in bed: One-person assist				
1. Have patient bend knees and place soles firmly on bed.				
2. Have patient grasp overhead trapeze, siderails, or headboard.				
3. Slide your hands and arms under patient's hips, facing foot of bed, outside foot ahead of inside foot.				
4. Instruct patient to move with you at count.				
5. On count, patient pulls with arms and pushes with feet as you pull.				

	Unsatisfactory	Needs more practice	Satisfactory	Comments
Moving a patient up in bed: Two- or three-person assist				
1. Move patient close to one side of bed.				
2. If able, have patient's knees bent and soles firmly on bed.				
3. Nurse 1 slides arms under patient's head and shoulders.				
4. Nurse 2 slides arms under patient's hips.				
5. Nurse 2 counts, and both move patient.				
Turning a patient in bed: Back to side				
1. Move patient to one side of bed.				
2. Raise rail and move to other side.				
3. Prepare pillows for support.				
4. Turn lower body using one of two methods described.				
5. Move patient's near arm out of patient's way.				
6. Place patient's far arm across chest.				
7. Grasp patient behind far shoulder.				
8. Roll patient toward you.				
9. Adjust position as needed.				
Turning a patient in bed: Back to abdomen				
1. Move patient to edge of bed.				
2. Raise side rail and move to other side of bed.				
3. Prepare pillows for support.				
4. Place patient's near arm close to body.				
5. Turn patient's face away from you.				
6. Roll patient onto side.				
7. Check arm and face positioning.				
8. Roll patient further onto abdomen.				
9. Adjust position as needed.				

	Unsatisfactory	Needs more practice	Satisfactory	Comments
Turning a patient: Logrolling				
1. With help, move patient to side of bed in one unit.				
2. Raise side rail on that side of bed.				
3. All assistants move to other side of bed.				
4. Place pillows correctly.				
5. Assistants reach across and grasp patient's body.				
6. At count, all turn patient in one unit.				
Note: All the movements described can be facilitated by using a turn sheet or pull sheet. See page 179.				
Supine position				
1. Place patient on back, with spine in straight alignment.				
2. Place low pillow under head.				
3. Place arms at side or elevated on pillow, with hands prone.				
4. Place handrolls if needed.				
5. Keep legs straight.				
6. Place trochanter or ankle roll on one or both sides.				
7. Position feet with toes pointed up and support with footboard, sandbags, or carton.				
Side-lying position				
1. Turn patient on side.				
2. Place low pillow under head.				
3. Undertuck pillow along back.				
4. Place lower arm forward of body.				
5. Flex and support lower arm on pillow used for head.				
6. Flex top arm and rest on pillow in front of body.				
7. Place handrolls if needed.				
8. Flex top leg and bring slightly forward.				
9. Place pillow lengthwise between legs.				
10. Support feet with positioning aids to prevent plantar flexion.				

	Unsatisfactory	Needs more practice	Satisfactory	Comments
Prone position				
1. Place patient on abdomen.				
2. Turn patient's head to one side.				
3. Straighten spine.				
4. Place folded towel under each shoulder.				
5. Place arms flat at side or flexed at elbow near patient's head.				
6. Place handrolls if needed.				
7. Position patient's feet in space between mattress and footboard or use roll under ankles.				
Positioning a patient in a chair				
1. Place feet flat against floor.				
2. Position knees and hips at right angle.				
3. Straighten spine.				
4. Support elbows on armrests.				
5. Place handrolls if needed.				
Fowler's position				
1. Place patient in supine position.				
2. Elevate head of bed 18 to 20 inches.				
High-Fowler's position				
1. Place patient in supine position.				
2. Elevate head of bed to greater than 45-degree angle.				
Orthopneic position				
1. Have patient sit up in bed with overbed table across lap.				
2. Pad table with pillows and elevate to comfortable height.				
3. Have patient lean forward with head and arms resting on table.				

	Unsatisfactory	Needs more practice	Satisfactory	Comments
Lithotomy position				
1. Position patient on back.				
2. Raise knees and separate legs.				
3. If on table, place feet in stirrups.				
Sim's position				
1. Use side-lying position, with single pillow only under head.				
2. Turn far enough onto abdomen so underarm extends behind patient's back.				
Knee-chest position				
1. Have patient kneel on bed or table with hips in air.				
2. If special table, have patient kneel on platform with head on table.				
Trendelenburg position				
1. Position patient on back with head lowered at 45-degree angle.				

QUIZ

Short-Answer Questions

1. What is the primary reason for having the bed in the flat position when moving a patient? _____

2. What two important functions are fulfilled by having the patient assist you whenever possible?

    a. _____

    b. _____

3. If a patient is grasped under the axillae by a nurse attempting to move the patient, a _____ may occur.

4. A turn sheet should be placed under which part of a patient's body?

    _____

5. List two reasons why patients should be checked after moving.

    a. _____

    b. _____

6. List three reasons for proper and frequent positioning of a patient in bed.

    a. _____

    b. _____

    c. _____

7. To prevent external rotation of the leg when a patient is in the supine position, you might use a _____

8. When a patient is in a side-lying position, the top leg is _____ over the lower leg.

9. When a patient is in the prone position, two methods can be used to keep the feet from plantar flexion—the possible development of footdrop. What are these two methods?

    a. _____

    b. _____

Multiple-Choice Questions

_____ 10. In all positions, the spine should be

       a. slightly flexed.
       b. straight.
       c. slightly extended.
       d. curved.

_____ 11. A patient's position should usually be changed

       a. every hour.
       b. every two hours.
       c. every four hours.
       d. once per shift.

Module 13 Applying Restraints

MAIN OBJECTIVE

To apply a variety of restraints taking into account both the comfort and safety of patients.

RATIONALE

Sometimes physical restraints are applied for the safety of patients and occasionally for the protection of the staff. All restraints must be applied with care to avoid damaging tissue and causing undue discomfort to patients. The nurse must use discretion in deciding when restraints should be applied and know the proper application of any restraints used.

PREREQUISITES

Successful completion of the following modules:

VOLUME 1
Assessment
Charting
Medical Asepsis
Basic Body Mechanics
Moving the Patient in Bed and Positioning

SPECIFIC LEARNING OBJECTIVES

	Know Facts and Principles	Apply Facts and Principles	Demonstrate Ability	Evaluate Performance
1. *Reasons for physical restraint*	List two reasons for applying restraints	Give reason in a particular situation	In a clinical situation, understand reason for application	
2. *Legal implications*	State reason for obtaining order		Check order before applying or take steps to obtain order	
3. *Choice of restraint*	Know various restraints used. State factors that decide use of particular restraint.	Adapt choice to patient's need	With an individual patient, choose appropriate restraint	Evaluate own performance with instructor
4. *Application of restraints*			Apply restraint chosen, taking into account comfort and safety factors	Evaluate own performance using Performance Checklist
5. *Safety*	Give rationale for releasing restraints at intervals		Remove restraints at proper intervals, and turn or exercise patient	Evaluate own performance using Performance Checklist
6. *Recording*	List data to be recorded		Make complete record of entire procedure, including assessment demonstrating need for restraint	

LEARNING ACTIVITIES

1. Review the Specific Learning Objectives.
2. Read the section on the effects of immobility (in the chapter on activity and rest) in Ellis and Nowlis, *Nursing: A Human Needs Approach,* or comparable material in another textbook.
3. Read through the module.
4. In the practice setting:
   a. Inspect the various physical restraints.
   b. Have a partner apply various restraints to you. Now, answer the following questions:
      (1) Which are the most comfortable?
      (2) Which are the least comfortable?
      (3) Why?
   c. Apply the various restraints to your partner. Check them for comfort and safety.
5. In the clinical setting:
   a. Observe any restraints being used. Have they been applied correctly and safely?
   b. When the opportunity arises, apply an appropriate restraint with your instructor's supervision.
   c. Using the Performance Checklist, evaluate your performance with the help of your instructor.

APPLYING RESTRAINTS

The decision to restrain a patient physically must always be made after *careful* assessment and with an order from a physician. However, if the immediate safety of a patient or of the staff is in question, apply restraints at once, and secure an order at the earliest possible moment. If this procedure is not followed, the patient could take legal action against you.

Often restraints are applied simply so a patient cannot move an extremity that has tubes or appliances connected to it. If restraints are being applied because a patient is extremely agitated or irrational, get extra help before you approach the patient.

Regardless of how irrational a patient may be, always explain what you plan to do and why. Never convey an attitude of punishment with regard to restraints. For example, you might say that the restraint is to "remind" the patient not to lean too far forward in the chair. This often makes the procedure more acceptable. Some facilities use the term *protective device*. Others commonly refer to them as *Poseys*, which is a brand name and not a descriptive term.

Never leave a restraint on for longer than two hours without checking and moving it.

Choosing a Restraint

Make the choice of restraint fit the need. Use the minimum restraint necessary to effectively protect the patient or staff. For example, if a patient were attempting to remove a nasogastric tube with the left hand, and the right upper extremity is paralyzed, you would need only a wrist restraint to the left wrist.

With the restraint chosen, give the patient the maximum mobility possible that still accomplishes the task. For the patient just described, you might leave the left wrist restraint loose enough so that some flexion of the elbow can take place, even though the patient cannot reach the nasogastric tube.

Kinds of Restraints

1. *Wrist or ankle restraint*   A canvas or cloth strap with a thread-through buckle device or opening in the strap. (See Figure 13.1.) Slip the restraint on patient's wrist or ankle, thread it, and tie to the bed frame (never to a side rail). The ties of wrist and vest restraints should be tied to the movable portion of the bed frame, so that if the head of the bed is raised the ties will not be pulled.

2. *Body restraint*   A back-to-back belted restraint (Figure 13.2). The top and smaller belt is fastened around the patient's waist; the lower belt is fastened to the bed frame.

3. *Vest restraint*   A canvas or mesh vest with tails that are crossed in the back through an opening in one and secured to the bed frame (Figure 13.3). See note about ties, above.

4. *Elbow or knee restraint*   A canvas or mesh wraparound restraint that has lengthwise rigid stays to prevent joint flexion. (See Figure 13.4.)

5. *Soft-tie restraints*   Some facilities make their own restraints. One of the most common is a soft tie, a long (5 to 8 feet)

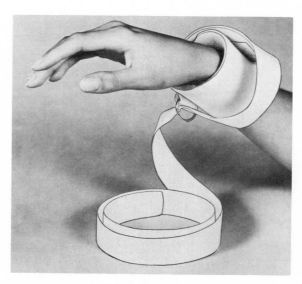

FIGURE 13.1   WRIST RESTRAINT
Courtesy J.T. Posey Company, Pasadena, California

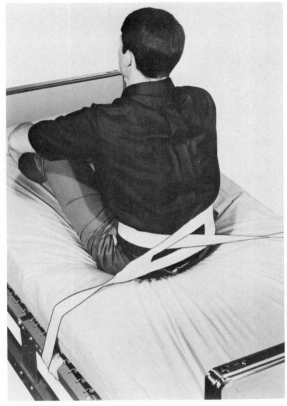

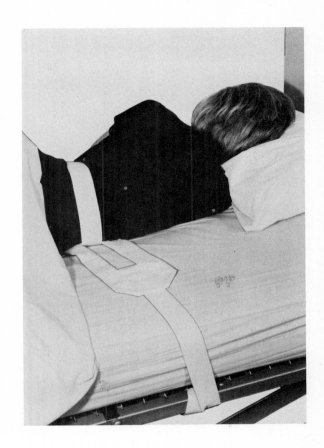

FIGURE 13.2   BODY RESTRAINT
Courtesy J.T. Posey Company, Pasadena, California

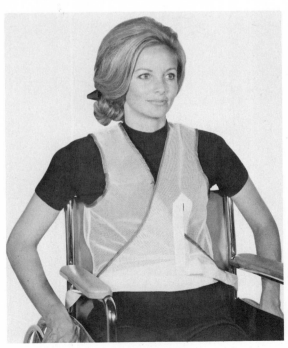

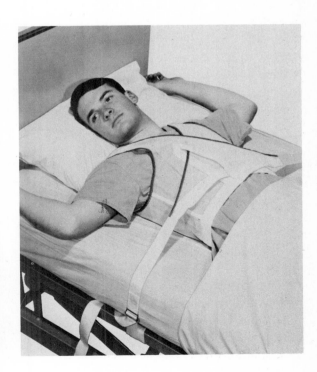

FIGURE 13.3   VEST RESTRAINT
Courtesy J.T. Posey Company, Pasadena, California

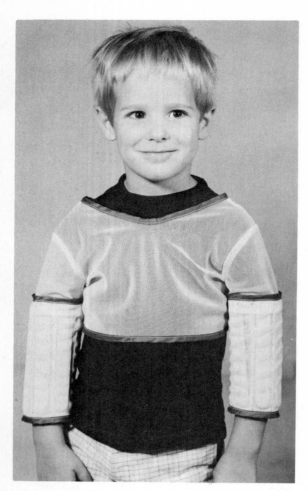

FIGURE 13.4   ELBOW RESTRAINT
Courtesy J.T. Posey Company, Pasadena, California

and narrow (approximately 3 inches) piece of fabric. It is often made from a worn bedspread or other heavy fabric.

The soft tie is used in a variety of ways. For a *waist restraint,* place it across the patient's lap and under the arms of the chair; then tie it securely behind the chair. If necessary, wrap the tie around the arm of the chair before tying it or wrap it around the back legs of the chair and tie it under the chair to keep the knot out of the patient's reach. (See Figure 13.5.)

This long tie may also be used as a *figure-8 restraint.* The purpose of this restraint is to keep a patient from sliding,

feet first, from under the restraint and out of the chair. You can substitute a large sheet twisted from opposite corners into a long tie for the soft tie in making a figure-8 restraint. Place the center of the tie across the top of the patient's thighs, just above the knees. Pass the ends behind each leg and bring them up between the legs at the knees. Then cross the two long ends and put them under the arms of the chair and around to the back of the chair, where they are tied together. Take care not to pull this restraint too tight, and check the inner aspects of the thighs and knees carefully for skin abrasion. This restraint is useful in maintaining a correct sitting posture.

6. *Mitt restraint*   A mitt restraint (Figure 13.6) is used for a patient who is

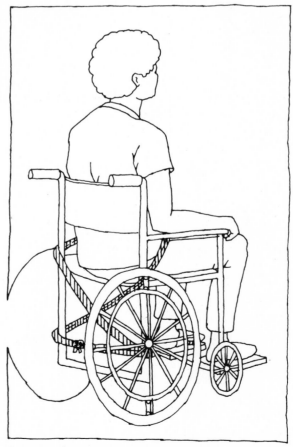

FIGURE 13.5   SOFT-TIE RESTRAINT

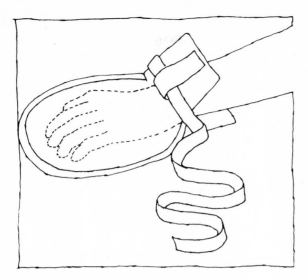

FIGURE 13.6 MITT RESTRAINT

abstractly pulling at tubes or appliances. This restricts only the hand and fingers, allowing the arm to move freely. Mitts are available commercially, or they can be made by wrapping the hands loosely with strips of soft fabric or rolls of dressing material. Secure the wrapping with paper tape. Remove the mitts periodically, as you would other restraints, to clean and exercise the hands and fingers.

Removing Restraints

Restraints must be removed every two hours or less, so that the patient's position can be changed or the restrained extremity exercised. If the patient's skin is fragile or the patient is extremely restless, add extra padding to the restraint.

Recording

Record on the nurses' notes the type and location of the restraint and the time and the reason for application. If you do not yet have a physician's order, note that the physician has been notified of your action.

Procedure

1. Assess the patient's need for restraint. Always restrain the patient as little as possible to accomplish your purpose. Occasionally you may overrestrain the patient initially, but it is best to be safe. You can modify a restraint later if necessary. When possible, provide for the patient's elimination needs before application.
2. Have or obtain a physician's order. A verbal order by telephone will suffice.
3. Wash your hands.
4. Select the appropriate restraint for accomplishing your purpose with the least limitation to the patient.
5. Explain what you are going to do and why. Showing the restraint to the patient is sometimes helpful in allaying the patient's fears.
6. Apply the appropriate restraint. *Never* knot the ties to the side rails. (If the rails were suddenly lowered, the patient's extremities could be injured.)
7. Add extra padding if necessary. Clean rags or washcloths can be used.
8. Wash your hands.
9. Record the type and location of the restraint, and the time it was applied as well as the reason for its application.
10. Remove the restraint in two hours or less, turn the patient, and exercise the restrained extremities.
11. Reapply if necessary.

PERFORMANCE CHECKLIST

	Unsatisfactory	Needs more practice	Satisfactory	Comments
1. Assess patient's need to be restrained.				
2. Have or obtain physician's order.				
3. Wash your hands.				
4. Select appropriate restraint.				
5. Explain to patient what you are going to do and why.				
6. Apply appropriate restraint.				
7. Add extra padding if necessary.				
8. Wash your hands.				
9. Record type and location of restraint, time, and reason for application.				
10. Remove in two hours or less, and turn patient or exercise extremity.				
11. Reapply if necessary.				

QUIZ

Short-Answer Questions

1. List two reasons why physical restraints are applied to patients.

    a. _____

    b. _____

2. To restrain a patient who is trying to remove a tube, such as a catheter, you could apply either a _____ or _____ restraint.

3. For a patient who is attempting to get up and out of bed, you would apply a _____ or _____ restraint.

4. List two reasons why restraints should be removed every few hours.

    a. _____

    b. _____

Multiple-Choice Question

_____ 5. A major reason a nurse should obtain a physician's order after restraining a patient is to

   a. determine the type of restraint to be used.
   b. determine the length of time to apply.
   c. legally protect the physician.
   d. legally protect the nurse.

Module 14 Range-of-Motion Exercises

MAIN OBJECTIVE

To perform range-of-motion exercises on patients' joints, using proper sequence and joint positioning.

RATIONALE

Within 24 hours, a joint that has not been moved can begin to stiffen and eventually become inflexible. With longer periods of joint immobility, the tendons and muscles can be affected as well. The strong flexor muscles pull tight, resulting in a contraction of the extremity or permanent position of flexion. This position is called a *contracture*. Many persons with an illness or injury become unable to move one or more of the body's joints themselves. Unless contraindicated by an order from a physician, the nurse must promptly take over this function. With skill in handling the various body parts and knowledge of their movements, the nurse can maintain joint and extremity function until a time when patients can move all joints independently. Performing range-of-motion (ROM) exercises can save patients undue and lengthy rehabilitation.

PREREQUISITES

Successful completion of the following modules:

VOLUME 1
Assessment
Charting
Medical Asepsis
Basic Body Mechanics

SPECIFIC LEARNING OBJECTIVES

	Know Facts and Principles	Apply Facts and Principles	Demonstrate Ability	Evaluate Performance
1. *Types of ROM*	Know three types of ROM	State reasons for selection of kind of ROM with individual patients	In the clinical area, select correct kind of ROM for patient	Check decision with instructor
2. *Joints to be exercised*	State rationale for deciding which joints need exercising	Given a patient situation, describe side of body or joints requiring ROM	In the clinical area, perform ROM on appropriate joints for particular patient	
3. *Sequence used for exercising various joints*	List order for exercising various joints		Use prescribed sequence, making adaptations for particular patients	Evaluate own performance using Performance Checklist
4. *Special attention to certain joints*	Explain rationale for exercise of particular functional joints	Determine mobility or lack of mobility of key joints	Emphasize functional joints when doing ROM	
5. *Performing ROM*	Give frequency of ROM for optimum effect to patient	Determine frequency of ROM for particular patient	Do ROM at predetermined frequency	Evaluate frequency by checking joint flexibility
6. *Recording*	List what data are needed for chart	Determine correct manner of charting data for facility	Chart procedure correctly, adding pertinent data	Evaluate own performance with instructor

LEARNING ACTIVITIES

1. Review the Specific Learning Objectives.
2. Read the section on range-of-motion and active and passive exercises (in the chapter on activity and rest) in Ellis and Nowlis, *Nursing: A Human Needs Approach,* or comparable material in another textbook.
3. Review the anatomy of the skeletal and muscular systems.
4. Look up the module vocabulary terms in the glossary.
5. Read through the module and study the figures.
6. In the practice setting:
   a. Standing, move the joints on one side of your body through range of motion. Begin with your neck. Use the Performance Checklist as a guide.
   b. Practice ROM, with a partner, for one side of the body.
   c. Change positions and have your partner perform ROM on one side of your body.
   d. Together, evaluate your performances of steps b and c.
7. In the clinical setting:
   a. Perform ROM on a patient with your instructor's supervision.
   b. Using the Performance Checklist, evaluate yourself with the help of your instructor.

VOCABULARY

abduction
adduction
circumduction
contracture
contraindicate
distal
dorsiflexion
eversion
extension
external rotation
flexion
internal rotation
inversion
opposition
plantar flexion
pronation
proximal
radial deviation
rotation
supination
ulnar deviation

RANGE-OF-MOTION EXERCISES

Range of motion (ROM) exercises are ones in which a nurse or patient moves each joint through as full a range as is possible without causing pain. Most persons, through activities of daily living, move and exercise their joints. When any joint cannot be moved voluntarily, the patient or nurse must take over this function and move the joint at regular intervals to maintain muscle tone and joint mobility.

Types of ROM

ACTIVE

In active ROM, instruct the patient to perform the movements on a nonfunctioning joint. Active ROM helps a patient feel independent because he or she is directing the activity. Not only can patients be taught a planned ROM program, but they can also carry out additional ROM by being encouraged to participate in their own care. Combing the hair exercises joints of the upper extremity; lifting the foot for bathing exercises joints of the lower extremity. Encourage other appropriate activities as well.

ACTIVE ASSISTIVE

Active-assistive ROM is carried out with both patient and nurse participating. Encourage the patient to carry out as much of each movement as possible, within the limitations of his or her strength and mobility. You may support or complete the desired movement.

PASSIVE

Passive range of motion is performed by a nurse on a patient's immobilized joints. Your assessment skills are needed to determine which parts or joints must be ranged and with what frequency.

Joints Needing Exercise

When a patient is completely paralyzed on one side of the body, ideally the joints should be ranged four to five times daily for full maintenance of joint flexibility. In reality, however, the staff's time restrictions may limit the exercise to only one or two times a day. Of course, limited ranging will not lead to the optimum patient rehabilitation.

It is difficult to assess need when extremities or joints are just weak or partially affected. Through the use of assessment skills, you should be able to determine which joints are not being moved sufficiently by the patient and therefore which must receive ROM. When a patient receives ROM for the first time, it is helpful to exercise both affected and unaffected joints to establish a baseline of normal functioning for the patient. With each ROM procedure, put each joint through the range six to eight times. If you are also bathing the patient, you will not have to range all the joints this many times because several of the bathing movements are the same. *Never* force a joint to the point of pain.

Sequence of Exercises

Joints are exercised sequentially, starting with the neck and moving downward. Remember that joints move in different ways: the knee and elbow move in just one direction; the neck, wrist, and hip move in several directions. Several movements can be accomplished at the same time. For example, flexion of the knee and external rotation of the hip (see Figure 14.6) can be done simultaneously, as can abduction and external rotation of the shoulder (see Figure 14.2). Never grasp joints directly. It is more comfortable for the patient, and better for ROM, if you grasp the extremities gently but firmly either distally or proximally to the joint. Do not grasp the fingernails or toenails; this can be very uncomfortable for the patient. When exercising extremities, work from the proximal joints toward the distal joints.

It is important for every joint to receive adequate exercise, but it is crucial that several particular joints remain functional.

For example, flexion of the thumb must be maintained so that there is opposition of the thumb to the other fingers, which will leave the patient with a useful rather than a nonuseful hand. Hip and knee extension allows the patient to walk successfully when he or she is again mobile, and maintaining ankle flexion helps to prevent footdrop.

Time of Exercise

Bath time is one of the appropriate times during the day to administer ROM. The warm bath water relaxes the muscles and decreases spasticity of the joints. During the bath, also, areas are exposed so that the joints can be both moved and observed.

Evaluate the effectiveness of the ROM regime by observing the flexibility and range of the joints. Then, adjust the regime to the individual needs of the patient.

Record Keeping

The date, time, and initials *ROM* must be recorded. If a patient is to receive ROM on a long-term basis, you may make notations about various joints. Notations about joint movement are usually made in degrees of movement possible; that is, a right angle would be 90 degrees.

ROM Procedure

Note: After each movement, return the part to its anatomical position. Each joint movement is described separately here. Remember that it is possible to move two joints, such as the shoulder and the elbow, at the same time.

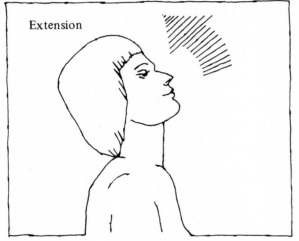

Extension

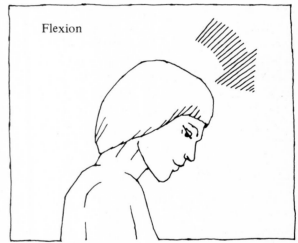

Flexion

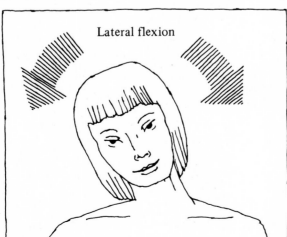

Lateral flexion

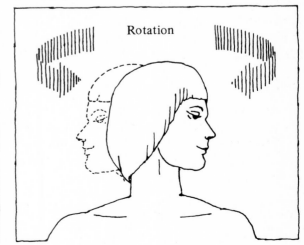

Rotation

FIGURE 14.1 EXERCISING THE NECK

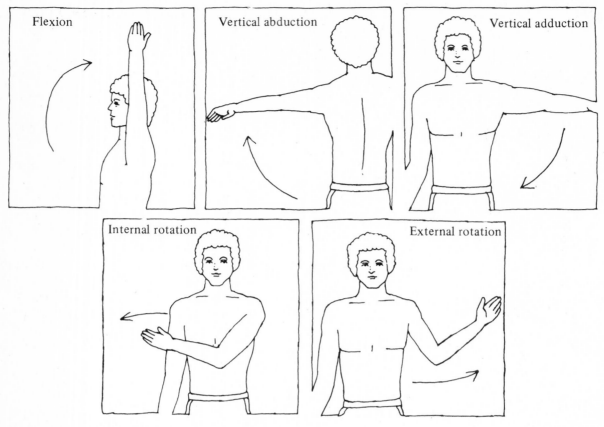

FIGURE 14.2   EXERCISING THE SHOULDER

1. Wash your hands.
2. Explain to the patient what you are about to do and ask for the patient's cooperation.
3. Lower the head of the bed so that the patient is in the supine position. Raise the entire bed to a comfortable working level for you. Remember to maintain your own proper body mechanics as you carry out the exercises for the patient.
4. Follow the procedure below in order to administer ROM to one side of the body.
   a. Neck (Figure 14.1)
      (1) *Extension*   Position the head as if looking upward.
      (2) *Flexion*   Position the head as if looking at the toes.
      (3) *Lateral flexion*   Move the head sideways from one side to the other, keeping the ear near the shoulder.
      (4) *Rotation*   Use a twisting motion, as though the patient were looking from one side to the other.
   b. Shoulder (Figure 14.2)
      (1) *Flexion*   Raise the arm forward and overhead. The elbow may be bent to prevent striking the head of the bed.
      (2) *Extension*   Return the arm to the side of the body.
      (3) *Vertical abduction*   Swing the arm outward from the side of the body and upward.
      (4) *Vertical adduction*   Return the arm to the side of the body.
      (5) *Internal rotation*   Swing the arm up and across the body.
      (6) *External rotation*   Rotate the

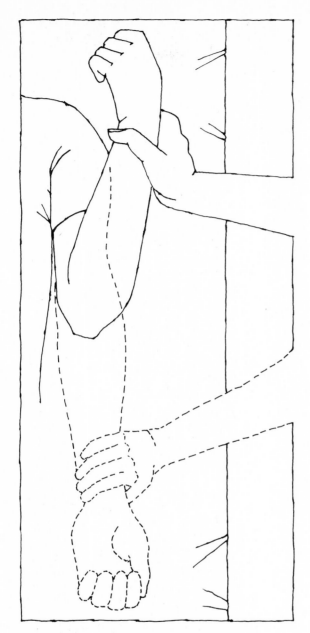

FIGURE 14.3   EXERCISING THE ELBOW

shoulder outward from the body, keeping the elbow at a right angle.

c. Elbow (Figure 14.3). These movements can be performed in conjunction with the shoulder movements.

   (1) *Flexion*   Bend the elbow.

   (2) *Extension*   Straighten the elbow.

d. Wrist (Figure 14.4)

   (1) *Flexion*   Grasping the palm and supporting the arm with your

other hand, bend the wrist forward.

   (2) *Extension*   Straighten the wrist.

   (3) *Radial deviation*   Bend the wrist toward the thumb.

   (4) *Ulnar deviation*   Bend the wrist toward the little finger.

   (5) *Circumduction*   Move the wrist in a circular motion.

e. Fingers and thumb (Figure 14.5). All three joints of each finger and the fingers and thumb can be moved through flexion and extension together. A hand can be partially functional if a patient is able to place the thumb and index finger or third finger in opposition to one another. Therefore, you should take special care to range these joints as thoroughly as possible.

   (1) *Flexion*   Bend the fingers and thumb onto the palm.

   (2) *Extension*   Return them to their original position.

   (3) *Abduction*   Spread the fingers.

   (4) *Adduction*   Return the fingers to the closed position.

   (5) *Circumduction*   Move the thumb in a circular motion.

f. Hip and knee (Figure 14.6). The hip and knee can be exercised together. Place one hand under the patient's knee and, with the other hand, support the heel.

   (1) *Flexion*   Lift the leg, bending the knee as far as possible toward the patient's head.

   (2) *Extension*   Return the leg to the surface of the bed and straighten.

   (3) *Abduction*   With the leg flat on the bed, move the entire leg outward toward the edge of the bed.

   (4) *Adduction*   Bring the leg back toward the midline or center of the bed.

   Note: Steps (3) and (4) can be performed with the knee bent. This allows you to give better

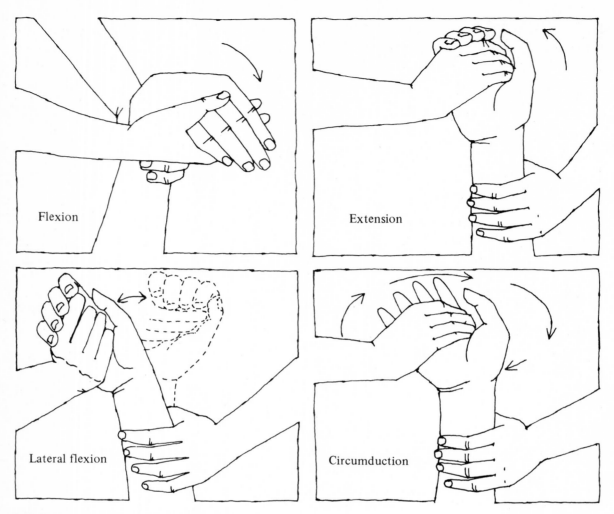

Flexion

Extension

Lateral flexion

Circumduction

FIGURE 14.4   EXERCISING THE WRIST

support to some patients and affords a greater range of movement.

(5) *Internal rotation*   With the leg flat on the bed, roll the entire leg in one unit inward, causing the toes to point inward. This will rotate the hip joint *internally*.

(6) *External rotation*   With the leg flat on the bed, roll the entire leg outward, causing the toes to point outward. This will rotate the hip *externally*.

g. Ankle (Figure 14.7)

(1) *Dorsiflexion*   Cup the patient's heel with your hand and rest the sole of the foot against your forearm. Steady the leg just above the ankle with your other hand. Put pressure against the patient's toes with your arm to flex the ankle.

(2) *Plantar flexion*   Change your hand from above the ankle to grasping the ball of the foot. Move the other arm away from the toes and push the foot downward to point the toes.

(3) *Circumduction*   Rotate the foot

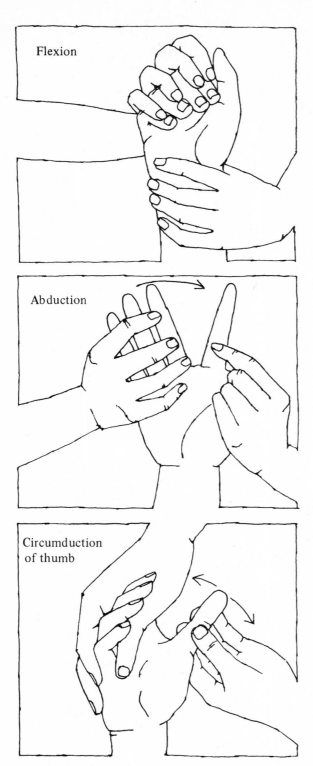

Flexion

Abduction

Circumduction
of thumb

FIGURE 14.5   EXERCISING THE FINGERS
AND THUMB

on the ankle, moving it circularly
first in one direction and then in
the other.
h. Toes (Figure 14.8)
(1) *Flexion*   Bend the toes downward.
Avoid grasping the nails because
this can be uncomfortable for
the patient.
(2) *Extension*   Bend the toes upward.
5. Wash your hands.
6. Record which body parts were ranged
and any significant limitations and
reactions of the patient.

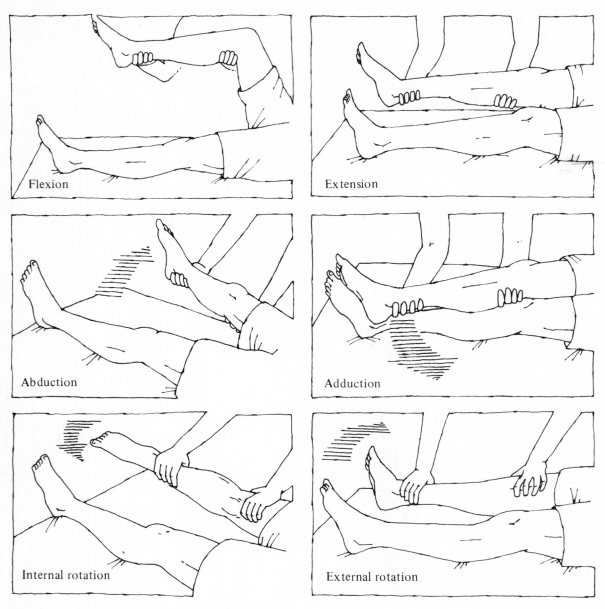

Flexion

Extension

Abduction

Adduction

Internal rotation

External rotation

FIGURE 14.6   EXERCISING THE HIP AND KNEE

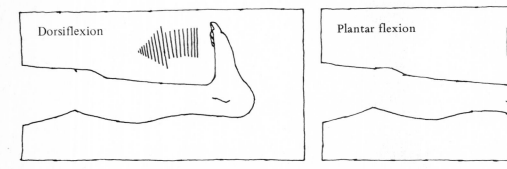

Dorsiflexion

Plantar flexion

FIGURE 14.7   EXERCISING THE ANKLE

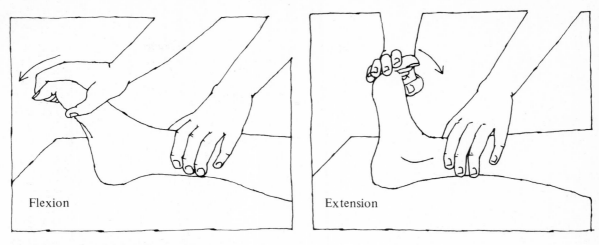

Flexion

Extension

FIGURE 14.8   EXERCISING THE TOES

PERFORMANCE CHECKLIST

	Unsatisfactory	Needs more practice	Satisfactory	Comments
1. Wash your hands.				
2. Explain to patient what you are going to do.				
3. If raised, lower head of bed. Raise entire bed to comfortable working level.				
4. Follow procedure below in order to administer ROM to one side of body. a. Neck: (1) Extension				
(2) Flexion				
(3) Lateral flexion				
(4) Rotation right				
(5) Rotation left				
b. Shoulder: (1) Flexion				
(2) Extension				
(3) Vertical abduction				
(4) Vertical adduction				
(5) Internal rotation				
(6) External rotation				
c. Elbow: (1) Flexion				
(2) Extension				
d. Wrist: (1) Flexion				
(2) Extension				
(3) Radial deviation				
(4) Ulnar deviation				
(5) Circumduction				
e. Fingers and thumb: (1) Flexion				
(2) Extension				
(3) Abduction				
(4) Adduction				
(5) Circumduction (thumb)				

	Unsatisfactory	Needs more practice	Satisfactory	Comments
f. Hip and knee: (1) Flexion				
(2) Extension				
(3) Abduction				
(4) Adduction				
(5) Internal rotation				
(6) External rotation				
g. Ankle: (1) Dorsiflexion				
(2) Plantar flexion				
(3) Circumduction				
h. Toes: (1) Flexion				
(2) Extension				
5. Wash your hands.				
6. Record essential data.				

QUIZ

Short-Answer Questions

1. List three purposes of ROM.

   a. _____

   b. _____

   c. _____

2. Contractures occur when the stronger muscle group of an extremity shortens or pulls. These muscles are the _____.

3. ROM that is performed by the patient is called _____.

4. When the hand is held in an outward, upward position, it is called

   _____.

5. To comb the hair, the shoulder assumes a position of _____.

Multiple-Choice Questions

_____ 6. ROM should be performed

   a. every time a patient is repositioned.
   b. at bath time.
   c. when ordered by the physician.
   d. four to five times a day.

_____ 7. Joints of the body should be exercised sequentially; that is,

   a. alternately, from one side to the other.
   b. from distal to proximal.
   c. from proximal to distal.

_____ 8. "Scissoring" one leg over the other may bring about

   a. hip flexion.
   b. hip extension.
   c. adduction.
   d. circumduction.

Module 15 Transfer

MAIN OBJECTIVE

To transfer a patient from a bed to a chair, wheelchair, commode, or stretcher, with a maximum of comfort and safety for both the patient and nurse.

RATIONALE

Having patients get out of bed has proved very beneficial to them. This activity not only maintains and restores muscle tone but also stimulates the respiratory and circulatory systems and improves elimination. Many patients are unable to move themselves or need assistance in moving. It is the nurse's responsibility to help (1) by moving patients, (2) by directing patients in the best techniques for self-movement, and (3) by seeing that there are sufficient persons on hand to ensure patients' safety during transfer.

PREREQUISITES

Successful completion of the following modules:

VOLUME 1
Assessment
Charting
Medical Asepsis
Basic Body Mechanics
Moving the Patient in Bed and Positioning
Applying Restraints

SPECIFIC LEARNING OBJECTIVES

	Know Facts and Principles	Apply Facts and Principles	Demonstrate Ability	Evaluate Performance
1. Reasons for transfer	List four reasons for patient's activity	Given a patient situation, relate purpose of activity	In clinical setting, state reasons for patient's activity	
2. Safety	List common hazards to patient	Recognize hazards in a patient situation	Provide safe setting for transfer	Determine that patient was not injured in transfer
3. Assessment of patient	State reasons for knowing patient's diagnosis and capabilities	Give examples of how different diagnoses and capabilities would affect plans for transfer	Gather data on patient's abilities and diagnoses before moving patient	After transfer, review procedure to find whether more data would have helped. Validate with instructor.
4. Transfer of patient a. Bed to chair b. Bed to stretcher c. Chair to chair	List steps of usual transfer procedures	Plan modification of procedures for particular patient situation. Identify best procedure to use in specific situation.	Successfully transfer patient a. from bed to chair or commode b. from bed to stretcher c. from chair to chair or commode	Evaluate own performance using Performance Checklist

LEARNING ACTIVITIES

1. Review the Specific Learning Objectives.
2. Read the section on posture and body mechanics and ambulation (in the chapter on activity and rest) in Ellis and Nowlis, *Nursing: A Human Needs Approach,* or comparable material in another textbook.
3. Look up the module vocabulary terms in the glossary.
4. Read through the module.
5. In the practice setting:
   a. Place a colored tie or scarf around your partner's left arm and another on the left leg (or right arm and right leg). This will be the nonfunctional side.
   b. Transfer your partner from a supine position in bed to an upright position sitting on the side of the bed.
   c. Transfer your partner from the bed to a chair using a one-person, minimal-assist transfer.
   d. Transfer your partner using a one-person, maximal-assist transfer.
   e. With a third person, transfer your partner using a two-person, maximal-assist transfer.
   f. Transfer your partner using a two-person lift transfer.
   g. Transfer your partner from a bed to a stretcher using a three-person horizontal lift.
   h. Change roles as "patient" and nurse, and repeat all of the transfers until each person participating has had an opportunity to be in each role.
   i. If a hydraulic lifting device is available:
      (1) Obtain the lift.
      (2) Review the specific directions.
      (3) Practice pumping up and lowering the device without a person in it.
      (4) Using the directions in this module, transfer another student from a bed to a chair and back to the bed using the lift.
      (5) Ask the student who was transferred to describe how it felt.

VOCABULARY

horizontal
hydraulic
supine
weight-bearing

TRANSFER

Moving patients out of bed has proved very beneficial to them. The movement strengthens muscles that have been weakened by inactivity, and respiration, circulation, and elimination are stimulated by the increased activity. Patients need only dangle their legs over the side of the bed or sit in a chair at the bedside for a few minutes to improve their well-being.

Properly helping a patient from the bed to a chair is an important nursing function, in which you play a vital role by giving the patient physical support and encouragement. Pay special attention to safety precautions, as well as to the basics of body mechanics, to ensure both your safety and the patient's.

The desired level of activity is usually determined by a physician's orders, but nursing assessment is necessary to determine the best method for carrying out the order.

Safety

Falls are the most common hazard to a patient being transferred. The patient may become dizzy or have less strength than expected, or the nurse may not be strong enough to accomplish the task. Consider these possibilities carefully before beginning. If a patient begins to fall, he or she should be lowered to the bed, the chair, or the floor in such a way as to prevent injury.

Another hazard in moving patients is the pull on indwelling tubings (catheters, IV tubing). Arrange to move tubings as necessary to avoid dislodging them. To avoid bruises from striking side rails or furniture, position the patient carefully. Also, be sure the patient is wearing shoes or slippers (with firm soles), so that he or she does not slide or bruise the feet.

Assessment

To facilitate a transfer, you must know the patient's diagnosis and any restrictions to be observed. For example, a patient with a repaired fractured hip may be allowed to have only 25 percent of his or her weight bearing on the affected side, whereas a post-op patient who has had an appendectomy may not be restricted in any way.

In addition, you should assess the capabilities of the patient. Is the patient capable of moving all extremities? If the patient is partially incapacitated, which is the stronger side? How was the patient transferred before? Asking the patient is not always the best way to get this information; some patients may not be able to provide accurate information. You should check with other nurses and/or consult the record and Kardex. You also must know what equipment is available for moving patients, as well as what persons are available to assist you.

Planning

With the data in hand, devise a plan to transfer the patient in the safest and most convenient manner, taking into account proper body mechanics for both you and the patient. Be realistic: you may need more than one person to transfer a severely disabled or heavy patient.

The position of the bed can help greatly in transfer. Raise the head of the bed and drop the patient's feet over the side to place the patient in an upright sitting position. Then, simply by lowering the entire bed, you often can put the patient's feet in contact with the floor. Some beds are lowered by an electrical control at the side or foot of the bed, while some are lowered manually by crank. Make these mechanical devices work for you.

Foot coverings are essential. Firm-soled shoes give the patient a sense of security and prevent slipping. If shoes are not available, leather-soled slippers can be used. Always put braces and appliances on a patient before he or she is transferred.

A transfer and ambulation belt is a very important assistive device. The belt is made of heavy twill with a positive buckle. It is placed around the patient's waist to give those assisting with the activity a way to hold onto the patient firmly. In the past, these belts were only available in physical therapy departments, so many nurses are not familiar with their use. But, once you have used one, you will be convinced of its value.

When a belt is not available, devise a substitute from items on hand. A drawsheet can be folded and wrapped around the patient's waist. If the sheet is thin, tie it; if it is too bulky to tie, cross it in back and grasp the ends along with the side when you use it for lifting. A patient's gown can be another substitute. Tie it around the patient's waist and use it as you would a transfer belt. A patient may even have a regular leather belt that can be used, but be careful that a narrow belt does not cut into the patient.

Procedure

As simply as possible, explain to the patient what you intend to do or how you intend to help, as well as what his or her participation will be. Ask if there are any questions.

It is essential that you appear confident. It is also important not to rush the patient.

BED TO CHAIR: ONE-PERSON MAXIMAL ASSIST

1. Angle the wheelchair or armchair to the bed so that the chair is on the patient's stronger side. If the footrests are removable, remove them at this time; otherwise, fold them out of the way. This arrangement will allow the patient to pivot on the stronger leg.
2. Lock the bed and wheelchair. Be sure the patient sees the chair and its position.
3. Begin with the patient in a supine position, with the hips placed where the bed will bend as the head of the bed is raised, and close to the edge of the bed.
4. Raise the head of the bed so that the patient is in a sitting position. (This decreases the effort for both you and the patient.) Raise the bed slowly so that the patient does not get dizzy.
5. Lower the bed so that the patient's feet will touch or be near the floor. If the

bed does not lower, obtain a footstool. The patient's feet must be firmly planted when the pivot is done.
6. Grasp the legs with one arm and place the other arm behind the patient's back. Swing the patient's legs over the side of the bed while swiveling the patient's body, so that the patient ends up sitting on the edge of the bed with the feet hanging down.
7. Allow the patient to sit for a few minutes to prevent lightheadedness or orthostatic hypotension, which can occur with any sudden change in circulation caused by lowering the legs. Support the patient if he or she feels dizzy.
8. Place a transfer and ambulation belt on the patient's waist.
9. Position the patient's feet slightly apart, with the patient's hands on the bed or on your shoulders. Do not let the patient hold you about the neck.
10. Bend your knees with a wide stance and grasp the patient at the belt. You may want to straddle the patient's weaker leg with your own legs, or to stabilize the patient's knees by supporting them with your own knees. (See Figure 15.1.)
11. Straighten your knees, assisting the patient to a standing position.
12. Stand close to the patient and pivot to the chair.
13. Instruct the patient to place both hands on the arms of the chair.
14. Lower the patient to the seat.
15. Be sure the patient's body is positioned firmly back in the seat.

This same technique can be used to transfer a patient from one chair to another.

BED TO CHAIR: ONE-PERSON MINIMAL ASSIST

Proceed as you would for the one-person, maximal-assist transfer, above, with two exceptions. It is not necessary to brace the patient's knees nor is a transfer belt usually necessary. You will be primarily providing balance, not lifting the patient's weight. (See Figure 15.2.)

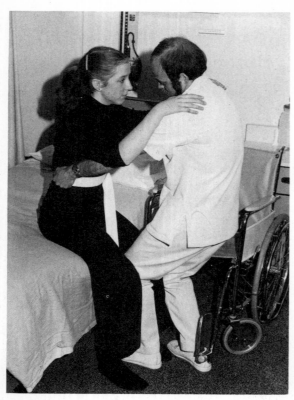

FIGURE 15.1   BED TO WHEELCHAIR: ONE-
PERSON MAXIMAL ASSIST
Courtesy Ivan Ellis

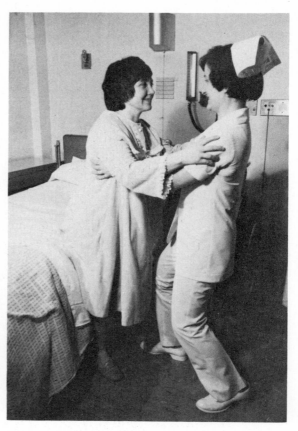

FIGURE 15.2   BED TO WHEELCHAIR: ONE-
PERSON MINIMAL ASSIST
Courtesy Lawrence Cherkas

BED TO CHAIR: TWO-PERSON MAXIMAL ASSIST

1. Put the bed flat.
2. Place a transfer belt around the patient. This is especially important in this transfer.
3. Help the patient to a sitting position on the edge of the bed as described in the one-person maximal assist, steps 6–7, page 223.
4. Position the wheelchair next to the bed, at a 45-degree angle, with the seat facing toward the bed. Secure the brakes.
5. Nurse 1 stands in front of the patient (one-person maximal assist, step 10, page 223), grasping the belt at the sides.
6. Nurse 2 stands between the wheelchair and the bed, with one knee on the bed, and grasps the transfer belt at the back. (See Figure 15.3.)

7. Nurse 1 signals, "One, two, three, *lift!*" Both assistants lift and pivot the patient at the same time, and then lower the patient into the wheelchair.

CHAIR TO CHAIR: TWO-PERSON LIFT

1. Place the chairs (or commode and chair) side by side, facing in the same direction.
2. Remove the footrests from the wheelchair or fold them out of the way, and lock or brace the chair (or commode).
3. The taller nurse (1) stands behind the chair.
4. The shorter nurse (2) stands facing the patient.
5. Nurse 1 folds the patient's arms across the patient's chest. The nurse then reaches around from behind the patient and grasps the opposite wrists while supporting under the patient's arms.

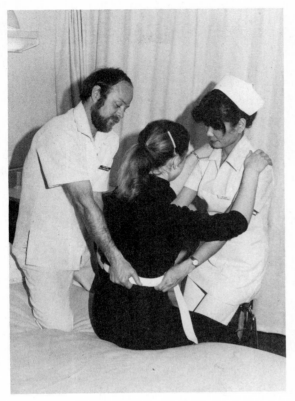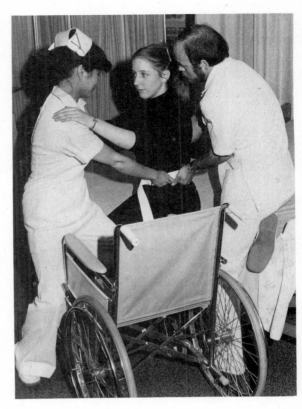

FIGURE 15.3 BED TO WHEELCHAIR: TWO-PERSON MAXIMAL ASSIST
Courtesy Ivan Ellis

6. Nurse 2 bends knees and hips into a squatting position and grasps the patient under the knees to support the legs. (See Figure 15.4.)
7. Nurse 1 counts ("One, two, three, *lift*!"), and both lift at the same time.

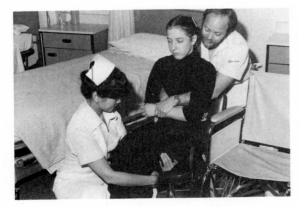

FIGURE 15.4 CHAIR TO CHAIR: TWO-PERSON LIFT
Courtesy Ivan Ellis

Nurse 1 controls the timing because he or she will bear the greatest weight.
8. When the word "lift" is said, both nurses lift the patient and move over to the second chair (or commode), lowering the patient immediately.

BED TO CHAIR: TWO-PERSON LIFT

1. Put the bed flat and lock it.
2. Set the wheelchair beside the bed and secure its brakes. If armrests are removable, remove the one next to the bed.
3. Slide the patient to the edge of the bed.
4. Nurse 1 slides one arm under the patient's shoulders and begins lifting the shoulders. The nurse places one knee on the bed and slides his or her arms around the patient until both arms are under the patient's arms and the patient is sitting, leaning on the nurse's chest.

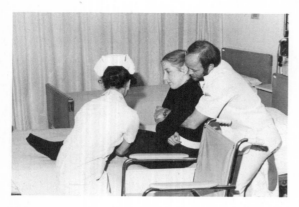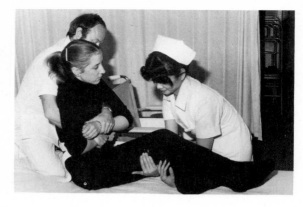

FIGURE 15.5   BED TO CHAIR: TWO-PERSON LIFT
Courtesy Ivan Ellis

5. The patient's arms are crossed on the patient's chest, and nurse 1 grasps the opposite wrists in front of the patient.
6. Nurse 2 squats beside the bed and slides both arms under the patient's thighs from the same side. (See Figure 15.5.)
7. Nurse 1 counts ("One, two, three, *lift!*"), and both nurses lift the patient into the wheelchair (or commode).

This lift can be augmented with a third person, who slides his or her arms under the patient's buttocks so that the three people can lift at one time.

BED TO CHAIR: HYDRAULIC LIFT
The hydraulic lift enables a nurse to lift a very heavy patient or one who is very incapacitated without relying on personal strength. (The Hoyer is one brand of hydraulic lift.) All lifts have a sturdy frame that supports the patient's weight; a canvas or nylon sling of some type, which is positioned under the patient; and a hydraulic pump. Consult the literature for specifics about the particular brand and model used in your facility, but the following should serve as a general outline of the procedure. Two people are usually needed to ensure the patient's safety; and two are essential for incapacitated patients who cannot support their own heads.

1. Explain to the patient the purpose of the lift and how it works. Emphasize

the safety of the procedure because the patient may be frightened by the large mechanical device.
2. Place the patient in the supine position.
3. Place the sling under the patient by rolling the patient side to side and slipping it under the body in the same way you would place a sheet under a patient in bed. If the patient is not clothed (transfer to a tub, for example), cover the patient with a bath blanket.

For the patient's safety, the sling must be positioned correctly. If the lower edge of the sling is too high, the patient could slip feet first out of the sling. If the lower edge is too low (on a two-part sling), the patient could "fold up" and slip out of the sling.
   a. *One-piece sling*   Place the bottom edge just above the knees. The top edge can extend behind the shoulders or to the head.
   b. *Two-piece sling*   Place one of the canvas strips behind the patient's thighs, so that it forms a seat for the sling. Position the second canvas strip under the patient's shoulder blades, so that it supports the patient's trunk in a semireclining position.
4. Lower the bed.
5. Position the lift itself by the bed, so that the lifting arm extends above the patient. If the support legs are adjustable, they

should be in their widest, most stable position.

6. Place the patient's arms across his or her chest, keeping them out of the way during the lift.

7. Fasten the chains of the lift to the sling. The chains to the seat section should be slightly longer than the chains to the trunk section, to create a semireclining position when the sling is lifted. When you fasten the chains, make sure hooks are pointed *away* from the patient to prevent them from jabbing the patient. Also be careful not to catch skin folds in the metal edges and chains.

8. Nurse 1 stands at the patient's head, to support the head and guide the patient during the lift.

9. Nurse 2 makes sure the valve on the hydraulic pump is closed and begins pumping, gradually lifting the patient off the bed. Lift *just* until the patient clears the bed and no higher. The higher the lift, the less stable its balance.

10. Nurse 1 guides the patient and nurse 2 guides the lift, as the lift is maneuvered away from the bed. (See Figure 15.6.)

11. Double-check the position of the bath blanket if you are transporting a patient to a tub. You may want to place additional coverings around the patient's buttocks and shoulders to keep the patient warm and to provide for modesty.

12. Slowly, keeping careful balance, move the lift to the chair, tub, or other bed.

13. Position the patient above the next resting place, with special attention to the correct positioning of the hips.

14. Release the hydraulic valve carefully, and lower the patient very slowly, correcting the positioning as the patient moves downward. Be careful not to open the valve too far, which would cause the patient to move down too abruptly.

15. Close the valve as soon as the patient's weight is on the chair. If you don't, the support arm will lower onto the patient.

16. Detach the chains from the sling and

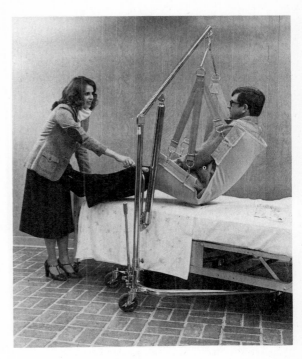

FIGURE 15.6   HYDRAULIC LIFT
Courtesy Ted Hoyer & Company, Inc., Oshkosh, Wisconsin

remove the lift. The sling usually remains under the patient in the new position, so that the reverse procedure, back to the bed, is easy. If you've transferred the patient to another bed, remove the sling by turning the patient side to side.

HORIZONTAL LIFT: THREE- OR FOUR-PERSON ASSIST

1. Place the stretcher at a right angle to the bed at the foot of the bed, with the brakes secured.

2. Move the patient to one side of the bed.

3. Nurse 1, the tallest nurse, stands at the patient's head and slides his or her arms under the patient's neck and shoulders.

4. Nurse 2, the next tallest nurse, stands at the patient's waist and hips and slides both arms under the patient.

5. The shortest nurse, nurse 3, stands at the patient's knees and slides both arms under the lower legs and thighs. If a fourth nurse is used, nurse 2 is at the waist and chest, nurse 3 is at the

hips, and nurse 4 is at the knees and legs.

6. On the count ("One, two, three, *lift!*"), given by the person with the heaviest weight (usually nurse 2), the nurses lift and roll the patient toward themselves in a hugging motion.

7. Holding the patient against their bodies, the nurses walk together, with synchronized steps, to the side and backward, until they are parallel to the stretcher. (See Figure 15.7.)

8. At the count ("One, two, three, *down!*") the patient is placed on the stretcher.

Recording

A record of the best means of transfer, the patient's ability to cooperate, and any aids or devices needed should be available to all health care team members. The Kardex or nursing care plan is usually used for this purpose.

Each time a transfer is carried out, note the exact nature of the activity, the time of the activity, and the patient's response to the activity on the patient's record. Evaluate the patient's response in light of pain, fatigue, pulse and respiration rate, blood pressure changes, and dizziness.

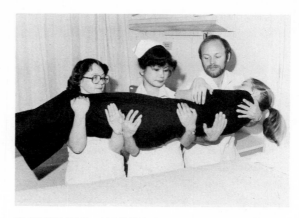

FIGURE 15.7 HORIZONTAL LIFT: THREE-PERSON ASSIST
Courtesy Ivan Ellis

PERFORMANCE CHECKLIST

General procedure	Unsatisfactory	Needs more practice	Satisfactory	Comments
1. Verify physician's order.				
2. Assess patient.				
3. Plan for modifications of usual procedure.				
4. Discuss plan with patient.				
5. Wash your hands.				
Bed to chair: One-person maximal assist				
1. Angle chair to bed on patient's stronger side.				
2. Lock or brace bed and chair.				
3. Have patient in supine position.				
4. Raise head of bed slowly.				
5. Lower bed.				
6. Swing patient's legs over side of bed while swiveling patient's body to achieve sitting position.				
7. Allow patient to sit for a few moments.				
8. Place transfer belt on patient.				
9. Put patient's feet slightly apart and position hands on your shoulders.				
10. Straddle patient's knees with your own, keeping wide stance and knees bent.				
11. Straighten your knees, lifting patient to a standing position.				
12. Stand close to patient and pivot to chair.				
13. Place patient's hands on armrests.				
14. Lower patient to seat.				
15. Be sure patient's buttocks are positioned in back of seat.				

	Unsatisfactory	Needs more practice	Satisfactory	Comments
Bed to Chair: Two-person maximal assist				
1. Put bed flat.				
2. Apply transfer belt.				
3. Assist patient to sit.				
4. Position wheelchair at 45-degree angle and lock.				
5. Nurse 1 stands in front of patient and grasps belt at sides.				
6. Nurse 2 stands between chair and bed, with one knee on bed and grasps belt at back.				
7. Nurse 1 signals, and both lift.				
Chair to chair: Two-person lift				
1. Place chairs side by side.				
2. Remove footrests from chair and lock or brace chair (commode).				
3. Taller nurse (nurse 1) stands behind chair with patient.				
4. Shorter nurse (nurse 2) stands facing patient.				
5. Nurse 1 crosses patient's arms and grasps wrists from behind.				
6. Nurse 2 squats and grasps patient around knees.				
7. Nurse 1 counts.				
8. On *"lift,"* both nurses lift patient and move to second chair (or commode).				
Bed to chair: Two-person lift				
1. Put bed flat and lock it.				
2. Position chair and secure brakes.				
3. Slide patient to edge of bed.				
4. Nurse 1 slides arm under patient's shoulders and maneuvers patient to sitting position.				
5. Nurse 1 crosses patient's arms over chest and grasps opposite wrists.				
6. Nurse 2 squats beside bed and slides arms under patient's thighs.				
7. Lift at nurse 1's signal.				

	Unsatisfactory	Needs more practice	Satisfactory	Comments
Bed to chair: Hydraulic lift				
1. Explain procedure to patient.				
2. Place patient in dorsal-recumbent position.				
3. Position sling correctly and drape patient if necessary.				
4. Place bed in low position.				
5. Position lift over patient.				
6. Place patient's arms across chest.				
7. Fasten lift's chains.				
8. Nurse 1 at patient's head.				
9. Nurse 2 begins pumping.				
10. Nurse 1 guides and supports patient's head while nurse 2 moves lift away from bed.				
11. Double-check draping.				
12. Slowly move lift to new position.				
13. Position patient above chair.				
14. Release valve and lower patient slowly.				
15. Close valve promptly.				
16. Detach chains from sling.				
Horizontal lift: Three- or four-person assist				
1. Place stretcher at right angle to bed.				
2. Move patient to edge of bed.				
3. Tallest nurse (1) stands at patient's head and shoulders.				
4. Second tallest nurse (2) stands at patient's waist and hips.				
5. Shortest nurse (3) stands at patient's legs.				
6. Lift and roll at signal.				
7. Nurses hold patient and walk to stretcher.				
8. At signal, nurses place patient on stretcher.				

Recording	Unsatisfactory	Needs more practice	Satisfactory	Comments
1. Record on Kardex: a. Time planned for activity				
b. Type of activity				
c. Best method and aids to use				
d. Patient's ability to participate				
2. Record on patient's chart: a. Activity carried out				
b. Time of activity				
c. Patient's response				

QUIZ

Short-Answer Questions

1. List four reasons for patient activity.

   a. _____

   b. _____

   c. _____

   d. _____

2. What should you do if a patient begins to fall during a transfer?

   _____

3. How would right-sided paralysis affect a patient's transfer?

   _____

4. What is the purpose of a transfer belt?

   _____

5. Why is a patient changed from a lying-down to a sitting position slowly?

   _____

Module 16 Ambulation

MAIN OBJECTIVE

To assist patients in ambulation, taking into account their capabilities as well as safety precautions.

RATIONALE

Having patients ambulate not only maintains and restores muscle tone and joint flexibility, but also stimulates the respiratory and circulatory systems. Activity improves appetite and elimination. In addition, it enhances the patient's psychological well-being, which for many represents a positive move toward good health.

PREREQUISITES

Successful completion of the following modules:

VOLUME 1
Assessment
Charting
Medical Asepsis
Basic Body Mechanics
Moving the Patient in Bed and Positioning
Applying Restraints
Transfer

SPECIFIC LEARNING OBJECTIVES

	Know Facts and Principles	Apply Facts and Principles	Demonstrate Ability	Evaluate Performance
1. *Reasons for ambulation*	List four reasons for patient's activity	Given a patient situation, relate purpose of activity	In clinical experiences, state reasons for patient's activity	
2. *Safety*	List common hazards to patient from ambulating and from use of assistive devices	Recognize hazards in a patient situation	Provide safe setting for ambulation. Maintain correct body mechanics for self and patient.	Determine that patient was not injured in ambulation
3. *Assessment of patient*	State reasons for knowing patient's diagnosis and capabilities	Give examples of how different diagnoses and capabilities would affect plans for ambulation	Gather data on patient's abilities and diagnoses before ambulating patient	After ambulation, review procedure to find whether more data would have helped. Validate with instructor.
4. *Ambulation of patient*	State ways of supporting patient while ambulating	Plan specific means of support for particular patient	Ambulate patient safely with supervision	Evaluate own performance using Performance Checklist
	Describe various gaits used for cane, walker, or crutches	Given a situation, describe gait that would be used for each assistive device	Correctly assist patient with use of assistive devices	
5. *Recording*	List data to be recorded on nursing care plan. List data to be recorded on patient's record.	Given a patient situation, determine what should be recorded on nursing care plan and what on patient's record	In the clinical setting, update nursing plan on patient's ambulation. In the clinical setting, chart activity and patient's response.	Evaluate own performance using Performance Checklist

LEARNING ACTIVITIES

1. Review the Specific Learning Objectives.
2. Read the chapter on activity and rest in Ellis and Nowlis, *Nursing: A Human Needs Approach,* or a comparable chapter in another textbook.
3. Look up the module vocabulary terms in the glossary.
4. Read through the module.
5. In the practice setting:
   a. Practice ambulation with a partner. Take turns being the patient and being the nurse. Use a tie to mark one of the "patient's" legs as the weaker leg.
   b. Using the procedures in the module, practice each ambulating technique. Be sure to go through the teaching and explanations for the "patient" each time. When you are the "patient," evaluate your partner's performance using the Performance Checklist. Do each of the following techniques:
      (1) Simple assisted ambulation
      (2) Using a cane
      (3) Using a walker
      (4) Using crutches (Include three-point gait, three-point-plus-one gait, four-point gait, and sitting down with crutches.)
   c. When you believe that you have mastered these skills, ask your instructor to check your performance.
6. In the clinical setting:
   a. Seek opportunities to ambulate patients.
   b. Ask your instructor to approve your plan and supervise you.

VOCABULARY

affected
ambulate
cane
crutch
crutch palsy
gait
quad cane
tolerance
walker
weight-bearing (partial-weight-bearing)

AMBULATION

There is a general approach you can use to help patients to walk which should be modified as needed for a specific patient.

General Procedure

1. Assess the patient's capabilities and the activity permitted. Be certain you know the patient's previous level of activity and response to that activity. Find out if any assistive devices have been used for ambulating this particular patient.
2. Plan the type of ambulation. From your knowledge, set a tentative goal as to how far you will ambulate the patient and the amount of help that will be needed. If you intend to increase ambulation progressively, you must be prepared with alternative plans if the patient is unable to increase the activity level.
3. Wash your hands.
4. Explain to the patient what you are planning to do, and encourage questions, so that the patient can participate fully in the activity.
5. If this is a new activity or an increase in activity, you may want to take the patient's pulse and blood pressure before ambulation to use as a baseline. If this has been done recently, it is not necessary to repeat these measurements.
6. Obtain a robe and shoes. It is important that the patient be covered for both warmth and modesty. Firm-soled supportive shoes are best for ambulation because they give the patient additional stability. If shoes are not available, use slippers. If at all possible, avoid "scuffs," which can easily slip off, and cloth slippers, which tend to slide on smooth floors.
7. Position the bed and help the patient to stand, using the appropriate techniques discussed in Module 15, Transfer, and later in this module regarding assistive devices.

8. Ambulate the patient for the distance or time ordered. Watch the patient carefully for signs of fatigue or faintness, or for other responses to the activity. Ask the patient to let you know if he or she begins to feel faint or dizzy. Stay *close*. If the patient is using a walker or crutches, stand behind the patient or slightly to the side. Use a belt around the patient's waist if he or she seems unsteady.

   If the patient loses balance slightly, help the patient regain balance. If the knees buckle and the patient makes no attempt to straighten up, control the descent to the floor. Do not try to hold the patient up: this is likely to cause you injury and is often unsuccessful anyway. Simply steady and support the patient, being sure that the patient's head does not strike anything, as you allow him or her to slide slowly to the floor. You will need help to return the patient to bed.

   It is wise to be familiar with the environment when you are ambulating a patient, so that you know where the patient can sit and rest if he or she becomes weak and unsteady. If the patient feels dizzy, sitting with the head down for a few minutes may be sufficient to restore stability, or you may have to get a wheelchair to return the patient to bed.

9. After you have returned the patient to bed, evaluate the patient's response in terms of fatigue level and feelings of well-being. You may have to retake pulse and blood pressure if these are significant parameters for this patient.
10. Wash your hands.
11. Record the activity as appropriate for your facility. In most instances, any new information regarding times planned for activity, the best method and aids needed, and the patient's ability to participate are recorded on the nursing care plan. The specific activity carried out, the time of the activity, and the

patient's response are usually noted on the patient's chart, either on a flow sheet or on the progress notes.

Simple Assisted Ambulation

This is the most common situation in which you will ambulate a patient. Follow the General Procedure, above, and use these directions for the ambulation itself.

1. In most cases, walk on the patient's weaker, or affected, side. Then if the patient falters, you can give assistance and support. However, if the patient has poor balance and tends to lean toward the person assisting, you should walk on the patient's strong side, so that the patient's weight is shifted to the strong leg, rather than the weak leg, when he or she leans.

2. Support the patient as you walk, but do not allow the patient to put an arm around your shoulders. If the patient should start to fall, the weight could strain your back and cause severe injury. Instead, offer support by extending an arm bent at the elbow with the palm up. The patient can then rest a hand on your arm. You can maintain firm support, and the patient can determine how much support is needed.

   Another method of providing safety with minimal support is to use a transfer and ambulation belt around the patient's waist. In this instance, you walk to the side and slightly behind the patient with one hand grasping the belt in the center back. The other arm may be extended at the patient's side for the patient to grasp (Figure 16.1).

3. Walk slowly and with an even gait. It is very difficult for a patient if your gait is uneven, speeding up and slowing down. Synchronize your steps with the patient's. Also try to make your steps the same size as the patient's, which will make your supportive arm feel more stable to him or her. By using smooth,

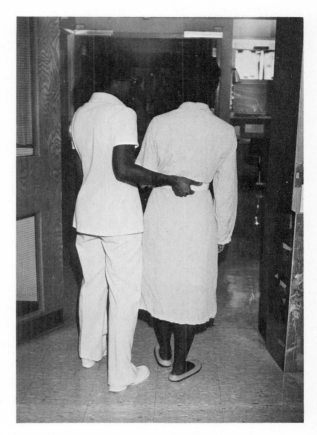

FIGURE 16.1 AMBULATION The nurse stands on the patient's weaker side and grasps the ambulation belt; the patient may also hold a cane on the stronger side.
Courtesy Lawrence Cherkas

coordinated movements, you instill the patient with confidence in you, as well as diminish his or her fear of falling.

4. Help the patient return to bed.

Using a Cane

A cane is used by persons who need additional help in balance, or by persons who are able to bear weight on both legs but one leg is weaker than the other. If the cane is used to help in balance, encourage the patient to use a normal gait and to go slowly enough so that the cane is easy to use. This does take time to perfect. A quad cane is used when maximum support is needed. When a cane is used to augment a weak leg, a specific gait tends to be more effective.

The gait usually is taught by a physical therapist, who is responsible for securing and measuring the cane. Then, you support the therapist's instruction and help the patient with its daily use.

1. The patient grasps the cane in the hand *opposite* to the affected leg.
2. The patient then slides his or her hips forward in the chair, to make standing easier.
3. The patient grasps the arm of the chair with the free hand, and the cane *and* the chair arm with the other hand if this is possible. If the patient cannot grasp both, then only the cane is grasped in order to stand.

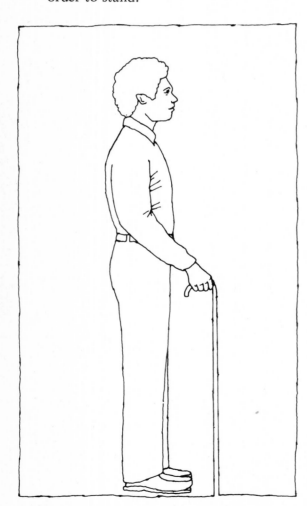

FIGURE 16.2 PROPER CANE STANCE Cane on strong side; elbow slightly flexed. Cane is to the side and 6 inches in front of the foot.

4. The patient pushes to a standing position using the arms of the chair for support. Encourage this type of independence. If the patient needs help to stand, give only the help that is needed and allow maximum independence. This will help to develop muscle strength and balance.
5. After the patient is standing, encourage him or her to pause in place, both to gain balance and to place the cane initially. This keeps the patient from tripping on the cane. Best balance is maintained if the cane is placed close to the foot, so that the patient remains erect, not bent over (Figure 16.2).
6. Gait pattern:
   a. The cane is moved ahead approximately 4 to 6 inches.
   b. The weak leg is then moved ahead opposite the cane.
   c. The weight is then placed on the weak leg and the cane.
   d. The strong leg is moved forward. The steps of both legs should remain equal to promote normal walking (Figure 16.3).
   e. Repeat the sequence.
7. The nurse walks to the side and slightly behind the patient, to provide support if needed.
8. Sitting:
   a. Using the cane, the patient turns around and backs up to the chair.
   b. The patient reaches behind and grasps the arm of the chair with the free hand. The other hand holds the cane and grasps the other arm of the chair at the same time, if possible; if not, it continues to hold the cane.
   c. The patient lowers himself or herself into the chair.

Using a Walker

Walkers are used by patients who have at least one weight-bearing leg and arms strong enough to bear some weight. They may also be used by patients who are generally weak and those with balance problems. They give

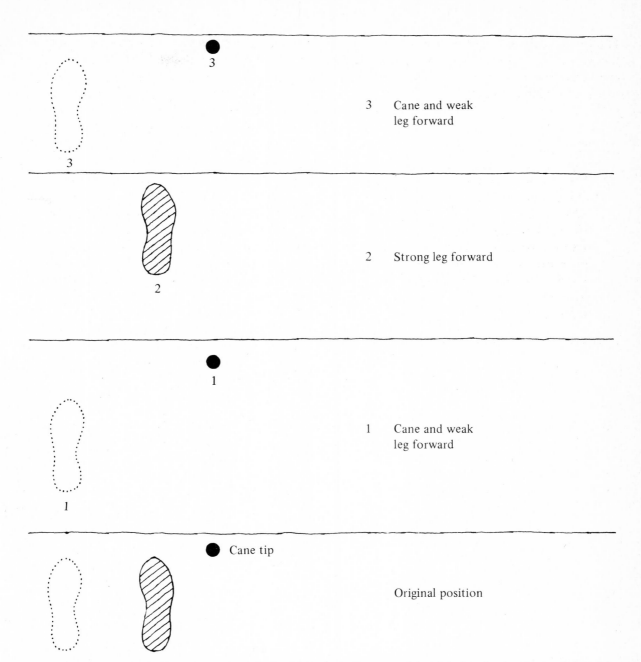

3   Cane and weak
leg forward

2   Strong leg forward

1   Cane and weak
leg forward

Cane tip

Original position

FIGURE 16.3   WALKING WITH A CANE   Dashed lines indicate partial weight bearing by the weak leg. A normal alternating stride is used, in the order shown.

greater support and stability than does a cane. The *pick-up walker* is the more stable; it does not slip when the patient leans on it (Figure 16.4). The *rolling walker* allows a smooth normal gait but is less steady. Usually, the physical therapist determines which style of walker will be used. When there is a question, generally the more stable, pick-up walker is recommended. Walkers can be

adjusted in height. Ideally, they should reach slightly below waist level, so that the handgrips can be grasped with comfort and so that the arms are slightly flexed to give strength to the support.

1. Place the walker in front of the seated patient.
2. The patient places both hands on the

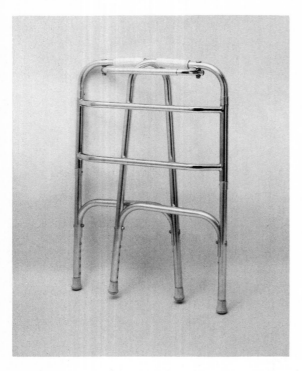

FIGURE 16.4   A FOLDING PICK-UP WALKER
Courtesy American Hospital Supply Corp.,
McGaw Park, Illinois

arms of the chair and pushes up to a standing position. The chair provides greater pushing force than does the walker, which is higher. In addition, the patient may pull the walker over by trying to use it to stand.

3. One at a time, the hands are moved to the handgrips of the walker, in order not to lose balance during the transfer.

4. Gait pattern for the pick-up walker:
   a. Move the walker and the weak leg ahead, 4 to 6 inches.
   b. Place weight on the arms for support and put some weight on the weak leg, if this is permitted. If no weight bearing is allowed on the weak leg, the arms must support all the weight.
   c. Move the strong leg forward.
   d. The pattern is then repeated.

5. You should walk closely behind and slightly to the side of the patient.

6. Sitting:
   a. The patient turns around in front of the chair and backs up until the legs

touch the chair. The walker is used for support during this maneuver.
   b. The patient reaches behind with one hand and then the other to grasp the arms of the chair.
   c. Using the arms of the chair, the patient lowers himself or herself into the chair.

Crutch Walking

The physical therapist is usually responsible for initiating the crutch-walking process. This includes correctly adjusting the length of the crutches, determining the appropriate gait based on the patient's condition, and initiating the patient teaching.

You must be aware of the basis for the therapist's decisions, so that you can reinforce the teaching. In addition, there may be settings in which you will be expected to carry out some of these functions because a physical therapist is not available.

ADJUSTING CRUTCHES FOR SIZE

Crutches are adjusted so that, when a patient stands straight, the tip of the crutch rests

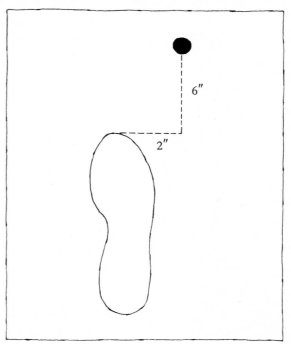

FIGURE 16.5   MEASURING CRUTCHES   Position the crutch tip 2 inches to the side of the foot and 6 inches ahead.

approximately 6 inches out in front of the foot and 2 inches to the side of the foot (Figure 16.5). The top of the crutch rests against the chest wall, with approximately 2 inches between the crutch top and the axilla (Figure 16.6). The patient should not rest on the crutches in a way that puts pressure on the axillae. This causes pressure on the nerves that control the hand and can lead to numbness, tingling, muscle weakness, and even paralysis from nerve damage (crutch palsy).

The handgrip should be placed so that the elbows are slightly flexed (approximately 30 degrees) when the hands grasp the grip. The

arm is stronger and more stable in this position than when fully extended. Also, if the arm is fully extended, the patient may experience discomfort from strain on the elbow joint.

DETERMINING THE APPROPRIATE GAIT

The gait is chosen according to the weight-bearing ability of both legs. As you read the directions for the various gaits, you will note that some allow no weight bearing, some allow for partial weight bearing, and one allows for full weight bearing on both legs (using the crutches for balance and stability). The patient's physician indicates whether full or partial weight bearing is allowed.

TEACHING THE PATIENT

Ideally, a person using crutches should be able to ambulate, with a safe gait, independently. In order for this to happen, the patient must understand how to use the crutches and must practice using them. Explain as you progress, encouraging the patient to ask questions about anything that is not clear.

Follow the General Procedure, page 238, and use the special steps below for crutch walking. To encourage independence, stand close beside and slightly behind the patient, ready to catch the patient if needed, but allowing the patient to proceed unaided. A transfer and ambulation belt may be used.

1. *Standing up from a sitting position* The patient holds both crutches in one hand on the strong side. The patient grasps the arm of the chair with the opposite hand or pushes on the bed, raising the patient to a standing position.
2. *Placing the crutches* The patient then balances on the strong leg, or on both legs if weight bearing is allowed, while carefully positioning the crutches under each arm, keeping the tips approximately 2 inches to the side and 6 inches in front of the feet. This is sometimes called the *crutch stance.*

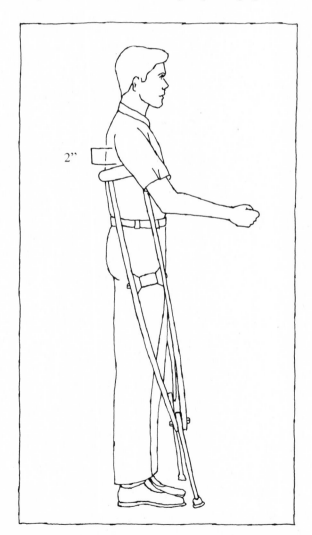

2"

FIGURE 16.6 MEASURING CRUTCHES The top of the crutch should fall 2 inches below the axilla.

3. Begin gait
   a. *Three-point gait* This gait is used for
      patients with only one leg able to
      bear weight; the other leg is held off
      the floor. (See Figure 16.7.)
      (1) The weight is supported on the
          strong leg.
      (2) Both crutches are lifted simul-
          taneously and placed forward 4
          to 6 inches.
      (3) The weight is shifted to the
          crutches.
      (4) The patient steps forward on
          the strong leg so that the
          foot is just behind the crutches.
      (5) The weight is shifted to the
          strong leg.

   (6) The pattern is repeated.
   Adaptations to the three-point gait
   Weaker patients may have to move
   one crutch forward at a time to
   maintain better balance and support.
   Very strong patients may swing the
   strong leg up past the crutches on
   each step. This is called a *swing-
   through gait.*
   b. *Three-point-plus-one gait* This gait
      is for patients who have one strong
      leg and one leg that can partially
      bear weight. This is also called the
      *three-point-with-partial-weight-
      bearing gait.* (See Figure 16.8.)
      (1) Patient stands in crutch stance
          with full weight on the strong

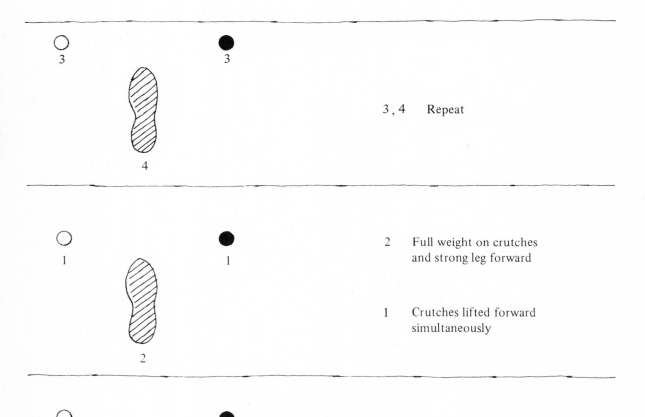

3 , 4   Repeat

2   Full weight on crutches
     and strong leg forward

1   Crutches lifted forward
     simultaneously

Crutch stance

FIGURE 16.7   THREE-POINT GAIT

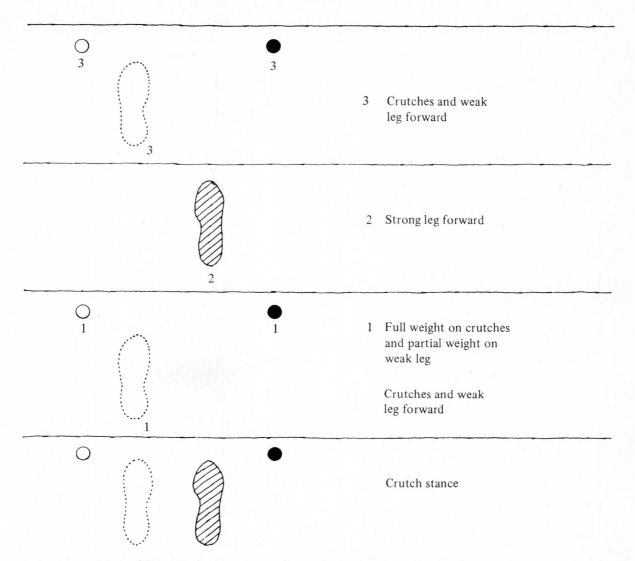

FIGURE 16.8   THREE-POINT-PLUS-ONE GAIT (PARTIAL WEIGHT BEARING)

3   Crutches and weak
    leg forward

2   Strong leg forward

1   Full weight on crutches
    and partial weight on
    weak leg

    Crutches and weak
    leg forward

    Crutch stance

leg, the affected side bearing only partial weight.

(2) The patient shifts all the weight to the strong leg.

(3) Both the crutches and the affected leg are then moved forward 6 to 12 inches.

(4) The patient then shifts the weight to the hands on the crutches, with some weight on the affected or weaker leg.

(5) The strong leg steps ahead in front of the crutches. The length of the steps for both legs should be the same to encourage a normal, even stride.

(6) The weight is shifted back to the strong leg.

(7) The pattern is repeated.

c. *Four-point gait*   This gait is used for patients with muscular weakness, lack of balance, or lack of coordination. (See Figure 16.9.)

(1) Start with the weight on both legs and both crutches. Each leg and each crutch is moved independently.

(2) Left crutch is moved forward.

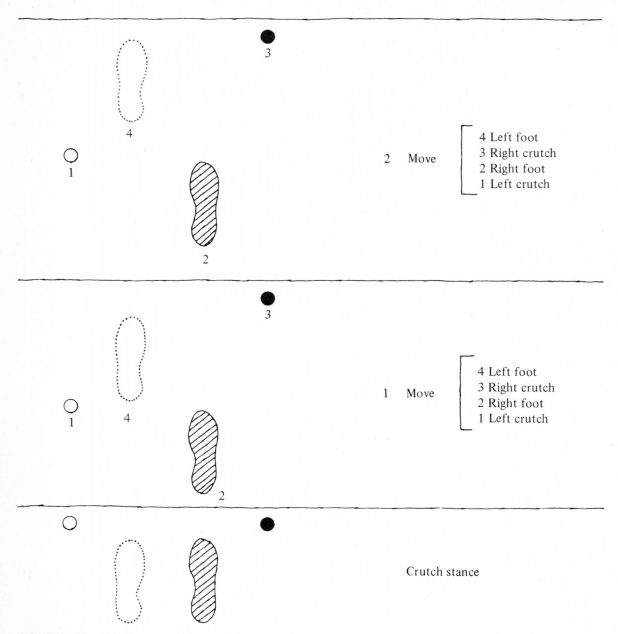

FIGURE 16.9   FOUR-POINT GAIT   Each foot and each crutch is moved independently, to achieve a smooth alternating gait.

(3)   Right leg is moved forward.
(4)   Right crutch is moved forward.
(5)   Left leg is moved forward.
(6)   The pattern is repeated.

4. *Sitting down with crutches*   No matter which gait has been used for walking,

when the patient is ready to sit down a single process is used.

a. The patient walks up to the chair, using the appropriate gait.

b. The patient should then turn around, so that his or her back is to the chair and the backs of the legs touch the seat of the chair. The crutches are used for support during the turning process. Care is taken not to step on the non-weight-bearing leg.

c. Both crutches are then grasped with one hand.

d. The other hand reaches back to grasp the arm of the chair.

e. The patient then lowers himself or herself into the chair, using the support of both the crutches and the chair.

PERFORMANCE CHECKLIST

	Unsatisfactory	Needs more practice	Satisfactory	Comments
General procedure				
1. Assess patient.				
2. Plan type of ambulation.				
3. Wash your hands.				
4. Explain plan to patient.				
5. Take baseline vital signs if necessary.				
6. Obtain robe and shoes.				
7. Position bed and assist patient to stand.				
8. Ambulate according to correct technique.				
9. Evaluate patient's response.				
10. Wash your hands.				
11. Record				
a. On nursing care plan:				
(1) Time planned for activity				
(2) Type of activity				
(3) Best method and aids to use				
(4) Patient's ability to participate				
b. On patient's chart:				
(1) Time of activity				
(2) Activity carried out				
(3) Patient's response				
Simple assisted ambulation				
1. Walk on appropriate side for patient's condition and ability.				
2. Provide support to patient.				
3. Walk slowly and with even gait.				
4. Assist patient to return to bed.				
Using a cane				
1. Patient holds cane in hand opposite weak side.				
2. Patient moves hips forward in chair.				
3. Patient grasps arms of chair.				
4. Patient pushes to standing position.				
5. Patient gains balance.				

	Unsatisfactory	Needs more practice	Satisfactory	Comments
6. Gait pattern: a. Cane held ahead 4 to 6 inches.				
b. Weak leg moved ahead, opposite cane.				
c. Weight on weak leg and cane.				
d. Strong leg moved ahead.				
e. Repeat sequence.				
7. Nurse stands to side of and behind patient.				
8. Sitting: a. Patient turns around and backs to chair.				
b. Patient grasps arms of chair.				
c. Patient lowers self into chair.				

Using a walker

	Unsatisfactory	Needs more practice	Satisfactory	Comments
1. Walker placed in front of seated patient.				
2. Patient puts both hands on arms of chair.				
3. Hands move to walker one at a time.				
4. Gait pattern for pick-up walker: a. Walker and weak leg moved ahead 4 to 6 inches.				
b. Weight placed on arms with some weight on weak leg if permitted.				
c. Strong leg moved forward.				
d. Repeat pattern.				
5. Nurse stands behind and slightly to side of patient.				
6. Sitting: a. Patient turns around and backs up to chair.				
b. Patient reaches behind to grasp arms of chair, one hand and then the other.				
c. Patient lowers self into chair.				

Crutch walking	Unsatisfactory	Needs more practice	Satisfactory	Comments
1. Patient stands with both crutches in one hand.				
2. Patient takes crutch stance, with crutch tips approximately 6 inches to side and slightly ahead of feet.				
3. Begin gait a. Three-point gait: (1) Weight is supported on strong leg.				
(2) Crutches and weak leg are lifted forward 6 to 12 inches simultaneously.				
(3) Weight is shifted to crutches.				
(4) Strong leg steps forward.				
(5) Weight is shifted to strong leg.				
(6) Repeat pattern.				
b. Three-point-plus-one gait (partial weight bearing): (1) Patient takes crutch stance, with full weight on strong leg and partial weight on weaker leg.				
(2) Weight is shifted to strong leg.				
(3) Crutches and affected leg move forward 6 to 12 inches.				
(4) Weight is shifted to hands on crutches, with some weight on affected leg.				
(5) Strong leg steps ahead with same-sized steps.				
(6) Weight is shifted to strong leg.				
(7) Repeat pattern.				
c. Four-point gait: (1) Patient takes crutch stance with weight on both legs and both crutches.				
(2) Left crutch is moved forward.				
(3) Right leg is moved forward.				
(4) Right crutch is moved forward.				
(5) Left leg is moved forward.				
(6) Repeat pattern.				

	Unsatisfactory	Needs more practice	Satisfactory	Comments
4. Sitting down with crutches: a. Patient walks to chair.				
b. Patient turns around so back is to chair and backs of legs touch chair.				
c. Patient grasps both crutches in one hand.				
d. Free hand reaches back and grasps arm of chair.				
e. Patient lowers self into chair using support of both crutches and chair.				

QUIZ

Short-Answer Questions

1. Give four reasons why ambulation is beneficial.

   a. _____

   b. _____

   c. _____

   d. _____

2. What is the major hazard of ambulation for patients? _____

   _____

3. Why are shoes better than most slippers for ambulation? _____

   _____

4. What types of assistive devices could be used for a person with one weak leg and one strong leg? _____

5. How is the length of crutches determined? _____

6. For which patient condition is a four-point crutch gait used?_____

   _____

7. When a patient is standing up from a chair to use a walker what should

   he or she hold on to? _____

8. On which side is a cane held? _____

9. When a patient using crutches sits down, what should he or she do with

   the crutches? _____

10. Which gait is appropriate for a patient who can bear no weight on one

    leg while using crutches? _____

Module 17 Postmortem Care

MAIN OBJECTIVE

To care for patients after death in a skilled and respectful manner.

RATIONALE

In addition to the important task of giving comfort and emotional support to bereaved families, the nurse also has the responsibility to care for patients' bodies after death. Postmortem care is but a continuation of the quality of care a nurse gives patients before death. Important to this task is an attitude of respect. In addition, a body is frequently viewed by survivors in the hospital environment, which makes postmortem care an even more essential task.

To have patients clean and in repose after death not only comforts the bereaved families, but is a nursing function that reflects personal involvement with individual patients.

Remember, patients are the nurse's responsibility from the time they enter the unit until the time they leave—whether in recovery or in death.

PREREQUISITES

Successful completion of the following modules:

> **VOLUME 1**
> Charting
> Medical Asepsis

256

SPECIFIC LEARNING OBJECTIVES

	Know Facts and Principles	Apply Facts and Principles	Demonstrate Ability	Evaluate Performance
1. *Pronouncement of death*	State criteria for pronouncing patient dead	In a situation, list steps in reaching pronouncement by physician		
2. *Autopsy*	Define autopsy. List reasons for performance of autopsy.	Given a situation, discuss reason for autopsy		
3. *Medical examiner's cases*	List instances in which death should be reported to medical examiner	Given a situation, discuss whether death is reportable	In the clinical setting, determine whether death should be reported	Evaluate by reviewing criteria of your locale
4. *Body changes after death*	State three changes that occur in body after death		In the clinical setting, describe body's changes after death	
5. *Caring for the body*				
a. *Privacy and the family*	Discuss ways to provide privacy for patient and family		In the clinical setting, provide privacy and demonstrate concern for patient's family	

b. *Positioning*	Describe proper positioning	In the practice setting, position body as if in death	With assistance, administer postmortem care to patient after death, including positioning body, cleaning body, caring for valuables and personal effects, and identifying body	Evaluate with instructor using Performance Checklist
c. *Cleaning and preparing*	Outline procedure for cleaning and preparing body			
d. *Care of valuables and personal effects*	State appropriate disposition of valuables and personal effects	Identify form used for disposition of valuables and effects		
e. *Identification of the body*	Describe method of body identification			
6. *Recording*	Identify essential information regarding death that must be included in patient's record	Given a situation, simulate final recording on chart	In the clinical setting, make correct and accurate final entry on patient's record	Evaluate completeness of recording with instructor

LEARNING ACTIVITIES

1. Review the Specific Learning Objectives.
2. Read the section on death care and grief (in the chapter on death) in Ellis and Nowlis, *Nursing: A Human Needs Approach,* or comparable material in another textbook.
3. Look up the module vocabulary terms in the glossary.
4. Read through the module.
5. In the practice setting:
   a. Demonstrate the proper positioning of a body by positioning a partner.
   b. Reverse roles, and have your partner position you.
   c. Discuss the reasons for positioning with your partner.
   d. With your instructor as facilitator, join in a small group with three or four classmates. Explore together some of your feelings concerning touching and caring for a patient after death.
6. In the clinical setting:
   a. Read the procedure and policy manuals provided by your facility with regard to the care of the patient after death and the responsibility and process for reporting death to a medical examiner.
   b. Examine the various forms (for autopsy, for release of body) used in your facility.
   c. If death occurs, assist the instructor or a staff nurse for your first experience in giving postmortem care.
   d. When a subsequent opportunity arises, give postmortem care with the assistance and evaluation of your instructor.

VOCABULARY

autopsy
coroner
edema
electroencephalogram
forensic medicine
funeral director
hyperalimentation
medical examiner
morgue
mortician
postmortem examination
repose
resuscitate
rigor mortis
sphincter
turgor

POSTMORTEM CARE

In many facilities, the physical aspects of postmortem care are carried out by nursing assistants. On some units, particularly in the area of critical care, postmortem care is given by nurses as part of the total-care concept. The nurse must possess those skills, as well as the sense of dignity necessary to care for a patient's body.

Pronouncement of Death

Death is usually defined as the complete cessation of respiration, heartbeat, and blood pressure. Because peripheral pulses can disappear long before the heart actually stops beating, check for apical heartbeat using a stethoscope. The heartbeat is usually the last vital sign to disappear. Once you have identified death in this manner, summon a physician. Only a physician can legally pronounce a person dead.

In delivering modern health care, many different situations can occur. Some patients, by the wishes of their families and physicians, are designated "no code"; that is, no heroic measures will be taken nor will resuscitation be employed in the event of their deaths. As a nurse, you must understand that "no code" does not mean "no care." "No code" patients are in the terminal stages of an illness. When such a patient is dying, you should continue the high quality of care you would give to any patient until the moment of death.

For the majority of patients, if you determine that respiration and heartbeat have stopped, you would initiate resuscitation according to your facility's procedure. (See Module 26, Cardiopulmonary Resuscitation.) Resuscitation measures would continue until the patient recovered vital function or the physician pronounced the patient dead.

A baffling situation is one in which the patient is having basic vital functions sustained by machines. Identifying death in these cases is very complex. Many facilities and some state laws use the Harvard De-

cision as a basis for identifying death in these situations. This requires a flat brain trace (electroencephalogram) for at least 24 hours. This criterion is now being questioned because of documented evidence that some persons who had a flat brain wave tracing for 24 hours did in fact recover. This was true, however, only in cases of diabetic coma and barbiturate poisoning. A complete discussion of this question is beyond the scope of this module. Only *after* death has been pronounced by a physician should machines supporting vital functions be turned off.

Autopsy (Postmortem Examination)

An *autopsy* is the examination of the body after death. Autopsies may be complete or partial. A complete autopsy consists of an examination of each of the body's organs including the brain. A partial autopsy consists of an examination of only those organs of interest to determine the cause of death. Autopsies serve a variety of purposes: to ascertain the exact cause of death (in some cases, this may help the family recover insurance benefits or a legal settlement), to add to scientific knowledge, and to help in statistical data gathering. If an autopsy is done in the hospital at a physician's request, there is usually no charge to the family. On occasion, the family will ask to have an autopsy performed and a charge will be incurred. You should check the specific policies in your facility.

It is the physician's responsibility to secure permission for an autopsy. Standard forms are available for this (Figure 17.1) and should be made out in duplicate with original signatures on each. The methods followed for autopsy permission are defined by state law, and again you should know the specifics of your state. A general guideline is to secure the consent of the closest blood relative, although some states have very broad guidelines, even allowing telephone permission with two witnesses on the line. For example, the guidelines of Washington State are presented in Figure 17.2. Your facility may have a policy about staff members'

PERMIT FOR AUTOPSY

I the undersigned, hereby request and authorize a complete _____

_____ including the removal, retention and disposal of such organs

and tissue as are deemed necessary by the physicians and surgeons of the staff of

Northwest Hospital to determine the cause of death and the furthering of medical

knowledge on _____

Name of Deceased

SIGNED: _____ Relationship _____

Person requesting

Examination

Date: _____

WITNESS: _____

Name of Mortician _____

Northwest Hospital
SEATTLE, WASHINGTON 98133

PERMIT FOR AUTOPSY

NWH M-135 REV. 11/76

FIGURE 17.1 PERMIT FOR AUTOPSY
Courtesy Northwest Hospital, Seattle Washington

witnessing an autopsy consent: some discourage the practice; others do not. Again, check the policy at your facility.

In certain deaths, an autopsy is required by law, in which case the permission of the next of kin is not necessary. These county or state laws may vary slightly in different

areas, and here too you should know the law of the jurisdiction in which you practice. These cases are called *coroner's cases* or *medical examiner's cases*. There is no charge to the family for an autopsy that is required by law.

The word *coroner* originates from the

Autopsy or postmortem may be performed in any case where authorization has been given by a member of one of the following classes of persons in the following order of priority:

1. The surviving spouse.
2. Any child of the decedent who is eighteen years of age or older.
3. One of the parents of the decedent.
4. Any brother or sister of the decedent.
5. A person who was guardian of the decedent at the time of death.
6. Any other person or agency authorized or under an obligation to dispose of the remains of the decedent. The chief official of any such agency shall designate one or more persons to execute authorizations pursuant to the provisions of this section.

If the person seeking authority to perform an autopsy or postmorten makes reasonable efforts to locate and secure authorization from a competent person in the first or succeeding class and finds no such person available, authorization may be given by any person in the next class.

FIGURE 17.2 WASHINGTON STATE LAW—PERMISSION FOR AUTOPSY

word *crown*. (A king would designate an appointee to oversee the disposition of bodies and estates.) A coroner need not be a physician and is either an elected or a political appointee. A medical examiner is appointed and is a physician, usually with a special degree in pathology or forensic medicine. Increasingly, counties are moving from having a coroner to having a medical examiner.

In addition to investigating unusual circumstances of death, the coroner or medical examiner also has jurisdiction over any real property of an unidentified or unclaimed deceased person. (See, for example, Figure 17.3.)

The Medical Examiner must be notified immediately in all cases of:

1. Patients pronounced "dead on arrival."
2. Deaths in the Emergency Ward (unless the patient has been ordered to the hospital by the attending physician).
3. Deaths occurring in surgery.
4. Those deaths, regardless of the time spent in the hospital, which occur within one (1) year following an accident.
5. Where death results from unknown or obscure causes.
6. Where death is caused by any violence whatsoever.
7. Where death results from a known or suspected abortion, whether self-induced or otherwise.
8. Where death results from drowning, hanging, burns, electrocution, gunshot wounds, stabs or cuts, lightning, starvation, radiation, exposure, alcoholism, narcotics or other addictions, tetanus, strangulations, suffocation or smothering.
9. Where death is due to premature birth or stillbirth.
10. Where death is due to a virulent contagious disease or suspected contagious disease which may be a public health hazard.
11. Where death results from alleged rape, carnal knowledge or sodomy.
12. Where death occurs in a jail or prison.
13. Where a body is found dead or is not claimed by relatives or friends, death must be reported before the body is removed.

FIGURE 17.3 MEDICAL EXAMINER'S CASES—KING COUNTY, STATE OF WASHINGTON

The particular person who is responsible for reporting applicable deaths to the coroner or medical examiner can vary from facility to facility. Read the policy manual where you practice, to know your role.

Organ or Tissue Donation

Be aware of the patient's wishes before death regarding the donation of certain tissues and organs, or the wishes of the family after death. Many families find some degree of consolation in knowing that some other person will benefit from a donated organ. In either case, signed permission is needed. Forms are available for this purpose. To ensure the viability of tissues, you should move ahead promptly on these requests. Most coroners and medical examiners honor these requests unless they need a particular organ for their purposes. It is important that you convey these wishes to the appropriate resource in your community.

The Death Certificate

You have no responsibility to file a death certificate. However, because you may serve as a resource person for the family, you should understand the process.

Federal law makes it mandatory that a death certificate be made out for each death. This document is kept on file with the local health department after it is completed by the mortician. It is signed by both the physician and the mortician. One to three copies are given to the family for insurance purposes and other legal matters, and the family may make additional copies if necessary.

Changes in the Body After Death

RIGOR MORTIS

Rigor mortis is a stiffening or hardening of the muscles caused by a chemical change in the protein of the muscles after death. It occurs quite rapidly, sometimes within an hour if the patient has died suddenly while active or exercising. In the chronically ill, bedridden patient, rigor mortis may not take place for some hours. The degree of rigor mortis differs greatly from one patient to another. It begins in the involuntary muscles but initially becomes noticeable in the muscles of the head and neck. It then travels downward to the trunk and finally to the lower extremities. Rigor mortis is most evident about 48 hours after death, and disappears gradually after about 96 hours (a time lapse in which you are not involved).

POSTMORTEM COOLING

The body gradually cools as circulation slows and stops.

SKIN DISCOLORATION

Skin discolors easily after death because the red blood cells are so fragile. The slightest pressure can rupture these cells and release hemoglobin, which spots the skin. Remember this when you work with the patient's body. Many times, you do not know whether the family plans to view the body later, so always handle the body gently, and apply both tags and gown loosely.

SKIN INDENTATION

Rough handling can also result in skin indentation. After death, the skin immediately loses its natural turgor and elasticity. Once this happens, the lightest pressure can indent the skin, a condition that is intensified if the patient had edema.

Caring for the Body

1. Provide privacy. Patients are not routinely moved to a private room when death is imminent. If the patient had required constant care that was disturbing another patient, and if a private room was available, a move might have taken place. Privacy should be provided for the patient, family, and staff who are sharing the death experience. In a nonprivate room, closing the door and pulling the bed curtains can give a sense of privacy. If there are other patients in the room, offer them an honest explanation.
2. Know the whereabouts of the patient's family. Members of the family may want to be present when death occurs.

Do not underestimate this: it is extremely important to some families. Usually, the patient's family has been called if death was expected, but they may not be in the patient's room at all times. If death was unexpected, the family will have been notified and be on their way to the hospital. In this case, it is important to give postmortem care so that the body is presentable for viewing.

3. Attend to the religious practices of the patient and the family. Since religious practices vary, you should know specific preferences before the patient dies. The rituals cover a broad spectrum, from the Orthodox Jewish practice of washing the body to the Roman Catholic rite of anointing the body by a priest.

4. Wash your hands.

5. Position the body using proper body alignment.
   a. Place the bed in the flat position.
   b. Use the supine position for the body.
   c. Place the arms at the patient's side. Do not cross the hands because the underlying hand will become discolored or indented. The mortician will reposition the hands later. (Rigor mortis does not prevent repositioning.)
   d. Place a low pillow under the head. This prevents blood from pooling in the face, which can cause discoloration.
   e. Close the eyes. Gently hold your index finger for a few seconds on each eyelid and the eyes will remain closed.
   f. Replace the patient's dentures if the body is to be viewed. This gives the face a more familiar and natural appearance for the family. If the dentures do not fit or do not remain in place, obviously this may not be possible.

6. Remove IVs, nasogastric tubes, urinary catheters, and oxygen equipment. These should be discarded.

7. If the patient had special indwelling lines or catheters, such as those used to take direct blood pressure readings, to deliver hyperalimentation solutions, or to dialyze the patient, cut approximately 1 inch from the body and tape to the skin. These do not interfere with the viewing, and their insertion sites and functioning may prove important medically or legally in cases of obscure causes of death.

8. Remove watches and jewelry. Make an itemized list of *all* possessions. Regardless of monetary worth, these items are often very important as mementos for the family. Ask the spouse or closest relative what to do with the patient's wedding band if one is worn. Some prefer that the band never be removed, in which case, tape it carefully in place. Others may want to keep the ring, in which case, remove it and give it personally to the family. *Always* chart the disposition of jewelry.

9. Wash the soiled areas of the body. Again, take care not to rub briskly.

10. Put a clean gown on the patient.

11. Use Chux under the patient if soiling occurs at the time of death. The sphincter muscles relax at death, and urine and feces may be expelled.

12. Replace soiled dressings, if the patient has surgical or other dressings.

13. Leave the wrist identification band in place. This is removed only if it is restricting the arm. It serves as an excellent method of identifying the body. All pieces of identification should have the patient's name, hospital number, and physician's name. The hospital band will have other data, including the date of admission.

14. Attach a second identification tag to the ankle. It is prudent to have two pieces of identification attached to the body in case one becomes detached and lost. The ankle is an appropriate spot because any marking on the skin there will not be noticeable when the body is viewed.

15. Replace the top linens (top sheet, spread, and pillowcase) to give the bed a fresh and clean appearance.

16. Tidy the unit. Dispose of any equipment. If the family is to visit, provide chairs so they can sit with the body if they wish. It is also thoughtful to rearrange any flowers that may be present.

17. Soften the lights. Turn off the ceiling lights and use the bedside lights, which will soften the features of the deceased for viewing.

18. Wash your hands.

19. Carefully list all jewelry and personal effects on the form provided by your facility. The disposition of these items should be recorded in the nurses' notes. Morticians request that dentures and eyeglasses be sent with the body. Later, if the body is to be cremated, the funeral director usually discards these items with the permission of the family.

20. Place personal effects in the container used by your facility. Include cards or letters received by the deceased. A variety of containers are available for this purpose (Figure 17.4), which are more appropriate than the paper and plastic bags often seen in practice. Follow the procedure of your facility for storing or giving the container to the patient's family.

21. After caring for the body or after the viewing, open the windows to cool the room until the body can be transported to the morgue. This retards the deterioration of the tissue. Many hospitals and convalescent centers do not have a morgue, and the mortician removes the body directly from the bed.

22. Transport the body out of the unit. The body is usually completely covered with a clean sheet. If the patient was isolated before death for an infection, you should attach a special tag to the body with this information. Some facilities have a striped covering for the body; some require that the body be encased in a large plastic bag. Check the policy in your facility. It is essential that you carry out some procedure, however, to protect all those coming in contact with the body.

    In many facilities, it is customary to shut the doors of all other patients' rooms as the cart passes out of the unit. This is done to protect the sensitivity of other patients. Observe the procedure used in your facility.

23. Wash your hands.

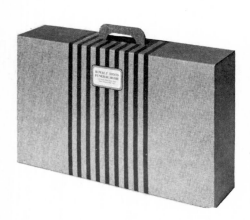
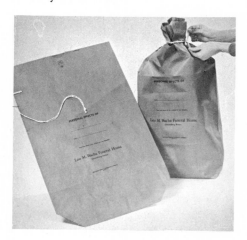

FIGURE 17.4   CONTAINERS FOR PERSONAL EFFECTS
Courtesy Kelco Supply Company, Minneapolis, Minnesota

24. Record on the chart. For example:

> 3:20 a.m. Vital signs ceased. Pro-
> nounced dead by Dr. Calhoun.
> Postmortem care given. Family
> viewed body. Wedding ring taped in
> place. Wristwatch and wallet given
> to wife.   S. Kelly, SN

PERFORMANCE CHECKLIST

	Unsatisfactory	Needs more practice	Satisfactory	Comments
1. Provide privacy.				
2. Know location of patient's family.				
3. Attend to religious practices of patient and family.				
4. Wash your hands.				
5. Position body: a. Bed flat.				
b. Supine position.				
c. Arms at side.				
d. Low pillow under head.				
e. Eyes closed.				
f. Dentures in place (if body is to be viewed in room).				
6. Remove IVs, nasogastric tubes, catheters, and oxygen.				
7. Cut special indwelling catheters or lines 1 inch from skin, and tape to skin.				
8. Remove watches and jewelry. If wedding ring is to remain in place, apply tape.				
9. Wash soiled areas of body.				
10. Put clean gown on patient.				
11. Use Chux under patient if soiling occurs.				
12. Change soiled dressings.				
13. Leave wrist identification band in place.				
14. Attach second identification tag to ankle.				
15. Replace top linens.				
16. Tidy unit.				
17. Soften lights.				
18. Wash your hands.				
19. On chart, list jewelry and personal effects given to family or locked up; list eyeglasses and dentures and state whether they were put in place or go with body.				

	Unsatisfactory	Needs more practice	Satisfactory	Comments
20. Place personal effects in appropriate container to be given to family. Make record or list.				
21. After viewing, cool room.				
22. Transfer body out of unit.				
23. Wash your hands.				
24. Record on patient's chart.				

QUIZ

Multiple-Choice Question

_____ 1. The last vital sign to disappear is usually the

    a. temperature.
    b. respiration.
    c. heartbeat.
    d. blood pressure.

Short-Answer Questions

2. What is the definition of an autopsy? _____
_____

3. Name three purposes for performing autopsies.

    a. _____
    b. _____
    c. _____

4. Describe the difference between a coroner and a medical examiner.

_____

5. Name five instances in your county when a death must be reported
   to the coroner or medical examiner.

    a. _____
    b. _____
    c. _____
    d. _____
    e. _____

6. Name three changes in the body after death.

    a. _____
    b. _____
    c. _____

7. Why should the arms be placed at the patient's side? _____

_____

8. Name four types of treatment equipment that are removed from the
   body after death.

    a. _____   c. _____
    b. _____   d. _____

9. List four of the special considerations you should take when the patient is to be viewed in the hospital room by the family.

   a. _____

   b. _____

   c. _____

   d. _____

Module 18 Collecting Specimens

MAIN OBJECTIVE

To collect and handle specimens correctly, with emphasis on the needs and comfort of patients.

RATIONALE

Specimens obtained by the nurse, or with the assistance of the nurse, may be the key to the diagnoses and therapies of the patients concerned. To handle the task well, the nurse must know the rationale for the test(s) involved, necessary preparation of the patients, correct methods of obtaining and handling specimens, and subsequent care of the patients.

PREREQUISITES

Successful completion of the following modules:

VOLUME 1
Assessment
Charting
Medical Asepsis

VOLUME 2
Sterile Technique
Catheterization

SPECIFIC LEARNING OBJECTIVES

	Know Facts and Principles	Apply Facts and Principles	Demonstrate Ability	Evaluate Performance
1. *Check order*	State two reasons to check order for collection of specimen	Given a patient situation, state rationale for laboratory test and nurse's involvement in securing specimen	Check order. In the clinical setting, state rationale for test ordered. Know and/or seek information about nurse's responsibility in securing specimen.	Evaluate with instructor
2. *Review procedure and gather equipment*	State review of procedure as integral part of activity	Given a patient situation, describe equipment necessary for obtaining specimen, handling specimen, and observing patient's response	In the clinical setting, review procedure involved and secure necessary equipment	Evaluate with instructor
3. *Prepare patient psychologically*	State two reasons for explanation to patient	Given a patient situation, describe what would appropriately be included in explanation to patient	In the clinical setting, prepare patient appropriately for obtaining of laboratory specimen	Evaluate with instructor
4. *Prepare patient physically*	List four aspects of physical preparation of patient	Given a patient situation, state aspects of physical preparation that would be appropriate	In the clinical setting, perform appropriate aspects of physical preparation for patient from whom specimen is obtained	Evaluate with instructor

5. *Perform procedure*	State four "rights" of obtaining laboratory specimen	Given a specific situation, state correct amount of given specimen and correct container	In the clinical setting, secure right amount of specimen at right time in right container from right patient	Evaluate with instructor using Performance Checklist
6. *Evaluate results and make patient comfortable*	State two appropriate observations to make in evaluating results	Given a specific situation, state observations and actions appropriate to procedure performed	In the clinical setting, evaluate results and make patient comfortable as appropriate to procedure	Evaluate with instructor
7. *Care for equipment and specimen*	State four aspects of caring for equipment and specimen	Given a specific situation, state care of equipment and appropriate handling of specimen	In the clinical setting, care for equipment and handle specimen appropriately	Evaluate with instructor
8. *Record data*	State six items of data to be included in charting	Given a patient situation, chart appropriate note	In the clinical setting, chart appropriately	Evaluate with instructor using Performance Checklist
9. *Special considerations* a. *Urine* b. *Blood* c. *Stool* d. *Sputum* e. *Drainage from wound* f. *CSF* g. *Ascitic fluid* h. *Fluid from pleural cavity*	State special handling, preparation, and positioning of patient; role of nurse; and special observations related to specific specimens	Given a specific situation, identify special considerations related to situation	In the clinical setting, secure laboratory specimens using special considerations as appropriate	Evaluate with instructor

LEARNING ACTIVITIES

1. Review the Specific Learning Objectives.
2. Read the section on performing treatments (in the chapter on direct care skills) and the section on collecting urine specimens (in the chapter on elimination) in Ellis and Nowlis, *Nursing: A Human Needs Approach,* or comparable material in another textbook. Also review the table regarding tests involving introduction of a large needle into an organ or body cavity in *Nursing: A Human Needs Approach.*
3. Look up the module vocabulary terms in the glossary.
4. Read through the module.
5. In the practice setting:
   a. Look over and compare available laboratory requisitions. Note the information required for different types of tests.
   b. With a partner as observer and "patient," simulate the collection of a urine specimen from a catheter for culture and sensitivity. Include all steps of the procedure except the actual securing of the specimen. Fill out a lab slip and chart. Have your partner evaluate you (using the Performance Checklist) with particular emphasis on your explanation to the "patient."
   c. Using your partner as the patient, practice positioning for a lumbar puncture. Have your instructor evaluate your performance.
6. In the clinical setting:
   a. Ask your instructor to help you obtain experience in filling out laboratory requisitions.
   b. Volunteer to obtain any specimen that can be secured by a nurse.
   c. Volunteer to assist the laboratory technician or physician with procedures to obtain specimens.

VOCABULARY

amoeba
ascitic fluid
cerebrospinal fluid (CSF)
culture and sensitivity (C & S)
cytology
incubate
lithotomy position
lumbar puncture (LP)
ova
paracentesis
parasites
thoracentesis

COLLECTING SPECIMENS

The basic points in the collection of any specimen are discussed below. Refer to the chart on pages 278 to 281 for special considerations related to specific specimens. The steps used are taken from the chapter on direct care skills in the section on performing treatments, in *Nursing: A Human Needs Approach*.

1. Check the order. Be certain you understand what the test is, why it has been ordered, and what your involvement in securing the specimen entails.
2. Review the procedure. If the test ordered is a routine one, this step may not be necessary. If, however, either the test itself or the procedure to be used in obtaining the specimen are unfamiliar, you must take steps to get the necessary information. Some hospitals maintain a guide to specific laboratory tests for use by the nurse as a quick reference. (See Figure 18.1.)
3. Gather the equipment. You may need equipment to obtain the specimen (catheterization set, lumbar-puncture tray), a container or containers in which to place the specimen (sterile test tube, jar, paper container), and equipment with which to observe the patient's response (blood pressure equipment).
4. Prepare the patient psychologically. Explain to the patient exactly what is going to happen to an extent that is appropriate and will enhance the patient's ability to cooperate. Allow the patient to express personal feelings and to ask questions as well.
5. Prepare the patient physically. Depending on the procedure to be performed, provide for privacy, adjust the lighting, and assist in positioning and draping.
6. Wash your hands.
7. Perform the procedure. Be certain that you obtain the right amount of specimen in the right container at the right time and, of course, from the right patient. Take care not to get any of the

ELECTROPHORESIS, SPINAL FLUID

Fasting not required

Requisition: Misc. (Blue)

Specimen: A <u>minimum</u> of 5 ml is required. If other tests are ordered as well, a larger volume is required. Check appropriate cards.

Test sent to Bio Science.

Turn-about Time: 1 week

FIGURE 18.1   SAMPLE LABORATORY TEST FILE
Courtesy Ballard Community Hospital, Seattle, Washington

specimen material on the outside of the container.

All of the above must be done while making observations of the patient appropriate to the procedure and offering support and reassurance as needed. (See the Special Observations column in the chart on pages 278–281.)

8. Evaluate the results. Essentially this means checking that the correct specimen was obtained in an amount adequate for the test to be performed, and observing the patient's responses, both physical and psychological, as appropriate.
9. Make the patient comfortable. This can include repositioning, changing or straightening the bedding, and administering medication for pain or discomfort. Again, this step depends almost entirely on the procedure you have performed.
10. Care for the equipment and the specimen. The care of the equipment is dictated by the type of equipment involved as well as the policies of your facility. Even with disposable equipment, you must be sure to dispose of particu-

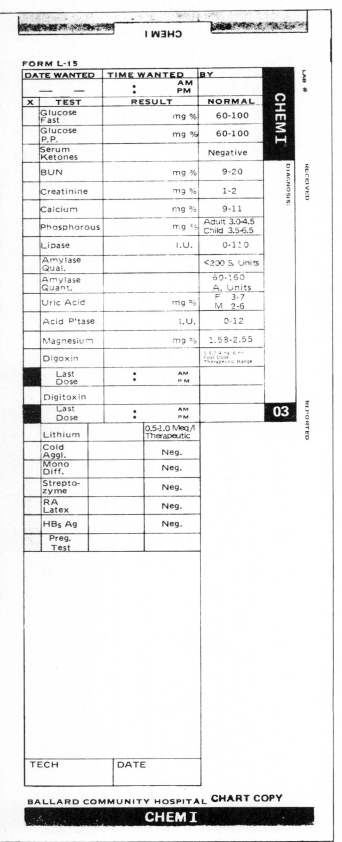

CHEM I

FORM L-15

X	TEST	DATE WANTED	TIME WANTED	BY
			AM PM	

X	TEST	RESULT	NORMAL
	Glucose Fast	mg %	60-100
	Glucose P.P.	mg %	60-100
	Serum Ketones		Negative
	BUN	mg %	9-20
	Creatinine	mg %	1-2
	Calcium	mg %	9-11
	Phosphorous	mg %	Adult 3.0-4.5 Child 3.5-6.5
	Lipase	I.U.	0-110
	Amylase Qual.		<200 S. Units
	Amylase Quant.		60-160 A. Units
	Uric Acid	mg %	F 3-7 M 2-6
	Acid P'tase	I.U.	0-12
	Magnesium	mg %	1.58-2.55
	Digoxin		0.8-2.4 ng 6 hr. Post Dose Therapeutic Range
	Last Dose	: AM : P M	
	Digitoxin		
	Last Dose	: AM : P M	
	Lithium		0.5-1.0 Meq/l Therapeutic
	Cold Aggl.		Neg.
	Mono Diff.		Neg.
	Strepto-zyme		Neg.
	RA Latex		Neg.
	HB$_S$ Ag		Neg.
	Preg. Test		

LAB #

CHEM I

DIAGNOSIS:

RECEIVED

REPORTED

03

TECH	DATE

BALLARD COMMUNITY HOSPITAL **CHART COPY**

CHEM I

lar items (needles, breakables) in appropriate ways.

A *very* important aspect of the nurse's role is to correctly handle and label a specimen. You must know if the specimen should be kept warm or refrigerated, taken immediately to the lab, or handled in some other special way. In addition, labeling must be *complete* and *accurate*. Although each facility will have its own procedure, the following information is often included: patient's name, identification number, age, room number (if in a health care facility), and physician's name. In most cases a laboratory requisition will accompany the specimen and must also be completely and accurately filled out. The patient's identifying information and diagnosis, as well as the date and time, are often included. (See Figure 18.2.)

11. Wash your hands.
12. Record the data. Date and time, as well as the procedure itself and the patient's emotional and physiological response, must be recorded on the patient's chart. Any drugs or solutions used and the amount, description, and disposition of the specimen obtained are also appropriately included. For example:

> 7/4/80 Catheterized with #16 straight catheter without difficulty. 60 ml cloudy yellow urine obtained and sent to lab. Patient continues to complain of burning on urination.
>   S. Penobscot, SN

FIGURE 18.2 A REQUISITION FOR SELECTED BLOOD CHEMISTRIES
Courtesy Ballard Community Hospital, Seattle, Washington

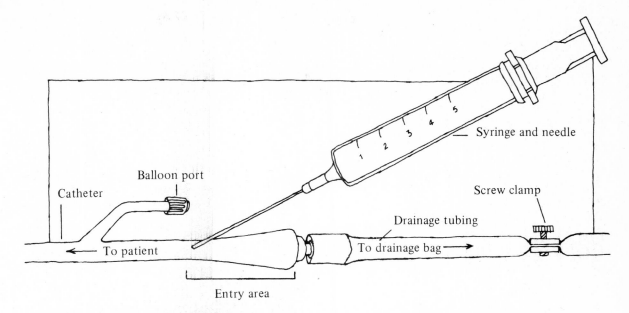

FIGURE 18.3 CLAMPING CATHETER AND REMOVING URINE FROM A CATHETER WITHOUT AN ENTRY PORT IN THE DRAINAGE TUBING

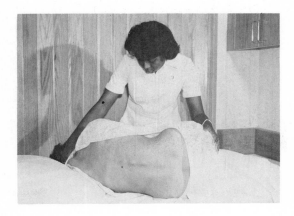

FIGURE 18.4 PATIENT POSITIONED FOR LUMBAR PUNCTURE
Courtesy Lawrence Cherkas

Specimen	Preparing the Patient	Positioning the Patient	Role of the Nurse	Special Observations Concerning the Patient	Handling the Specimen
Urine a. Voided	Instruct how to obtain clean voided specimen.	Up to bathroom or commode or on bedpan.	Obtain specimen. Clean voided specimen: 1. Clean vulva or penis thoroughly with soap and water. 2. Hold vulva apart while voiding to decrease contamination of urine. 3. Initial part of voiding passed into commode, bedpan, or urinal; pass next part into clean or sterile container (disposable kits are available). 4. Do not allow container to touch body.		Specimen may be clean or sterile: routine urinalysis is clean; culture and sensitivity is sterile. If not sent immediately to lab, refrigerate except in special cases.

Specimen	Preparing the Patient	Positioning the Patient	Role of the Nurse	Special Observations Concerning the Patient	Handling the Specimen
b. Catheter in place	Inform patient of procedure.	Supine, with top linen draped back to expose catheter.	To remove urine from indwelling catheter: 1. Obtain sterile 5-ml syringe with needle and alcohol swab. 2. Wipe entry port on tubing thoroughly with alcohol swab. If there is no entry port, wipe portion of catheter itself between balloon port and connecting end. 3. Insert needle into prepared portion of tubing and withdraw urine (Figure 18.3). If there is no urine in the catheter, clamp it off for 15 to 20 minutes before trying to obtain sample. 4. Remove syringe from catheter. 5. Expel urine from syringe into sterile container. 6. Dispose of equipment safely.	None	Related to purpose (see above).

Specimen	Preparing the Patient	Positioning the Patient	Role of the Nurse	Special Observations Concerning the Patient	Handling the Specimen
c. Catheter to be inserted	Explain procedure.	See Module 39, Catheterization	See Module 39, Catheterization, if urine from an indwelling catheter is necessary.	See Module 39, Catheterization.	Related to purpose (see above).
Blood	Instruction as to what to expect, as well as fasting directions if appropriate.	Babies may have to be mummied. (See Module 9, Basic Infant Care.)	Depending on setting, can be to prepare patient and assist physician or laboratory technician; can be to prepare patient only.	Apply pressure to puncture site to stop bleeding. If blood is obtained from an artery, apply pressure for full five minutes following procedure.	Procedure is sterile. For serology or chemical analysis, or if not immediately examined, refrigerate; for culture, incubate; for other tests, leave at room temperature.
Stool	Provide commode or bedpan.		Obtain specimen. Transfer from commode or bedpan to specimen container with tongue blade.	Patient may be embarrassed. Be reassuring and provide privacy.	Small amount usually adequate. If tests are for ova, parasites, or amoebas, send to lab immediately (while it is warm).
Sputum	Explain why specimen is needed and show container in which to expectorate.	Usually patient will be sitting up; splinting may help. Postural drainage can be used. (See Module 33, Care Procedures.)	Obtain specimen and/or assist respiratory therapist to obtain specimen through coughing.	Nausea may occur. Mouth care is indicated after a large amount of sputum is coughed up.	Specimen is clean for cytology; sterile for culture and sensitivity. Best collected in morning. Keep at room temperature until examined.

Specimen	Preparing the Patient	Positioning the Patient	Role of the Nurse	Special Observations Concerning the Patient	Handling the Specimen
Cerebrospinal fluid (CSF), usually done by lumbar puncture	Explain.	On side with back near side of bed, knees brought up, head forward (Figure 18.4); or sitting on edge of bed, with feet supported, leaning over overbed table. (The objective is to enlarge the intravertebral spaces.)	Assist patient to maintain position. Be reassuring. Assist physician in terms of setting up equipment, holding and labeling tubes for specimens, and cleaning up.	Signs of shock, nausea, and vomiting. Headache occasionally. Physician may order patient to lie flat for 1 to 24 hours after procedure.	Specimen is sterile, usually in several tubes. Be sure to number tubes sequentially (tube 1, tube 2, and so on). Send to lab immediately.
Ascitic fluid, done by paracentesis.	Explain. Have patient void before procedure to prevent puncture of bladder.	Sitting position.	Reassure patient. Assist physician by setting up equipment, measuring fluid, and cleaning up.	Signs of shock. Monitor vital signs for four to eight hours after procedure.	Specimen is sterile.
Fluid from pleural cavity, done by thoracentesis.	Explain. Warn patient not to cough or move suddenly during procedure or needle may puncture lungs.	Sitting position with arms over head or in front of chest. (The objective is to increase the size of the intercostal spaces.)	Reassure patient. Assist physician by setting up equipment, measuring fluid, and cleaning up.	Respiratory distress (cyanosis, dyspnea). Blood-tinged sputum. Monitor for four to eight hours after procedure for signs of respiratory embarrassment or shock.	Specimen is sterile.

PERFORMANCE CHECKLIST

	Unsatisfactory	Needs more practice	Satisfactory	Comments
1. Check order.				
2. Review procedure.				
3. Gather equipment: a. To obtain specimen				
b. To handle specimen				
c. To evaluate patient's response				
4. Prepare patient psychologically.				
5. Prepare patient physically: a. Privacy				
b. Lighting				
c. Positioning				
d. Draping				
6. Wash your hands.				
7. Perform procedure: a. Right amount of specimen				
b. Right container				
c. Right time				
d. Right patient				
8. Evaluate results: a. Right specimen in adequate amount for specific test				
b. Physical and psychological response of patient				
9. Make patient comfortable.				
10. Care for equipment and specimen: a. Dispose of equipment correctly.				
b. Refrigerate or keep warm, as appropriate.				
c. Label completely and accurately.				
d. Fill out lab requisition completely.				
11. Wash your hands.				
12. Record data.				

QUIZ

Short-Answer Questions

1. List three types of equipment that might be necessary when collecting a specimen.

   a. _____

   b. _____

   c. _____

2. List four aspects that might be included in the physical preparation of the patient.

   a. _____

   b. _____

   c. _____

   d. _____

3. List the four "rights" of obtaining laboratory specimens.

   a. _____

   b. _____

   c. _____

   d. _____

4. List five pieces of information usually included when a specimen is labeled.

   a. _____

   b. _____

   c. _____

   d. _____

   e. _____

5. Chart a mock note for a patient from whom a sputum specimen was collected for culture and sensitivity. _____

   _____

True-False Questions

_____   6. When blood is obtained from a vein, pressure must be applied to the puncture site for a full five minutes following the procedure.

_____   7. Sputum specimens are best collected in the morning.

_____   8. It is important that the patient void prior to a thoracentesis.

_____   9. Headache is a common complication of a lumbar puncture.

Module 19 Administering Enemas

MAIN OBJECTIVE

To give enemas to patients in a safe effective manner.

RATIONALE

Enemas are frequently given to hospitalized patients. There are many types of enemas and purposes to be accomplished by their administration. The nurse must understand the various kinds of enemas that may be ordered, their purpose, and how to administer them. In modern practice, the nurse may also be expected to make decisions as to which type of enema is most appropriate in an uncomplicated situation.

PREREQUISITES

Successful completion of the following modules:

VOLUME 1
Assessment
Charting
Medical Asepsis

SPECIFIC LEARNING OBJECTIVES

	Know Facts and Principles	Apply Facts and Principles	Demonstrate Ability	Evaluate Performance
1. *Types of enemas and indications for use*	List types of enemas and purpose for each type	Given a patient situation, identify whether enema is needed and appropriate type to be used	In the clinical area, identify purpose of enema ordered for specific patient	Evaluate own teaching by quizzing patient regarding knowledge
2. *Patient teaching*	State what patient needs to be taught regarding procedure	Given a patient situation, plan appropriate teaching	In the clinical area, explain procedure to patient	
3. *Procedure* a. *Equipment* b. *Temperature* c. *Patient's position* d. *Distance to insert tubing* e. *Lubrication* f. *Pressure*	Describe equipment used in enema procedure. Know correct temperature for solution. Describe correct patient position. State distance tip of device should be inserted. Know lubricant to be used. Explain how pressure is controlled. State how appropriate pressure is determined.	Given a patient situation, plan appropriate action to alleviate problems or to stop procedure if necessary. Select correct equipment. Plan procedure.	In the clinical area, carry out procedure correctly	Evaluate own performance using Performance Checklist
4. *Observations*	List observations to make before, during, and after procedure	Given a patient situation, identify observations that are significant	Identify what observations are significant. Institute corrective action if needed.	Evaluate own performance with clinical instructor
5. *Recording*	State what needs to be recorded	Given a patient situation, record data as though on chart	Record procedure and observations correctly	

LEARNING ACTIVITIES

1. Review the Specific Learning Objectives.
2. Read the sections on the intestinal system and defecation problems (in the chapter on elimination) in Ellis and Nowlis, *Nursing: A Human Needs Approach,* or comparable material in another textbook.
3. Look up the module vocabulary terms in the glossary.
4. Read through the module.
5. In the practice setting:
   a. Inspect and become familiar with the types of enema equipment available.
   b. Using equipment in the laboratory, go through the entire procedure as you would with a real patient without actually giving the enema. Use a mannequin if available or improvise a substitute.
   c. Have another student check your performance using the Performance Checklist.
   d. Evaluate your own performance.
   e. Compare your evaluation with your partner's.
   f. Have your partner do the procedure, and you evaluate his or her performance.
   g. Practice recording information regarding an enema.
   h. Repeat this section until you have gone through the procedure correctly.
   i. When you feel you have mastered the procedure, have your instructor evaluate your performance.
6. Consult with your clinical instructor regarding an opportunity to give an enema to a patient in the clinical area.

VOCABULARY

anal sphincter (external and internal)
ascending colon
descending colon
distention
electrolyte
feces
flatus
Harris flush
hypertonic
hypotonic
instillation
peristalsis
reflex contraction
sigmoid flexure
Sim's position
transverse colon

ADMINISTERING ENEMAS

Cleansing Enemas

The most common enema is the cleansing enema. This is given for the purpose of cleaning the lower bowel of fecal material. Standard equipment used in a cleansing enema is shown in Figure 19.1.

A large-volume enema is commonly used for a cleansing enema. Approximately 500 to 1000 ml fluid is instilled into the colon of the adult patient. The patient is encouraged to retain the fluid as long as possible, allowing it to loosen and soften fecal material in the colon. The large volume infused stimulates peristalsis and causes massive bowel evacuation.

A common solution for a cleansing enema is tap water. Occasionally, a mild, liquid castile soap is added to the tap water (this is called a soapsuds enema). A soapsuds enema irritates the colon, creating stronger peri-

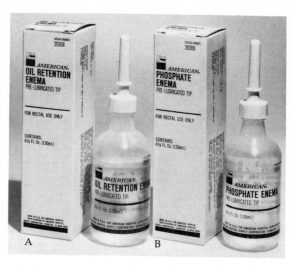

FIGURE 19.2 DISPOSABLE ENEMAS *A:* Oil retention enema; *B:* medicated cleansing enema. *Courtesy American Hospital Supply Corp., Evanston, Illinois*

stalsis. Normal saline can also be used. In fact, because it does not create electrolyte disturbances as readily as does plain water, it is preferred for patients who are vulnerable to electrolyte imbalances (elderly, very young, or severely debilitated patients). Saline enemas should also be chosen whenever several enemas must be given to an individual. Although a commercially prepared irrigating solution is preferred, it is possible to mix an acceptable substitute by using 1 teaspoon salt to each 500 ml water.

The small-volume, commercially prepared disposable enema is also used for cleansing (Figure 19.2). This type of enema contains a small amount (90 to 120 ml) of medicated solution: sodium phosphate is most frequently used. The solution is hypertonic, and thus draws fluid into the bowel, softening and lubricating the fecal mass. The medication is also an irritant, causing strong peristalsis and subsequent evacuation. The patient should retain the enema as long as possible (20 minutes is best) to allow the fluid from the body to enter the colon. This type of enema is especially useful for patients who cannot hold a large volume; and it does not create the electrolyte depletion caused by tap water. Because the hypertonic enema

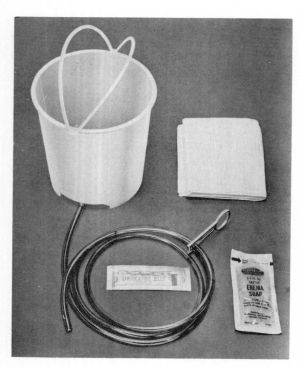

FIGURE 19.1   EQUIPMENT FOR A CLEANSING ENEMA   Some sets have a plastic bag instead of a bucket.
Courtesy American Hospital Supply Corp., Evanston, Illinois

uses the body's own fluid supply to moisten and lubricate the feces, it is inappropriate for a patient who is dehydrated. It is also less appropriate in a situation where immediate evacuation is desired. However, many patients prefer this type of enema because (1) it is given more rapidly and with less fuss and (2) it causes less abdominal distention and discomfort than does a large-volume enema. It is also very convenient for the nurse. When you use a commercially prepared enema, read and follow the package directions. The general directions for giving an enema still apply.

Oil-Retention Enemas

When fecal material has hardened, an oil-retention enema may be given to soften the feces. Oil-retention enemas are available in commercially packaged form containing 90 to 120 ml. (See Figure 19.2.) Instill approximately 90 to 120 ml into the patient's colon and have the patient retain it for as long as possible—an hour is needed to be effective. This enema is usually followed by a cleansing enema. If a commercially prepared oil enema is not available, use mineral oil. It is instilled using an asepto-syringe barrel attached to a rectal tube. Pour the oil into the open asepto barrel and allow it to flow by gravity.

Rectal Instillation of Medications

A variety of medications can be instilled into the colon by enemas. Dissolve the medication needed in 30 to 50 ml solution so that the volume of fluid will not cause peristalsis and loss of the medication. The medication is then absorbed through the intestinal wall. A cleansing enema to clear the colon may be needed before a medicated enema is given.

Cooling Enemas

Occasionally, an enema of cool fluid (cold tap water) is used to lower body temperature rapidly. This is done only when a patient's body temperature is dangerously high; it is not a common procedure. There are some differences of opinion as to the safety of this procedure because it can cause a shock-like reaction. When this enema is used, check the patient's temperature both before and after the procedure.

Return-Flow Enemas

A return flow enema, sometimes called a *Harris flush,* is used to remove intestinal gas and to stimulate peristalsis. Use a large volume of fluid, as you would in a cleansing enema, but instill the fluid in small increments (100 to 200 ml). Then, by lowering the container below the level of the bowel (Figure 19.3), siphon it out. This brings the gas out with the fluid. Continue this procedure until no more flatus is returned.

Using tap water, it is possible to deplete the patient's electrolytes, especially if a return-flow enema is needed several times a day. Although saline will lessen electrolyte depletion, you must first determine that the absorption of the sodium will not be detrimental to the patient.

Procedure

1. Verify the order. It is your responsibility to check the physician's order for the enema to be sure that the correct type is being administered to the correct patient.
2. Gather the equipment. Collect the appropriate equipment for the type of enema to be given and carry it, covered, to the patient's bedside.
   a. You will need an enema container with tubing and rectal tip for a cleansing enema. (See Figure 19.1.) Rectal tubes are sized using the French method: the larger the number, the larger the tube. The disposable enema set usually has a number 18–22 French tip. Oil-retention and Fleet's enemas commonly have a number 14 French tube. Tubes are available as small as number 10 French. This equipment may be

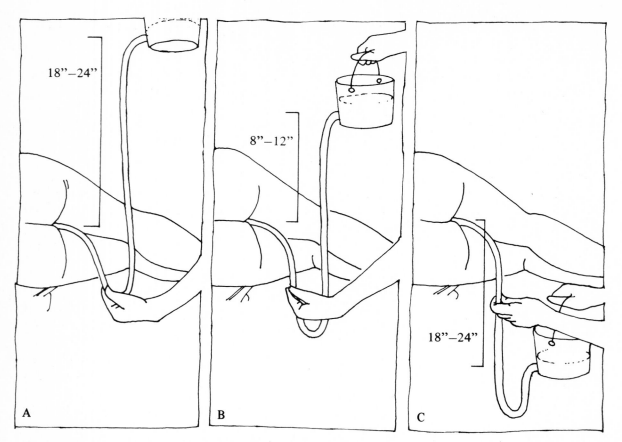

FIGURE 19.3   REGULATING FLUID PRESSURE BY HEIGHT OF CONTAINER   *A:* Moderate pressure;
B: low pressure; *C:* negative pressure, for siphoning.

disposable, depending on the facility.
The correct, commercially prepared
enema may be obtained from the
central supply unit or the pharmacy.
Check your facility's procedures.
Always check the tip of the tubing
for irregularities that could damage
tissue.

b. To mix an enema, use warm water
from the faucet for a solution that is
just slightly warmer than body temperature—100° F–105° F is appropriate. Use a bath thermometer to
check the solution's temperature. If
one is not available, estimate the
temperature by testing it on the
inner aspect of your forearm, as you
would check a baby's formula. It
should feel comfortably warm but
not hot. Then, by the time the solution is instilled through a tubing, it

will be approximately at body temperature.

A commercially prepared enema
may be warmed by immersing the
entire container in a basin of very
warm water. The correct temperature
helps to preserve homeostasis by eliminating the body's need to use large
amounts of energy to compensate
for heat lost into the enema solution.
Also, warmth stimulates peristalsis
and is more comfortable for the
patient.

c. You will need a bath blanket or
sheet to drape the patient, a waterproof pad to slide under the patient's
hips (these are usually provided in
commercial enema kits), and adequate lighting.

d. Use a lubricant to facilitate the insertion of the tube and to prevent

trauma to anorectal tissue. A water-soluble lubricant is most commonly used because it is easy to remove; however, a mineral-based lubricant is acceptable.

   e. Provide a bedpan or commode.

3. Identify the patient.

4. Explain the procedure. Although some persons have had enemas or are familiar with them, many have their first experience with an enema in the hospital setting. Your first task is to ascertain what the patient knows about the procedure and how he or she feels about it. Then you can teach the patient what is necessary to know. The patient particularly needs to know what to expect in terms of his or her own body's responses. Allow time for the patient to express personal feelings regarding the procedure.

5. Wash your hands.

6. Prepare the patient. Close the curtains or drapes to provide privacy. Raise the bed to a comfortable working height for you. Place the patient in left Sim's position. This position allows the fluid to flow by gravity and fill the descending colon. When an extreme, complete cleansing is necessary (for example, before a barium enema) after 300 to 400 ml have been administered, position the patient on the back for the next 300 ml. Then turn the patient to the right side while another 300 ml are instilled. This procedure helps the fluid fill the transverse and ascending colon. However, this can be difficult for the patient and is not done routinely.

   Enemas can also be administered with a patient on the right side or on the back, either for comfort or as indicated by the patient's condition. These positions are successful, but the patient may experience pressure at the anus with a smaller amount of fluid.

   Cover the patient with a drape of some kind (often a bath blanket) so that only the rectal area is exposed. This lessens the patient's embarrassment and

prevents chilling. Then place a waterproof pad under the patient's hips to protect the bed. Occasionally, a patient may ask to have an enema given while sitting on the toilet. This practice is undesirable because the fluid is inserted against gravity, making it difficult for the patient to retain the fluid and resulting in a less-effective cleaning of the bowel.

   Patients receiving large amounts of solution (750 to 1000 ml) are not usually able to retain the solution for more than five minutes, so it is comforting for them to have the commode or bedpan close at hand.

7. Administer the enema. For a commercially prepared enema, follow the directions carefully. For the conventional enema, continue as follows:

   a. Remove air from the enema tubing by allowing fluid to flow through to the tip and then clamping it.

   b. Lift the upper buttock to expose the anus. Insert the lubricated enema tip 3 to 4 inches. This places it past the internal anal sphincter and well into the rectum, so that the fluid does not put immediate pressure against the sphincter or create as much potential for trauma to the intestinal wall as further insertion would. It is possible to severely traumatize the intestinal mucosa, especially if the tubing is inserted into the sigmoid flexure or even the descending colon. Have the patient breathe through the mouth to relax the anal sphincter. Another technique for relaxing the sphincter is to touch the tip to the sphincter, wait for the reflex contraction to subside, and then insert it. If you encounter an obstruction, stop the procedure and report it.

   c. Raise the enema container above the patient's hips and unclamp the tubing. The higher the enema container is held above the level of the patient's hips, the greater the pressure.

Negative pressure is achieved by holding the fluid below the level of the patient's hips (Figure 19.3).

The pressure created by holding the enema container 12 to 18 inches above the patient's hips is enough to instill the fluid without being so great as to cause damage to the intestinal mucosa or to cause intestinal perforation. Use a lower pressure if the patient has excessive discomfort or cramping. However, you may have to use a higher pressure again, briefly, if the fluid is partially blocked by fecal material. This is determined when the fluid does not flow with the usual pressure. If cramping occurs despite the use of low pressure, stop the inflow of fluid temporarily, to allow the bowel to accommodate the fluid already given, before continuing. If severe cramping does not subside, the enema is usually discontinued.

If the patient has a large amount of gas, it is sometimes helpful to use a return-flow enema to remove the gas first. Then the patient is better able to hold the enema fluid and the evacuation will be more effective.

Sometimes a patient is unable to retain the fluid because of weakness or lack of control of the anal sphincter. You can hold the buttocks firmly together around the tube to help the patient retain the fluid, or you can place a baby bottle nipple over the tubing and hold it at the sphincter. If small amounts dribble back constantly, place the curved side of an emesis basin against the buttocks. This will catch the fluid as it dribbles out, and the patient will not end up lying in a puddle of enema fluid.

d. Once the correct amount of fluid has been given, clamp the tubing and remove it. By clamping first, you prevent the fluid from dripping out of the tube after the tube is removed.

e. Encourage the patient to hold the fluid as long as possible.

f. Assist the patient onto the bedpan or commode or to the bathroom. If the patient can be left alone, provide a call light and toilet tissue, and leave. Make sure you are close to help the patient if necessary.

8. Observe and evaluate the results. During the procedure, observe the patient for his or her response to the enema as well as for skin color and respiratory rate. The patient's pulse rate may be checked before and after the procedure. Also watch for signs of excessive fatigue. If the patient's response is adverse, discontinue the procedure and consult the physician. If the procedure is completed, observe the results. Estimate the quantity of fecal material expelled (small, moderate, or large), and describe its color and consistency (soft, hard, particles).

If the patient is able to use the bathroom following an enema, give instructions that the toilet not be flushed until you have had an opportunity to evaluate the results of the enema. You can place a piece of tape across the flushing handle as a reminder to the patient not to flush. Again, note the amount (estimated), and the consistency.

9. Make the patient comfortable. The patient may need help cleaning the anorectal area after receiving an enema. Also, you should provide an opportunity for handwashing. And, because an enema is often tiring, make arrangements for the patient to rest, including assistance with positioning and other comfort measures.

10. Clean or dispose of the equipment. Some enema equipment is disposable, but even a disposable enema container may be thoroughly cleaned and reused for the same patient. Dry it carefully to prevent the growth of microorganisms. Label the container with the date and

the patient's name. If nondisposable equipment is used, you must sterilize the equipment between patients.

11. Wash your hands.
12. Record the data on the patient's chart. These data include the type of enema, the amount administered, and the time given. Also record the results of the enema along with a description of the patient's response to the procedure.

PERFORMANCE CHECKLIST

	Unsatisfactory	Needs more practice	Satisfactory	Comments
1. Verify order.				
2. Gather equipment: a. Enema bucket with tubing and tip				
b. Solution at correct temperature				
c. Bath blanket or drape and waterproof pad				
d. Lubricant				
e. Bedpan or commode				
3. Identify patient.				
4. Explain procedure and purpose to patient.				
5. Wash your hands.				
6. Prepare patient: a. Privacy				
b. Position				
c. Draping				
7. Administer enema: a. Clear tubing of air and lubricate tip.				
b. Insert proper distance (3 to 4 inches).				
c. Give fluid with safe pressure (maximum height 18 inches above patient's hips).				
d. Stop if patient has discomfort.				
e. Use return-flow enema if needed.				
f. Clamp tubing before removing.				
g. Encourage patient to hold fluid as long as possible.				
h. Assist patient with bedpan or commode.				
i. Provide toilet tissue and call light.				
8. Evaluate results of enema.				
9. Make patient comfortable: a. Assist patient with cleaning and washing.				
b. Position patient for comfort and rest.				
10. Clean up equipment.				
11. Wash your hands.				

	Unsatisfactory	Needs more practice	Satisfactory	Comments
12. Record: a. Type of solution				
b. Amount of fluid				
c. Results				
d. Patient's response				

QUIZ

Short-Answer Questions

1. List four types of enemas and give the purpose for each type.

   Type   *Indication for use*

   a. _____   _____

   b. _____   _____

   c. _____   _____

   d. _____   _____

2. List three reasons why enemas are upsetting to many persons.

   a. _____

   b. _____

   c. _____

3. List four observations to be made of the patient while administering an enema.

   a. _____

   b. _____

   c. _____

   d. _____

4. How is fluid siphoned out of the bowel when giving a return-flow enema?

   _____

5. If a patient complains of severe cramping while an enema is being administered, what action should you take?

   _____

Module 20 Temperature, Pulse, and Respiration

MAIN OBJECTIVE

To measure and record patients' TPR[1] accurately and safely, recognizing deviations from the norm.

RATIONALE

Because temperature, pulse, and respiration (TPR) are basic measurements that are helpful in assessing patients' conditions, it is essential that the practicing nurse have the ability to take and record these signs accurately. TPRs are taken by both professional and nonprofessional staff in health care settings. Both can perform the mechanics of the procedure equally well. However, it is within the responsibility of the professional nurse to understand the deviations from normal on which assessments and interpretations are based.

After completing this module, you should be able to define, carry out, record, and assess these signs. You will have the ability to adapt this procedure to both well and ill individuals of any age group and make appropriate interpretations suggested by your findings. Then you will be ready to move on to Module 21, Blood Pressure, thus completing vital signs.

PREREQUISITES

1. Successful completion of the following modules:

   VOLUME 1
   Assessment
   Charting
   Medical Asepsis

2. Availability of a watch with a sweep second hand.
3. Familiarity with the use of the stethoscope.

[1]TPR is the symbol for one procedure measuring temperature, pulse, and respiration. VS stands for *vital signs,* which includes the measurement of blood pressure as well as TPR.

299

SPECIFIC LEARNING OBJECTIVES

	Know Facts and Principles	Apply Facts and Principles	Demonstrate Ability	Evaluate Performance
1. *Body temperature* *a. Normal body temperature* *b. Methods of measurement* *c. Temperature procedure* *d. Recording*	State normal temperature range in both Celsius and Fahrenheit measurements for oral, rectal, and axillary	Give examples of factors that can cause deviations in body temperature	Demonstrate taking patient's temperature using both Fahrenheit and Celsius thermometers, observing proper technique and safety precautions. On both graphic and nurses' notes, record data clearly and accurately.	Evaluate own performance using Performance Checklist
2. *Pulse* *a. Normal pulse rate* *b. Pulse rate procedure* *c. Recording*	Define normal pulse ranges	Point out factors that influence pulse rate	Count patient's pulse accurately, both radial and apical. On graphic, record in proper location; on nurses' notes, record pulse in numerical and descriptive terms.	Evaluate own performance using Performance Checklist
3. *Respiration* *a. Normal respiratory rate* *b. Respiratory rate procedure* *c. Recording*	Identify normal respiratory rate ranges	Relate factors influencing respiratory rates	Determine patient's respiratory rate using correct technique. Record rate and character of respiration on graphic and nurses' notes.	Evaluate own performance using Performance Checklist

LEARNING ACTIVITIES

1. Review the Specific Learning Objectives.
2. Read the chapter on oxygenation, circulation, and neurological function in Ellis and Nowlis, *Nursing: A Human Needs Approach,* or a comparable chapter in another textbook.
3. Look up the module vocabulary terms in the glossary.
4. Read through the module, taking note of the vital signs graphic form (Figure 20.1).
5. Review the steps of the procedure in the Performance Checklist.
6. In the practice setting:
   a. Inspect and become familiar with the TPR equipment.
   b. Select a partner. Take your partner's oral and axillary temperatures and compare the two findings.
   c. Record the oral temperature reading on the vital signs graphic form. (See Figure 20.1.)
   d. Have your partner drink a glass of cold water and repeat the oral temperature in five minutes. How does this reading compare with the one taken previously?
   e. If an electric thermometer is available, retake your partner's temperature and compare this reading with the reading from the conventional thermometer.
   f. With your partner in a supine position, count his or her radial pulse and record it. Record the quality of the pulse felt on a progress sheet or a piece of paper.
   g. After your partner has exercised briskly (running in place) for three minutes, retake his or her pulse and compare the rate and quality with the radial pulse taken previously.
   h. Choose another student in the practice setting. Then, you and your partner take an apical-radial pulse on the student. What would you consider normal? Why?
   i. Repeat steps f, g, and h, this time measuring respiration.
   j. Complete the vital signs graphic and turn it in to your instructor.
7. In the clinical setting:
   a. Check the form used by your facility, the type of equipment being used, and the cleaning method for thermometers.
   b. Take a TPR on a patient. Follow the procedure with supervision and record your results.
   c. If possible, repeat the TPR procedure four hours later on the same patient and compare the two readings. Which of the measurements has changed? What might this indicate relative to the patient's condition?

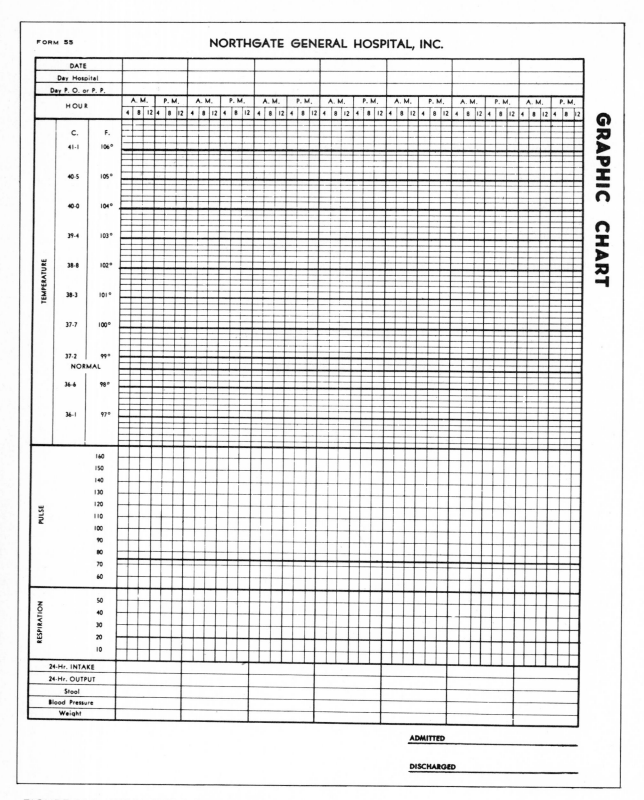

FIGURE 20.1   VITAL SIGNS GRAPHIC FORM
Courtesy Northgate General Hospital

VOCABULARY

Temperature

- axilla
- Celsius
- centigrade
- Fahrenheit
- febrile
- fever
- intermittent
- metabolism
- remittent
- Sim's position

Respiration

- apnea
- Cheyne-Stokes
- dyspnea
- Kussmaul's respirations
- orthopnea
- rhythm
- stertorous
- symmetry

Pulse

- apical pulse
- bounding pulse
- bradycardia
- carotid artery
- dorsalis pedis artery
- femoral artery
- midclavicular line
- pedal pulse
- pulse deficit
- radial artery
- tachycardia
- temporal artery
- thready pulse

TEMPERATURE, PULSE, AND RESPIRATION

The taking of TPR is important because it serves as an indicator of a patient's status. Most institutions have routine times for taking TPR—often, q.4 h. (every four hours) —but a patient's illness or certain other conditions may dictate more frequent measurement. For example, you would make an independent nursing decision to take the temperature of a flushed patient who complains of feeling warm. Routine TPR is usually taken on a number of patients at one time, and the readings are recorded on paper at the bedside. These readings are then transcribed either to a central clipboard at the nurses' station or directly on the graphic record in the patient's chart.

Temperature

Body temperature shows the balance between heat produced and heat lost by the body. It is surprisingly consistent in healthy individuals; that is, a normal oral reading is 98.6° Fahrenheit or 37° Celsius (sometimes called *centigrade*). Many factors—time of day, age, presence of infection, temperature of the environment, amount of exercise, metabolism, and emotional status—can raise or lower a patient's temperature. If a patient has been drinking liquids that are either hot or cold, delay taking the patient's temperature for at least five minutes.

If the temperature is elevated, the patient is *febrile,* that is, has a fever. Depending on the fluctuations of the elevation, the temperature can be described as *remittent* or *intermittent.* (See Glossary.)

EQUIPMENT

Temperature can be measured with a glass mercury thermometer orally, rectally, or by placing it in the axilla.

Glass thermometers can have a mercury bulb that is either slender or blunt (Figure 20.2). The slender bulb is designed to provide a larger surface for exposure when placed underneath the tongue. This type of thermometer is not safe for rectal or axillary use because of the danger of injury. The blunt, bulb thermometer is appropriate for individual use orally, rectally, or in the axilla. Some glass thermometers are color-coded: blue for oral or axillary use and red for rectal.

Electric thermometers (Figure 20.3) are now available for oral and rectal use. They are protected by disposable covers for aseptic reasons. These thermometers use metal sensing devices. With some, the sensor is placed directly on a vessel under the tongue while the patient holds the mouth open; others are placed under the tongue with the patient's mouth closed. The temperature registers almost instantly on a small display panel. Thermosensing tape is sometimes used with infants to obtain a more general reading.

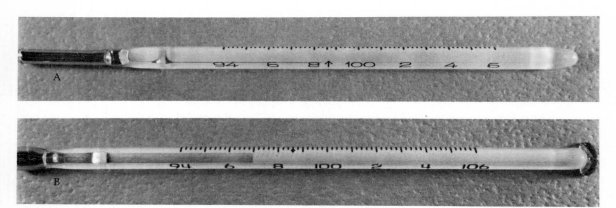

FIGURE 20.2   ORAL AND RECTAL THERMOMETERS   *A:* Oral thermometer; *B:* rectal thermometer.
Courtesy Ivan Ellis

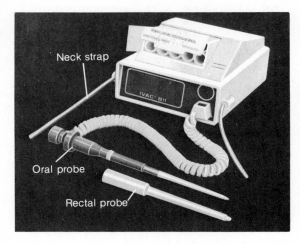

FIGURE 20.3   ELECTRIC THERMOMETER
IVAC 811 Electronic Clinical Thermometer System
Courtesy IVAC Corporation,
11353 Sorrento Valley Road, San Diego, California

A new chemical thermometer is available that is composed of a flat plastic stick holding multiple temperature-sensing chemical "dots" (Figure 20.4). Among the advantages of this device is that it is disposable, fast (registers in 30 seconds), and unbreakable.

An individual glass thermometer can be kept in a container at the patient's bedside, or a clean one may be obtained from the facility's central supply area each time TPR is taken. Occasionally, thermometers are cleaned on the unit using one of a number of cleaning methods. The electric thermom-eter is carried from one patient to another with a sufficient supply of disposable probe covers.

METHODS OF MEASURING TEMPERATURE

The most accurate temperature reading is the rectal one because the rectal cavity is closed and has high vascularity. A rectal reading is usually 1 to 1½ degrees higher than an oral reading. An oral temperature provides the next most accurate reading; axillary readings are the least reliable, and should only be taken if the other two routes are contraindicated. It is usually your decision to choose the appropriate method. Most often, you will use the oral route, but temperature should be taken rectally for infants, young children, and confused or unconscious patients, as well as for patients who have nasal packing or have had oral surgery. Also, if tubes or oxygen cause a patient to mouth-breathe, take a rectal temperature. And, if you have any doubt about the accuracy of an oral reading, again, take a rectal temperature.

Shake down glass thermometers with a quick snap of the wrist. They should register below 95° F or 36° C before you begin.

Oral Temperature   Provide adequate lighting so that when you obtain the temperature you can clearly read the measurement. Place a clean oral thermometer under the patient's

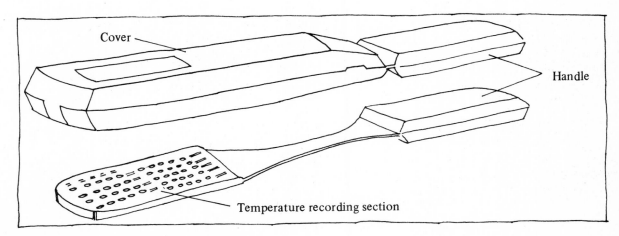

FIGURE 20.4 CHEMICAL THERMOMETER

tongue and instruct the patient to gently close the lips and breathe through the nose. Leave the thermometer in place for a full eight minutes. Studies show that oral thermometers left in the mouth for less than eight minutes can give incorrect readings: maximum temperature (highest reading) was reached in only 77.2 percent of the patients studied after six minutes; 88.4 percent, after seven minutes; and 94.6 percent, after eight minutes. In the past, a much shorter time was recommended, and some persons still follow the old guidelines. But, if you explain the need for the full eight minutes to patients, they are usually quite cooperative. Remove the thermometer and wipe it, with a twisting motion, from your fingers to the bulb—from clean to dirty. Discard the tissue. Hold the thermometer at eye level, read it without touching the bulb end, and write down your finding on paper. Then, shake down the thermometer.

Rectal Temperature So as not to damage the mucosa, first lubricate a clean rectal thermometer. Then insert it 1 to 1½ inches into the rectum, with the patient lying on his or her side. Always hold the thermometer with your hand to prevent displacement or breakage if the patient moves suddenly. Leave the thermometer in place for a full three minutes: only 92.6 percent of subjects studied measured maximum temperature after two minutes; the figure increased to 97.8 percent when the rectal thermometer remained in place for three minutes. Remove, clean, and read the thermometer as before. When you transfer the patient's temperature to the graphic form, mark (*R*) next to it, to indicate it was taken rectally.

Axillary Temperature Take axillary temperatures using the same general procedure. Place the thermometer in the patient's axilla with the bulb in the upward position. The patient's arm must be held close to the body with his or her forearm resting diagonally across the chest. Leave the thermometer in place for ten minutes.

Again, when you transfer the patient's temperature to the graphic form, mark (*A*) next to it, to indicate axillary measurement.

CLEANING THERMOMETERS

To clean a glass thermometer, carefully wipe it, with a twisting motion, from the tip held by the fingers to the mercury bulb (from clean to dirty). In this way, saliva and mucus are removed so that cleansing solutions will be effective. The thermometer can be kept at the patient's bedside after it has been washed with soap and cool water or soaked in solution. If you use a solution, thoroughly rinse it from the thermometer. In some facilities, wiped thermometers are collected and cleaned in a central supply area.

A product, a *thermometer sheath,* is available. The sheath keeps the thermometer itself from direct contact with the patient. The sheath is a very thin plastic tube that comes wrapped in a paper strip. To use, partially strip back the paper, according to directions, to expose the open end of the sheath. Insert the glass thermometer into the sheath and push downward, until it is completely protected except for the tip that you will hold in your hand. Then discard the paper covering. Insert the sheath-covered thermometer into the patient's mouth or rectum. Wait the appropriate time and then remove the thermometer. Pull the sheath downward over itself and discard. Read the thermometer. Because any microorganisms are enclosed in the sheath, you need only use a simple soap and cool water to wash the thermometer for reuse.

Pulse

Pulse rates vary greatly among adults. The American Heart Association states that a normal adult pulse rate may be 50 to 100 beats per minute. Also, the pulse rate can increase or decrease as a result of changes in body temperature. Exercise, the application of heat or cold, medications, emotions, hemorrhage, and heart disease can all affect pulse rates as well. The term *bradycardia* describes an adult pulse rate below 60 per minute; *tachycardia* refers to an adult pulse rate above 100.

RADIAL PULSE

Usually, you will use the radial artery at the wrist for taking the pulse. With some patients, this pulse may be indiscernible, and you will have to choose an alternate site, such as the temporal, femoral, or carotid artery. (See Figure 20.5.) Exert only light pressure, so that the artery is never completely occluded. Because a patient's position can modify the pulse, a resting pulse is usually taken with the patient in supine position for consistency.

Position the patient's arm alongside his or her body with the palm downward. Place your first three fingers lightly over the radial pulse and take the count for 15 seconds; then, multiply by 4 for a full-minute count. It has been shown that a 15-second count is as accurate, or more accurate, than a 30- or 60-second count. You can check pulse rate by repeating or extending the time period if necessary. Also determine pulse quality at this time. Use terms like *regular, irregular, bounding, thready,* and *weak.* Any pulse that is irregular should be taken for a full minute.

PEDAL PULSE

You can feel a pedal pulse by exerting light pressure with your fingers over the dorsalis pedis artery. This pulse is important in patients with compromised circulation or with possible restriction of the circulation of the lower extremities, as might be caused by tight dressings or casts.

APICAL-RADIAL PULSE

Apical-radial pulse, recorded *A/R,* is sometimes required for patients suffering cardiovascular disorders. It is always taken before the administration of cardiac drugs.

Two persons are necessary to take this pulse. Nurse 1 counts using the stethoscope

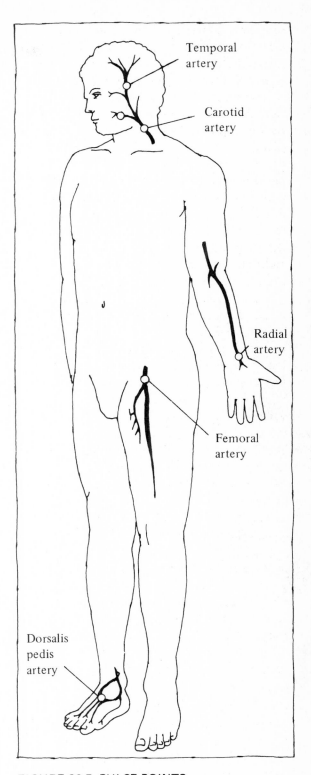

FIGURE 20.5 PULSE POINTS

over the apex of the heart below the nipple and slightly inside of the midclavicular line, while nurse 2 counts at the same time over the radial artery. Count for one full minute, using a single watch placed in a convenient location for both nurses to see.

If the radial pulse is lower than the apical, the difference is the *pulse deficit.* This means that some of the contractions of the heart are not sufficiently strong to push a wave of blood that can be felt at the radial site.

Respiration

All the factors that affect pulse rate will also cause the respiratory rate to vary. Normal adults breathe 16 to 20 times per minute. The rate as well as the rhythm may change when the patient is suffering from respiratory disorders. Also, the sides of the chest may not rise and fall symmetrically. Any difficulty in breathing is called *dyspnea.* (For more specific terms such as *stertorous, Kussmaul's respirations,* and *Cheyne-Stokes,* see Glossary.)

It is best to count respirations after taking the pulse. By using this sequence, you can keep your fingers on the patient's wrist and place the patient's arm across his or her chest. The patient should be unaware that you are doing another procedure and thus will continue to breathe naturally. Feeling the rise and fall of the patient's chest, you count for the required 30 seconds. Multiply the result by 2 to determine the rate for a full minute. If a patient's respirations are very irregular, you may choose to count for a full minute for accuracy.

Don't forget to record the patient's breathing characteristics.

Recording Vital Signs

Whether you take temperature, pulse, and respiration at the same time with a particular patient depends on your facility. Pulse and respiration are usually taken as a single procedure.

When you are assigned to several patients, you'll find the readings are sometimes difficult to remember. Keep a piece of paper in your pocket, so that after you have washed your hands, you can jot down the figures. Then transfer these numbers onto a team vital signs clipboard or notebook and, later, onto a graphic form in the patient's chart. Check with your facility for the routine to be used.

PERFORMANCE CHECKLIST

	Unsatisfactory	Needs more practice	Satisfactory	Comments
Electric thermometers				
Read manufacturer's handbook for variations in use.				
Oral temperature				
1. Wash your hands.				
2. Explain procedure and elicit patient's cooperation.				
3. Obtain proper thermometer.				
4. Check for adequate lighting.				
5. Shake down below 95° F or 36° C.				
6. Place thermometer under patient's tongue.				
7. Instruct patient to gently close mouth.				
8. Leave in place eight minutes.				
9. Remove and wipe thermometer with a downward twisting motion, clean to dirty.				
10. Read at eye level.				
11. Record finding on slip of paper.				
12. Replace in container in patient's unit or in appropriate receptacle labeled "dirty thermometers."				
13. Wash your hands.				
14. Transfer record to graphic form in patient's chart.				
Rectal temperature				
1. Wash your hands.				
2. Explain procedure and elicit patient's cooperation.				
3. Check for adequate lighting.				
4. Obtain equipment: a. Rectal thermometer				
b. Lubricant on tissue				
5. Position patient in Sim's position.				
6. Drape for privacy.				
7. Shake down below 95° F or 36° C.				
8. Insert lubricated thermometer 1 to 1½ inches, lifting buttocks slightly.				
9. Hold on to thermometer.				

	Unsatisfactory	Needs more practice	Satisfactory	Comments
10. Leave in place three minutes.				
11. Remove and wipe clean with tissue, clean to dirty.				
12. Read at eye level.				
13. Place in container or in utility room.				
14. Wash your hands.				
15. Transfer temperature to graphic, marking (*R*).				
Axillary temperature				
1. Wash your hands.				
2. Explain procedure and elicit patient's cooperation.				
3. Obtain proper thermometer.				
4. Check for adequate lighting.				
5. Shake down thermometer below 95° F or 36° C.				
6. Place thermometer in dry axilla, directed upward. Place patient's arm across chest.				
7. Hold end of thermometer.				
8. Leave in place ten minutes.				
9. Remove and read at eye level.				
10. Record finding on slip of paper.				
11. Place thermometer in container or in utility room.				
12. Wash your hands.				
13. Transfer temperature to graphic, marking (*A*).				

	Unsatisfactory	Needs more practice	Satisfactory	Comments
Radial pulse				
1. Wear watch with sweep second hand.				
2. Wash your hands.				
3. Explain procedure and elicit patient's cooperation.				
4. Place patient's arm next to body with palm downward.				
5. Place your first three fingers against radial artery.				
6. With gentle pressure, feel for pulsation.				
7. Count for appropriate time period; 15 seconds, 30 seconds, or full minute.				
8. Wash your hands.				
9. Record. Note unusual rate or quality.				
Apical-radial pulse				
1. Obtain stethoscope and watch with sweep second hand.				
2. Wash your hands.				
3. Explain procedure and elicit patient's cooperation.				
4. Drape left side of chest.				
5. Place watch between two nurses performing procedure, within view of both.				
6. Nurse 1 places stethoscope over apex of heart; nurse 2 places fingers over radial artery.				
7. Decide on start of counting time.				
8. Silently, but simultaneously, count for full minute: one person over apex, one person using radial artery.				
9. Wash your hands.				
10. Record as *A/R*.				
Respiration				
1. With fingers still in place after taking pulse rate, note rise and fall of patient's chest with respiration.				
2. Count for 30 seconds and multiply by 2 for full-minute count.				
3. Wash your hands.				
4. Record, noting unusual characteristics.				

QUIZ

Short-Answer Questions

1. The normal oral temperature for the average adult is _____ 37° C or _____ 98.6° F.

2. Four factors that may significantly change body temperature are

   a. _Time of day._

   b. _Presence of infection._

   c. _Emotional status_

   d. _If pt was drinking hot/cold liquids._

3. The bulb of the rectal thermometer should be lubricated in order to

   _____

4. The oral thermometer should be held in place _____ 8 _____ minutes; the rectal thermometer, _____ 3 _____ minutes; the axillary thermometer, _____ 10 _____ minutes; and the electric thermometer, _30 sec._ .

5. Place a *1* beside the most accurate method of obtaining a temperature reading, a *2* beside the next most accurate method, and a *3* beside the least accurate method.

   _____ 3 _____ Axillary

   _____ 1 _____ Rectal

   _____ 2 _____ Oral

6. Normal pulse range for the adult at rest is _____ 60 _____ to _____ 100 _____ .

7. Four common factors that can alter pulse rate are

   a. _Exercise_

   b. _Heat or cold application_

   c. _Emotions_

   d. _Medications_

8. Three arteries that can be conveniently used for counting the pulse rate are

   a. _Temporal_

   b. _Radial_

   c. _Carotid_

9. The normal rate of respiration for the adult at rest is _____ 16 _____ to _____ 20 _____ .

10. Four factors that cause changes in respiration are

   a. _Emotions_____

   b. _If pt. was exercising, walking_____

   c. _Type of disease_____

   d. _Medications_____

Module 21 Blood Pressure

MAIN OBJECTIVE

To accurately measure and record blood pressure using a cuff, sphygmomanometer, and stethoscope.

RATIONALE

Blood pressure is the pressure exerted by the blood in the arteries of the body. It serves, in combination with other observations, as an indicator of the circulatory status of patients.

The nurse must be able to measure and record blood pressure accurately, and to interpret that measurement in light of individual patients. To do this effectively, the nurse must know the norms and variables that affect blood pressure.

PREREQUISITES

Successful completion of the following modules:

VOLUME 1
Assessment
Charting
Medical Asepsis
Temperature, Pulse, and Respiration

SPECIFIC LEARNING OBJECTIVES

SPECIFIC LEARNING OBJECTIVES	Know Facts and Principles	Apply Facts and Principles	Demonstrate Ability	Evaluate Performance
1. *Definition* a. *Systolic BP* b. *Diastolic BP* c. *Normals* d. *Variables*	Define systolic and diastolic blood pressures. State norms for adults and children. List variables that affect blood pressure.	Given a patient situation, identify variables that might affect blood pressure. Given a patient situation, identify potential relationships between blood pressure and pulse. State rationale for taking blood pressure.	Promptly report blood pressures not within textbook norms as well as significant variations from baseline for particular patient	
2. *Equipment* a. *Cuff* b. *Bladder* c. *Hand bulb and valve* d. *Sphygmomanometer (mercury gauge and aneroid gauge)* e. *Stethoscope*	Identify equipment involved in taking blood pressure. State use for equipment involved in taking blood pressure.	Identify missing or malfunctioning equipment		Evaluate own performance with instructor using Performance Checklist
3. *Procedure* a. *Placement of cuff* b. *Estimation of systolic pressure* c. *Korotkoff sounds* d. *Systolic pressure* e. *Diastolic pressure*	State how blood pressure is correctly measured	Given a patient situation, identify correct and incorrect aspects of procedure	In the clinical setting, accurately measure patient's blood pressure	Blood pressure measurement by student is within 4 mm Hg of that taken by instructor
4. *Charting*	Know how to chart blood pressure on graphic and narrative records	Given a patient situation, identify correct charting of blood pressure	Accurately chart blood pressure on appropriate records	Evaluate own performance with instructor

LEARNING ACTIVITIES

1. Review the Specific Learning Objectives.
2. Read the section on circulation (in the chapter on basic vital functions) in Ellis and Nowlis, *Nursing: A Human Needs Approach,* or comparable material in another textbook.
3. Look up the module vocabulary terms in the glossary.
4. Read through the module.
5. In the practice setting:
   a. Look over and identify the parts of the blood pressure equipment in the practice setting and the clinical facility. How are they alike? Are there ways in which they differ?
   b. After reading over the procedure carefully, practice it, using another student as a patient, until you feel you can perform it adequately.
   c. Using a double, or "teaching," stethoscope (if one is available), measure the blood pressure of your partner with your instructor. If no teaching stethoscope is available, have your instructor check your blood pressure measurement on the same arm two minutes later. Repeat, using palpation. Repeat, doing a thigh pressure if equipment is available.
   d. Chart the arm blood pressure measurement on a graphic record as well as on a narrative record, including some mock observations of your "patient." Have your instructor look it over and make comments.
6. In the clinical setting:
   a. Under your instructor's supervision, measure the blood pressure of a patient and record it appropriately.

VOCABULARY

aneroid manometer
antecubital space
brachial artery
diaphragm
diastolic blood pressure
Korotkoff sounds
palpation
popliteal artery
radial artery
sphygmomanometer
stethoscope
supine position
systolic blood pressure

BLOOD PRESSURE

Norms and Variables

Generally speaking, blood pressure increases with age, being lowest in the newborn (approximately 40/20) and gradually increasing during childhood and adolescence to adult level (approximately 120/80). Blood pressure, however, varies considerably with the individual. Hence, a normal reading is usually identified as being within a certain range. For example, the normal range for adults is 110-140/60-90. A systolic blood pressure over 160 or a diastolic blood pressure over 100 is termed *hypertensive*; a systolic blood pressure below 100 is termed *hypotensive.* Blood pressure, however, is only one piece of data and must be evaluated in the context of an entire situation, not as an isolated event.

Many factors can affect blood pressure. Activity, anxiety, strong emotion, recent intake of food, disease, pain and drugs can all cause a *rise* in blood pressure. A *fall* in blood pressure is caused by blood loss or anything that causes blood vessels to dilate.

Equipment

What is commonly referred to as the *blood pressure cuff* really consists of an oblong rubber bag, or *bladder,* covered with a non-expandable fabric called the *cuff.* (See Figure 21.1.)

The *hand bulb* is a device attached to the bladder by a rubber tube through which air is pumped. The valve on the hand bulb opens, closes, and is regulated with a thumbscrew, allowing air to escape from the bladder at the desired rate.

The *mercury manometer* is manufactured in a variety of models, including a floor model (which can be moved from one place to another), a portable model that comes in a box, and a wall model (which is probably the most common). The mercury rises in a calibrated glass tube as the cuff is inflated with air and then falls as the air is released.

Rubber tubing connects the mercury reservoir with the cuff.

The *aneroid manometer* is an air pressure gauge that indicates the blood pressure by a pointer on a dial. The dial generally attaches to the cuff by hooks that fit into a small pocket.

The *stethoscope* is an instrument used for listening to body sounds. The *diaphragm* (flat surface) of the stethoscope is usually used for listening when blood pressure is measured.

WIDTH OF THE CUFF

Surprisingly, the width of the blood pressure cuff is important. If it is too narrow, it may yield a reading that is higher than the correct one; if it is too wide, it may yield a reading that is lower than the correct one. According to the American Heart Association, the cuff should be 20 percent wider than the diameter of the limb on which it is being used. Most facilities have at least three sizes: child, adult, and thigh (which is also used for arm pressures in obese persons). A child's cuff could be used for a very thin adult as well.

Procedure

1. Wash your hands.
2. Take the necessary equipment to the patient's bedside. Some facilities have a wall-mounted mercury gauge and a cuff at the bedside, and sometimes even a stethoscope. In other places, you will have to bring all the necessary equipment with you.
3. Introduce yourself to the patient and explain what you plan to do. Allow the patient to ask questions. Remember that many variables can affect blood pressure; be aware of such things as medications, recent activity, position, emotional state, recent meals, and pain.
4. Diminish room noise (radio, television, visitors' conversation). Also remind the patient not to talk to you while you are listening for the blood pressure.

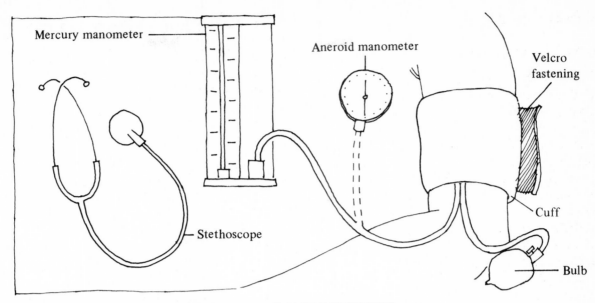

FIGURE 21.1   EQUIPMENT FOR MEASURING BLOOD PRESSURE

5. Position the patient. Blood pressure is usually measured with the patient in the supine position, but it can be measured using the sitting or standing position if so ordered. The patient's arm should be in a position of comfort, either stretched out beside the body in bed or on the arm of the chair, palm up. Usually either arm can be used, although the presence of a cast, bandage, or intravenous are some reasons why you might choose one arm over the other. In the rare cases where it is not possible to take an arm pressure, you can use the patient's leg instead of an arm. In any case, you should either remove any clothing in the way or roll up the patient's sleeves or pant legs. Do not attempt to apply the cuff over any bulky materials.

6. Wrap the blood pressure cuff around the arm above the elbow, making sure the rubber bladder is centered over the brachial artery. The lower edge of the cuff should be about 1 inch above the antecubital space (fossa). Wrap the cuff neatly and snugly, and attach it securely. There are many ways to secure the cuff, but Velcro is currently the most common method. If there is an aneroid gauge attached, place it where it can be easily read. Otherwise, the mercury manometer should be at eye level.

7. Place the stethoscope earpieces in your ears. This is a little sooner than is necessary, but it is handier if you are ready ahead of time. If you are not using your own stethoscope, wipe off the earpieces with alcohol before you use it.

8. Feel for the brachial artery, which is located near the center of the antecubital space, toward the little finger.

9. Keeping your fingers over the brachial artery, turn the valve on the hand bulb clockwise until it is tight.

10. Pump the hand bulb to fill the rubber bladder in the blood pressure cuff with air. As you pump, the gauge will register. Pump until you no longer feel a pulse and continue for 30 mm mercury beyond that point. (The radial artery can also be used for this purpose.)

11. Place the diaphragm of the stethoscope over the brachial artery. Wipe the diaphragm with an alcohol swab between patients to maintain medical asepsis.

12. Open the valve on the hand bulb (turning it counterclockwise) gradually, releasing the air from the rubber bladder, and watch the pressure registered on the gauge decrease.

13. Note the pressure at which you hear the first *regular* tapping sounds gradually getting louder. Sometimes you will hear sounds that you will think are first sounds, but they will not be regular nor will they get louder, so they are considered extraneous. The pressure at which you hear the first sound is called the *systolic blood pressure,* the point at which the heart is beating *(systole)* and exerting its greatest force.

14. Continue to open the valve gradually, listening for a muffling sound. Note both the point of muffling and the point at which the sound disappears. Facilities differ as to which of these two sounds they consider the *diastolic pressure* (the point at which the heart is relaxing and filling with blood).

15. If you want to double-check the blood pressure measurement, wait two minutes and then repeat on the same arm.

16. Remove the cuff from the patient's arm and remove the stethoscope earpieces from your ears. (Wipe the earpieces with an alcohol swab unless it is your personal stethoscope.) Store the equipment properly.

17. Wash your hands.

18. Record your findings on the patient's chart. In some facilities, only two numbers are recorded. In such instances, you will have to know which of the two lower sounds is considered the diastolic pressure and, hence, recorded. The American Heart Association recommends recording all three pressures, as follows:

140 / 80 / 68

If you do not hear all three points, use a dash to indicate the sound that was not heard, as follows:

140 / — / 68

If you hear beats all the way to zero, record your finding as follows:

140 / 80 / 0

The graph shown in Figure 21.2 demonstrates one method of display.

Measurement at the Thigh

There will be times when it is necessary to measure blood pressure using the thigh. In such an instance, use an appropriately larger cuff (usually 18 to 20 cm, which is 6 cm wider than the arm cuff) and position the patient on his or her abdomen. If the patient cannot lie on his or her abdomen, the knee may be slightly flexed with the patient in the supine position.

Place your stethoscope over the popliteal artery, and measure the patient's blood pressure, as you did in the preceding procedure, with the cuff applied at midthigh. "Comparison of intra-arterial blood pressure in the arms and legs in humans shows that the femoral systolic pressure is only a few millimeters of mercury higher, and the diastolic a few millimeters lower, than comparable arm pressure." [1]

Measurement During Shock

It may be very difficult to hear Korotkoff sounds when a patient is in a state of clinical shock. When you cannot hear Korotkoff sounds, measure systolic blood pressure by palpation. (The diastolic pressure cannot be measured in this manner.) The procedure is the same except that no stethoscope is used and the first pulsation felt is considered the systolic pressure. Direct arterial blood pressure monitoring is also appropriate in these cases. This type of blood pressure monitoring requires sophisticated equipment, which is usually available only in intensive-care settings.

[1] Kirkendall, Walter M., *et al.,* "Recommendations for Human Blood Pressure Determination by Sphygmomanometers" (New York: American Heart Association, 1967).

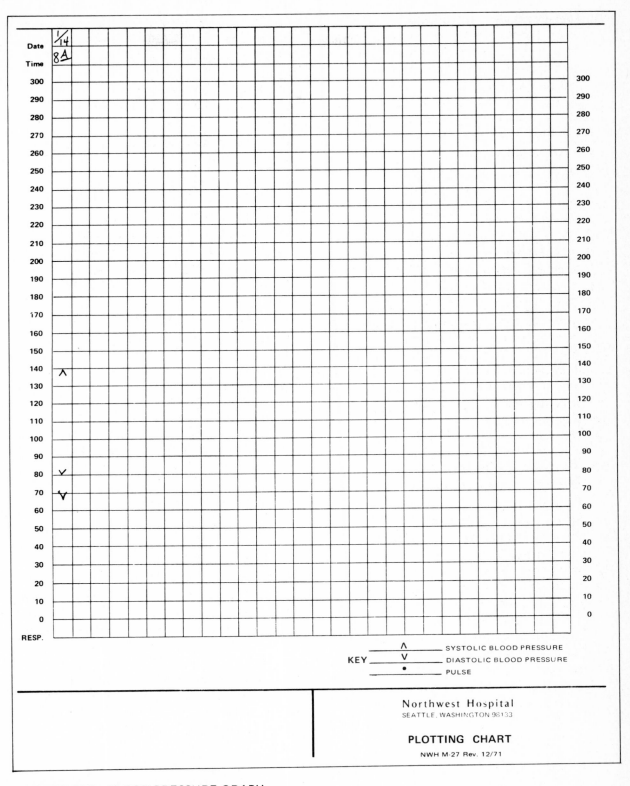

FIGURE 21.2 BLOOD PRESSURE GRAPH
Courtesy Northwest Hospital

PERFORMANCE CHECKLIST

	Unsatisfactory	Needs more practice	Satisfactory	Comments
1. Wash your hands.				
2. Gather equipment.				
3. Explain procedure to patient.				
4. Diminish room noise.				
5. Position patient.				
6. Apply blood pressure cuff.				
7. Place stethoscope earpieces in your ears.				
8. Locate patient's brachial artery.				
9. Close valve on hand bulb, and pump hand bulb to 30 mm mercury above last pulse felt.				
10. Place diaphragm of stethoscope over brachial artery and release valve.				
11. Note first sound, muffling, and last sound heard.				
12. Remove cuff from patient's arm and earpieces from your ears.				
13. Wash your hands.				
14. Record appropriately, including narrative as necessary.				

QUIZ

Multiple-Choice Questions

_____ 1. Factors that can affect blood pressure include (1) age; (2) height; (3) recent activity; (4) position; (5) recent meals; (6) pain.

    a. 1 and 3
    b. 1, 2, 3, and 5
    c. 1, 3, 4, 5, and 6
    d. 3, 4, 5, and 6

_____ 2. The usual position for a hospitalized patient to assume during blood pressure measurement is

    a. sitting.
    b. prone.
    c. supine.
    d. lateral.

_____ 3. The diaphragm of the stethoscope should be placed over which artery to measure blood pressure in the arm?

    a. Radial
    b. Brachial
    c. Femoral
    d. Carotid

_____ 4. The first sound you hear on release of the hand bulb valve indicates

    a. systolic pressure.
    b. diastolic pressure.
    c. pulse pressure.
    d. You cannot tell by one sound.

_____ 5. The point at which the heart is beating and exerting its greatest force is called

    a. systolic pressure.
    b. diastolic pressure.
    c. pulse pressure.
    d. basal pressure.

_____ 6. If you want to double-check a blood pressure measurement, how long should you wait before remeasuring on the same arm?

    a. 30 seconds
    b. One minute
    c. Two minutes
    d. It makes no difference.

Short-Answer Question

7. If the systolic pressure is heard at 140, the point of muffling is heard at
   80, and the last sound heard is at 70, what would the correct form for

   recording the blood pressure be? _____

Module 22 Isolation Technique

MAIN OBJECTIVE

To carry out correct isolation technique, placing emphasis on safety for patients, visitors, staff, and self.

RATIONALE

The isolation of hospitalized patients becomes necessary for a variety of reasons. Whatever the reason, the nurse must understand the rationale and be able to correctly carry out the procedure. This is true, not only to perform correctly, but so that explanations can be given to the patient, patient's family, and auxiliary staff regarding the procedures and the reasons for them.

There are a number of isolation procedures: one that protects the patient and several that protect the hospital staff. In this module, we will discuss the preparation of the isolation room and the procedure for entering the isolation room as well as give some consideration to sensory deprivation and its implications for the nurse.

PREREQUISITES

Successful completion of the following module:

VOLUME 1
Medical Asepsis

SPECIFIC LEARNING OBJECTIVES

	Know Facts and Principles	Apply Facts and Principles	Demonstrate Ability	Evaluate Performance

1. *Purpose*
   a. To protect patient
   b. To protect environment
	Know two major purposes of isolation	Given a patient situation, identify which of two major purposes of isolation should be utilized		

2. *Types*
   a. Rationale
   b. Protective
   c. Strict
   d. Respiratory
   e. Wound (dressing)
   f. Enteric
	Discuss various types of isolation and rationale for use of each	Given a patient situation, identify type of isolation procedure appropriate	In the clinical area, choose appropriate type of isolation for use with patient	Evaluate own performance with instructor

3. *Procedures*
   a. Preparing room
   b. Entering room (gown, mask, gloves)
   c. Bagging out
   d. Leaving isolation room
   e. Transporting patient in isolation
	Describe various procedures necessary for patient isolation	Given a patient situation, state which procedure would be appropriate to carry out	Carry out various types of isolation procedures correctly	Evaluate own performance with instructor using Performance Checklist

4. *Teaching*	List important facts to teach patient, family, and auxiliary staff	Given a patient situation, plan teaching appropriate for type of isolation	Instruct patient, family, and auxiliary staff on isolation procedure	Evaluate own performance with patient, family, staff, and instructor
5. *Sensory deprivation*	State causes and effects of sensory (social) deprivation. List techniques that can be used to prevent and/or decrease effects of sensory deprivation.	Given a patient situation, identify possible effects of sensory deprivation and list nursing techniques that could be used to decrease them	Recognize potential and real effects of sensory deprivation and use nursing techniques to intervene	Evaluate own performance by sharing experience with instructor and/or classmate

LEARNING ACTIVITIES

1. Review the Specific Learning Objectives.
2. Read the section on isolation (in the chapter on infection) in Ellis and Nowlis, *Nursing: A Human Needs Approach,* or comparable material in another textbook.
3. Look up the module vocabulary terms in the glossary.
4. Read through the module.
5. In the practice setting:
   a. With a partner, practice preparing to enter and leave the various types of isolation rooms: protective, strict, respiratory, wound (dressing), and enteric. Evaluate each other's performance, using the Performance Checklist.
   b. With a partner, practice double-bagging, alternating so that each of you has a turn being the person inside the room and outside the room. After you have done the procedure the first time, evaluate yourselves using the Performance Checklist. Then switch roles and repeat the procedure. Again, evaluate yourselves and repeat the procedure as necessary.
   c. When you are satisfied that you can carry out the procedure, have your instructor evaluate your performances.
6. In the clinical setting:
   a. Consult your clinical instructor for an opportunity to carry out isolation procedure.

VOCABULARY

isolation
microorganisms
sensory deprivation

ISOLATION TECHNIQUE

Types of Isolation

There are four types of isolation generally used to protect other people from the pathogens infecting a given patient; strict isolation, respiratory isolation, wound and skin precautions, and enteric precautions. Protective isolation is used to protect the patient from pathogens in the environment.

Strict isolation is used when the identified pathogens are transmitted through the air and by contact. Precautions to be taken include placing the patient in a private room with the door *closed;* wearing a gown, mask, and gloves when entering the room; washing hands on entering and leaving the room; and double-bagging (for decontamination) linens and other articles used in the care of the patient.

Respiratory isolation is used when the pathogens involved are airborne. A private room with the door closed is desirable. Gowns and gloves are not necessary, but masks *are* necessary, and hands should be washed on entering and leaving. Any article contaminated with secretions from the patient must be disinfected or double-bagged for disposal or decontamination.

Wound and skin precautions are used when the patient has a wound infected with microorganisms that can be spread by contact. Actual isolation is not required, but a private room is desirable. Gowns must be worn when in direct contact with the patient, masks are necessary during dressing changes only, and gloves should be used when in direct contact with the infected area. Hands are washed on leaving and entering the room. Instruments, dressings, and linens must be double-bagged for decontamination or disposal.

Enteric precautions are used when the pathogens involved are transmitted by direct contact with the gastrointestinal system. A private room is necessary for the pediatric patient. Gowns must be worn when in direct contact with the patient, gloves when in direct contact with the patient or

with contaminated material. Masks are not necessary, and hands are washed on entering and leaving the room. Linen should be double-bagged. Urine, feces or vomitus should be discarded in an adjoining *private* bathroom, and any articles contaminated with them must be discarded or disinfected. (Urine is included because of the proximity of the urinary and intestinal tracts.)

Protective isolation is used when a patient is particularly susceptible to infection and needs protection from the pathogens in the environment. A private room with the door closed is required. Gowns and masks must be worn by all who enter the room. Gloves need be worn only by those having direct contact with the patient. Hands are washed on entering and leaving the room. All items taken into the room should be individually evaluated for their potential to contaminate and harm the patient. Since the room and its contents are considered clean, no special measures are needed when removing articles and linens.

Preparing the Room

The preparation of a room for isolation procedure varies somewhat depending on the type of isolation that is needed. In general, you should remove all items of furniture and equipment that are not necessary to the care of the patient and collect and include all items that are necessary. In addition to routine health care items, you will need the following:

1. A private room with running water.
2. A sign on the outside of the door, preferably indicating what preparation is necessary to enter the room as well as what type of isolation is being carried out. (See Figures 22.1–22.6.)
3. An extra stand of some sort (often extra bedside stands are used), placed immediately outside the door to hold isolation laundry bags, gowns, masks, gloves, and other items specific to the care of individual patients. In some hospitals, these stands are prepared and

Protective Isolation
Visitors—Report to Nurses' Station Before Entering Room

1. **Private Room**—*necessary;* door must be kept closed.

2. **Gowns**—must be worn by all persons entering room.

3. **Masks**—must be worn by all persons entering room.

4. **Hands**—must be washed on entering and leaving room.

5. **Gloves**—must be worn by all persons having direct contact with patient.

6. **Articles**—*see* manual text.

FIGURE 22.1 PROTECTIVE ISOLATION SIGN
Courtesy Shamrock, Inc., Bellwood, Illinois

Respiratory Isolation
Visitors-Report to Nurses' Station Before Entering Room

1. **Private Room**—*desirable;* door or curtain should be kept closed whenever possible.

2. **Gowns**—not necessary.

3. **Masks**—must be worn by all persons entering room if susceptible to disease.

4. **Hands**—must be washed on entering and leaving room.

5. **Gloves**—not necessary.

6. **Articles**—those contaminated with secretions must be disinfected.

7. **Caution**—all persons susceptible to the specific disease should be excluded from patient area; if contact is necessary, susceptibles must wear masks.

FIGURE 22.2 RESPIRATORY ISOLATION SIGN
Courtesy Shamrock, Inc., Bellwood, Illinois

Wound & Skin Precautions
Visitors—Report to Nurses' Station Before Entering Room

1. **Private Room**—desirable.

2. **Gowns**—must be worn by all persons having direct contact with patient.

3. **Masks**—not necessary except during dressing changes.

4. **Hands**—must be washed on entering and leaving room.

5. **Gloves**—must be worn by all persons having direct contact with infected area.

6. **Articles**—special precautions necessary for instruments, dressings, and linen.

NOTE: *See* Manual for Special Dressing Techniques to be used when changing dressings.

FIGURE 22.3   WOUND AND SKIN PRECAUTIONS SIGN
Courtesy Shamrock, Inc., Bellwood, Illinois

Enteric Precautions
Visitors-Report to Nurses' Station Before Entering Room

1. **Private Room**

2. **Gowns**—must be worn by all persons having direct contact with patient.

3. **Masks**—not necessary.

4. **Hands**—must be washed on entering and leaving room.

5. **Gloves**—must be worn by all persons having direct contact with patient or with articles contaminated with fecal material.

6. **Articles**—special precautions necessary for articles contaminated with urine and feces. Articles must be disinfected or discarded.

FIGURE 22.4   ENTERIC PRECAUTIONS SIGN
Courtesy Shamrock, Inc., Bellwood, Illinois

Strict Isolation
Visitors-Report to Nurses' Station Before Entering Room

1. **Private Room**—*necessary;* door must be kept closed.
2. **Gowns**—must be worn by all persons entering room.
3. **Masks**—must be worn by all persons entering room.
4. **Hands**—must be washed on entering and leaving room.
5. **Gloves**—must be worn by all persons entering room.
6. **Articles**—must be discarded, or wrapped before being sent to Central Supply for disinfection or sterilization.

FIGURE 22.5   STRICT ISOLATION SIGN
Courtesy Shamrock, Inc., Bellwood, Illinois

Hepatitis Precautions
Visitors and Non-Unit Personnel Report to Nurse Before Entering Room

1. **Hands Must Be Washed**—before and after patient contact.
2. **Gowns and Gloves**—necessary when in direct contact with the patient's excretions.
3. **Excretion Precautions**—necessary.
4. **Linen and Dish Precautions**—(disposable dishes) necessary.
5. **Contaminated Needles and Syringes**—handle with extreme care.
6. **Aftercare of Equipment and Terminal Disinfection**—necessary.

FIGURE 22.6   HEPATITIS PRECAUTIONS
Courtesy Shamrock, Inc., Bellwood, Illinois

and kept in the central supply department and simply requisitioned when needed.

4. A laundry hamper for inside the room.
5. A wastebasket (preferably large) lined with plastic.
6. A thermometer and blood pressure equipment, which should be left in the room.
7. Special containers as needed for used needles, syringes, and instruments.

Entering the Room

One component of care that will prove very helpful as you prepare to enter an isolation room is *organization*. See that you have all the equipment you need before you are gowned and in the room. To stand helpless in the room waiting for someone else to bring you forgotten items is frustrating to you and other workers, not to mention the patient.

You will need some or all of the following equipment as you prepare to enter any kind of isolation room to care for a patient.

GOWN

1. Wash your hands. (See Module 3, Medical Asepsis.) It is a good idea to remove any rings you usually wear because the regular handwashing procedure may not remove microorganisms that lodge beneath rings. If there is no wall clock in the room and you need a watch to care for the patient, remove your watch and place it in a plastic bag, so that it is protected but still visible.
2. Put on a gown, making sure that all parts of your uniform are covered and that the ties are tied securely. (Some of the paper gowns use tapes.)

MASK

1. If they are necessary for the care of the patient, there should be a supply of masks outside the room. Masks can be made of cloth or of one of a variety of the disposable materials currently available. Most have time limits for usage and must be changed periodically if you are in the room for an extended period of time. In any event, they should be worn only once. If you wear a nursing cap, remove it.
2. Fasten both sets of ties securely.
3. If you wear glasses, tuck the mask under the lower edge of your glasses (the disposable masks sometimes have a metal strip that can be molded to fit snugly over the bridge of your nose and under your eyes) to prevent the glasses from steaming up.

GLOVES

1. There should be a supply of gloves outside the room if they are necessary for the care of the patient. They will be *clean* gloves. If sterile gloves are needed for a special procedure, take them into the room and don them there.
2. There is no special way to put on nonsterile gloves. You should, however, tuck the cuffs of your sleeves in securely. Paper gowns sometimes do not have cuffs and tend to slide out of gloves easily. Use masking tape to keep the gown secure in the gloves. Let a second person do the taping for you.

Double-Bagging

1. Use a double-bagging technique for all items coming out of an isolation room (except for a protective isolation room). If you are inside the room caring for a patient, place used items into appropriate containers: linen into the linen hamper, glass bottles and jars into a brown paper bag, and paper garbage into a wastebasket lined with plastic. Take care not to fill the bags too full because full bags are difficult to double-bag without breaking technique.

2. To carry out this procedure, you will need another nurse outside the room. The outside nurse forms a cuff with the upper edge of the appropriate bag, a laundry bag (usually with special markings) for linen and paper and/or plastic bags for glass and trash. The cuff protects the hands of the outside nurse from the contaminated articles.
3. Carefully close the inside bag and place it directly into the bag held by the outside nurse, being careful to touch only the inside of that bag (Figure 22.7).
4. The outside nurse then folds over and carefully secures the top of the outside bag, marking it in the manner prescribed by the facility. Isolation linen bags are often red (as opposed to another color for regular linen) or have a red stripe sewn on them. Brightly colored plastic tape can be used to mark the paper

and/or plastic bags. A felt-tipped marking pen is often used to indicate the contents of the bag, so that proper sterilization or destruction processes can be carried out. Check the procedure book at your facility for any special procedures related to the care of non-disposable equipment.

Note: If glass jars or bottles are being sent to be sterilized or incinerated, do not put lids or caps on them. A bottle or jar with a cap or lid in place will explode in an autoclave or incinerator, possibly causing injury to hospital staff.

Leaving the Room

This procedure assumes you are wearing a gown, mask, and gloves. It can be modified if all three are not being used.

1. Complete your work in the room.
2. Remove your gloves. With your left hand, peel the right glove off from the cuff, being careful not to touch your skin with your left glove. Then remove the left glove by placing one or two fingers of your right hand *inside* the glove and pulling it off. This procedure can be reversed if you are left-handed. Discard the gloves in the appropriate container.
3. Wash your hands.
4. Untie your mask and discard it carefully in a wastebasket or, if it is a cloth mask, in a laundry hamper, touching the *ties only.*
5. Wash your hands.
6. Untie your gown. Touching it only on the *inside,* pull it off, turning it inside out as you work, and carefully fold it with all outside surfaces toward the center (Figure 22.8). Place it in the laundry hamper.
7. Open the door, using a paper towel as a barrier on the doorknob. Discard the paper towel *inside* the room.
8. Wash your hands outside the room.

Note: The "reuse" technique for gowns is seldom used, except perhaps in protective-

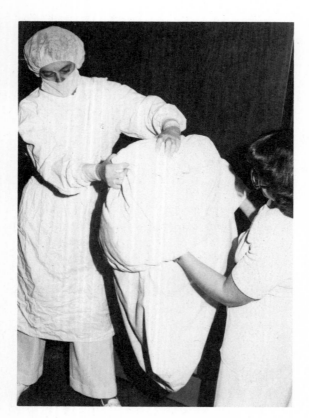

FIGURE 22.7   DOUBLE-BAGGING
Courtesy Ivan Ellis

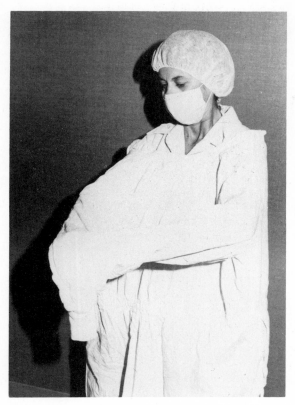

FIGURE 22.8   REMOVING AN ISOLATION GOWN
Courtesy Ivan Ellis

isolation situations. If it is used in your facility, check the procedure book to be certain you are following the exact procedure.

Cleaning or Disposing of Food Trays

Disposable eating containers and utensils for use by isolated patients are quite common now. In this case, dispose of excess liquids and soft foods in the toilet and the containers and utensils in the wastebasket. If the equipment is *not* disposable, *clean* dishes and silverware before double-bagging them and sending them for sterilization.

Transporting the Patient in Isolation

Although there may be times when a patient in isolation must be transported to another area, this should be done only when absolutely necessary. The necessary precautions vary according to the type of isolation in use.

In general, however, it is essential to keep in mind *who* you are protecting and from *what.* A patient in protective isolation must be protected from all those with whom he or she comes in contact; therefore, all who care for the patient in another department must wear gowns and masks. A patient in respiratory isolation must wear a mask; a patient in wound isolation should wear a gown outside his or her room. A patient on strict isolation must wear a gown and mask and should be covered by a sheet or bath blanket during transport. In addition, all items that are touched by the patient must be disinfected. Consult your facility procedure book for specific instructions.

Patient, Family, and Staff Cooperation

Among your many responsibilities with regard to isolation procedure is making certain that the patient and the patient's family understand the reasons for the type of isolation being carried out and that they respond to this knowledge with appropriate actions. This responsibility extends to the hospital staff and the physician as well. Remember that the chain will only be as strong as its weakest link.

It is probably true that *no one* likes isolation procedures, perhaps the patient least of all. For this reason, emphasize the do's rather than the don'ts: a positive approach may yield more in terms of observable results.

Combating Sensory Deprivation

Closely related to the idea that isolation procedure is extra work that no one really likes doing is the idea that patients in isolation feel that no one really wants to take care of them. This may be communicated by the fact that they are always the last to be cared for (and cold meals communicate a lot!), by careless remarks made outside doors but within hearing, and by countless nonverbal exchanges. In addition, those who *do* come in to see isolated patients (family, friends, staff) are often covered from head to toe, making normal communication impossible. Isolation rooms have generally been stripped of pictures, plants, and all other decorative items, making the total picture rather dismal. The variety of stimulation isolated patients receive is less, and it can be less meaningful too. There is usually a reduction in the amount of interaction these patients have with others. As a result, the patients can develop any one or combination of the following problems: decreased alertness and motivation, increased complaints, loneliness, depression, and anger.

There are some positive ways in which you can intervene in this process: give care to an isolated patient first, answer the call light promptly, stop by for a wave in the door. Provide the patient with puzzles, paperback books, and other paper items that can be burned. Often, the family can provide such items.

PERFORMANCE CHECKLIST

	Unsatisfactory	Needs more practice	Satisfactory	Comments
Entering the room				
1. Remove rings and watch, and wash your hands.				
2. Put on gown, making certain that all parts of your uniform are covered.				
3. Put on mask, tying both sets of ties securely.				
4. Put on gloves, tucking in cuffs of sleeves securely.				
Double-bagging				
1. Inside nurse: a. Place linen bag and/or paper bag inside bag being held by outside nurse. Be careful to touch only inside surface of outer bag.				
2. Outside nurse: a. Hold laundry bag or large paper bag, protecting hands with cuff formed at top edges.				
b. Carefully fold and secure top of bag, marking it in prescribed manner.				
Leaving the room				
1. Remove gloves, touching bare hands to *inside* surfaces only.				
2. Wash your hands.				
3. Untie mask ties and discard mask carefully, touching ties only.				
4. Wash your hands.				
5. Untie gown and remove it, touching only inside.				
6. Carefully fold gown with all outside surfaces toward center and place in laundry hamper.				
7. Open door, using paper towel as barrier.				
8. Wash your hands outside room.				

QUIZ

Short-Answer Questions

1. What are the two major purposes of isolation?

   a. _____

   b. _____

2. The organism that is causing Mr. Paulson's illness can be transmitted either by air or by contact. What type of isolation would be appropriate for him? _____

3. Mrs. Raymond is a post-op patient whose care has been complicated by the presence of a pathogen transmitted by direct contact, the mode of transmission being the gastrointestinal system. What type of isolation would be appropriate for her? _____

4. List three items required in the preparation of a room for isolation procedure.

   a. _____

   b. _____

   c. _____

5. How are items removed from a protective isolation room? _____
   _____

6. If you are the outside nurse bagging outside an isolation room and the inside bag touches your hand, what should you do? _____
   _____

7. A patient with severe leukemia has been ordered placed in isolation. What is the purpose of isolation for this patient? _____
   _____

   Situation: Mrs. Rogers has been in isolation for ten days. She seems irritable and shows no interest in eating or the activities ordered by the physician.

8. What could be the source of her problem? _____

9. List at least three nursing actions that might help Mrs. Rogers.

   a. _____

   b. _____

   c. _____

Module 23 Assisting with Examinations and Procedures

MAIN OBJECTIVE

To assist the examiner with the physical examination or diagnostic and therapeutic procedures, with emphasis on the preparation and support of patients.

RATIONALE

Although the sophistication of laboratory and radiological tests has increased remarkably in recent years, the foundation of diagnosis remains the physical examination. Examinations are also used to establish a baseline of patients' health status, as well as to rule out concurrent disease. The nurse who has special training in primary care may perform a physical examination as an important part of assessment; however, in most facilities, this remains the responsibility of the physician. Therefore, the nurse should gain knowledge that will make him or her a skillful and effective assistant.

PREREQUISITES

Successful completion of the following modules:

VOLUME 1
Assessment
Charting
Medical Asepsis
Range-of-Motion Exercises
Collecting Specimens
Temperature, Pulse, and Respiration

VOLUME 2
Inspection, Palpation, Auscultation, and Percussion
Sterile Technique

341

SPECIFIC LEARNING OBJECTIVES

	Know Facts and Principles	Apply Facts and Principles	Demonstrate Ability	Evaluate Performance
Assisting with a physical examination				
1. Equipment	List common equipment used to perform physical examinations	Identify each piece of equipment for part being examined	Gather appropriate equipment for examination	Evaluate own performance using Performance Checklist
2. Nurse's role in assisting	State two responsibilities of nurse and physician when performing physical examination			
3. Physical and psychological preparation of patient	Explain methods for preparing patient physically and psychologically	In the practice setting, prepare partner physically and psychologically	In the clinical setting, prepare patient physically and psychologically for test	Evaluate preparation through patient interview after procedure
4. Procedure a. Positioning for system being examined b. Sequence of physical examination	Name usual sequence for carrying out physical examination and position used with each step	With partner, simulate physical examination using sequence and position variations	Under supervision, assist physician in performing physical examination on patient	Evaluate with instructor
c. Findings	Briefly describe several findings from each part of examination		In the clinical area, relate to instructor signs and symptoms found	
d. Recording	List observations to be recorded	Practice recording of assisting with physical examination	Record procedure correctly on chart	Evaluate own performance using Performance Checklist

Assisting with diagnostic and therapeutic procedure				
1. Equipment	Name equipment needed for six procedures described	Identify equipment needed for each of six procedures	In the clinical setting, select appropriate equipment for procedure to be performed	Evaluate own performance using Performance Checklist
2. Nurse's role in assisting	State the role of the nurse in each procedure	In the practice setting, carry out nurse's role in simulated situation	Under supervision in the clinical setting, assist physician with any of six procedures. Collect specimens and record correctly.	Evaluate performance with instructor
3. Procedure a. Positioning b. Observation c. Specimen collection d. Recording	With each of six procedures, describe procedure, including position, necessary observation, specimen collection, and recording			

LEARNING ACTIVITIES

1. Review the Specific Learning Objectives.
2. Read the section on performing treatments (in the chapter on direct care skills) in Ellis and Nowlis, *Nursing: A Human Needs Approach,* or comparable material in another textbook.
3. Look up the module vocabulary terms in the glossary.
4. Review anatomy and physiology that relate to the system being studied. This can be very helpful.
5. Read through the module.
6. Become familiar with the equipment that is available in the practice laboratory.
7. In the practice setting:
   a. Using a partner for a patient, simulate the sequence of the physical examination, reassuring and explaining as you proceed. You may leave out the genital portion of the examination but be sure to include it in your explanation.
   b. Reverse roles, and you take the role of the patient.
   c. Evaluate each other's performance. Were the explanations sufficient? Was emotional support offered? Did you have any feelings about the experience?
   d. Practice the various positions for diagnostic procedures with your partner.
8. In the clinical setting:
   a. Consult with your instructor for an opportunity to assist with a physical examination and/or a diagnostic or therapeutic procedure. Do this under supervision.

VOCABULARY

antecubital fossa
asymmetry
bone marrow
bruit
caries
cerumen
concurrent
cranium
dorsal recumbent position
dorsiflexion
edema
gooseneck lamp
Homan's sign
hypovolemic shock
lesion
lithotomy position
lumbar puncture (spinal tap)
liver biopsy
manometer
nares
nasal speculum
ophthalmoscope
otoscope
paracentesis
patellar tendon
pectoralis muscles
periphery
pinwheel
proctoscope
ptosis
reflex hammer (percussion hammer)
sigmoidoscope
stab wound
stethoscope
stopcock
stylet
thoracentesis
trocar
tuning fork
turgor
uvula
vaginal speculum

ASSISTING WITH EXAMINATIONS AND PROCEDURES

Physical Examinations

The physical examination remains one of the most valuable data-gathering procedures. By using methods of inspection, palpation, auscultation, and percussion, often with the help of instruments, the examiner can obtain an overview of the patient's general health as well as data concerning specific systems. An examination can be performed as part of a yearly checkup, or it can be performed when a person has sought help because of signs or symptoms of illness. In the latter case, the physical assessment may suggest or even establish a diagnosis. Abnormal findings of other related or non-related systems may confirm the extent of the presenting illness or reveal a different, concurrent disease process altogether.

Usually, a physical examination is the second part of a standard two-part procedure called the HP, or history and physical. First, the examiner takes a detailed verbal history from the patient, which consists of demographic information, family medical history, and the patient's past history of injury or illness. A complete description by the patient of the current signs and symptoms completes the history. In some facilities, the history is taken and the physical is done by a skilled nurse.

SEQUENCE

Before beginning, the vital signs have usually been taken and recorded by the nurse. However, some physicians will retake the pulse, respiration, and blood pressure. Rarely do physicians measure a patient's temperature, but the nurse may be asked for such information. It is best to take the vital signs shortly before the physical examination, so that this information is at hand. Follow the procedure in the facility or office where you work.

Most examiners perform the physical examination in approximately the same sequence—from head to toe—perhaps be-cause this is the way it is taught. More importantly, the sequence lends a structure to the examination, so that you can assist more effectively by anticipating the sequence and so that the written data can be read more easily by health personnel. Occasionally, one part of an examination is more detailed or lengthy because specific pathology has been found that needs closer inspection.

NURSE'S ROLE

The nurse fulfills two major functions: (1) meeting the psychological and physical needs of the patient throughout the examination and (2) obtaining the necessary equipment and assisting the examiner.

The Psychological Factor Most persons have experienced a physical examination in a doctor's office, clinic, or hospital. Nevertheless, most patients commonly experience a degree of embarrassment or fear that brings about anxiety.

Certainly embarrassment can arise from having the entire body inspected. You can help overcome this by exposing the patient as little as is necessary. The element of fear is also understandable: a patient may worry that a disease process will be discovered. Most people greet the completion of a physical examination in which no disease is found with great relief.

You can help by clearly explaining to the patient what is about to take place and, in general terms, the parts of the examination. Use words the patient can understand. Your presence during the examination—and assuring the patient of it—also provides a degree of comfort. In fact, most male examiners request that a female nurse be present when they perform a vaginal examination, both for the patient's comfort and because of possible legal implications.

Assisting the Examiner By knowing what is physically expected of and psychologically comforting for the patient, your presence as an assistant to the examiner during a physical examination or the performance of procedures is important. For example, if the examiner is using sterile technique, you must provide items to the sterile field. Also, certain procedures can be performed more quickly and effectively with your help. It falls to you, the nurse, to make the examination as comfortable as possible for the patient and as effective as possible for the examiner.

PROCEDURE

1. Wash your hands. Observe medical asepsis throughout.
2. Gather the equipment. You will find it convenient to assemble the items on a tray. The specific items may vary: some physicians carry certain instruments in their bags; others do not, so you will have to obtain these from a storage area on the unit. The following are the most commonly used; delete or add to this list as the examiner indicates.
   a. Tongue depressor, or tongue blade
   b. Ophthalmoscope (Check that the batteries and bulb are working.)
   c. Otoscope (Check that the batteries and bulb are working.)
   d. Flashlight (Check that the batteries and bulb are working.)
   e. Reflex hammer, or percussion hammer
   f. Pinwheel
   g. Tuning fork
   h. Nasal speculum
   i. Vaginal speculum
   j. Clean gloves
   k. Lubricating jelly
   l. Gooseneck lamp
   m. Bath blanket (for draping)
3. Explain to the patient, in general, the steps of the examination. If the patient is female, tell her whether a vaginal examination will be performed.
4. Provide for the patient's privacy. Close the door of the room and pull the bed curtains.
5. Raise the bed to the high position, so that the examiner has a good working level. If the patient is immobile or not totally responsible, keep the side rails up until the examiner is ready to begin the examination, for reasons of safety.
6. Help the patient into a clean gown with the ties toward the front, to allow for easier access to the chest. In a clinic or office, you may use a special examination cover-up. Usually, this is a straight piece of fabric with an opening for the head, which drapes poncho-style over the patient, covering the patient's chest and back.
7. If the patient is able, help him or her to a sitting position on the side of the bed. Use sheet to cover the patient's lower body.
8. Because you should know the signs that the examiner is assessing, a brief summary is given below for your use. The necessary equipment is in italic.
   a. *Head and neck*
      (1) *Head* The cranium is palpated with the fingers for lumps, abrasions, asymmetry, and condition of the hair.
      (2) *Neck* The neck is palpated for asymmetry, distended veins, abnormal lymph nodes, and enlarged thyroid. Range of motion of the neck is performed to detect any limitations. The *stethoscope* is placed over the carotid artery to listen for bruits (abnormal sounds resulting from circulatory turbulence).
      (3) *Face* The face is inspected for asymmetry, ptosis (drooping of the eyelids), and skin condition.
      (4) *Eyes* Using a *flashlight* or *ophthalmoscope* (Figure 23.1), the eyes are observed for pupillary response (accommodation in a darkened room). With the ophthalmoscope, each eye is inspected, while the patient gazes straight ahead, to observe for corneal, lens, or vitreous abnormalities. The optic disc is assessed for size and color; each lower eyelid is pulled down for

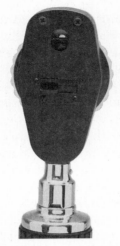

FIGURE 23.1 OPHTHALMOSCOPE HEAD
Courtesy Burton Division/Cavitron Corp.,
Van Nuys, California, and American Hispital
Supply Corp., McGaw Park, Illinois

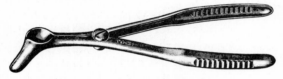

FIGURE 23.2 NASAL SPECULUM
Photograph courtesy of Sklar Manufacturing Co.,
Long Island, New York, and American Hospital
Supply Corp., McGaw Park, Illinois

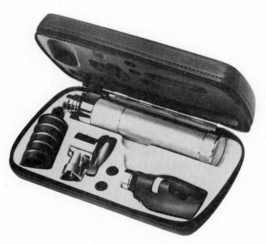

**FIGURE 23.3 COMBINATION OTOSCOPE-
OPHTHALMOSCOPE**
Photograph courtesy of Welch Allyn, Inc.,
Skaneateles Falls, New York, and American
Hospital Supply Corp., McGaw Park, Illinois

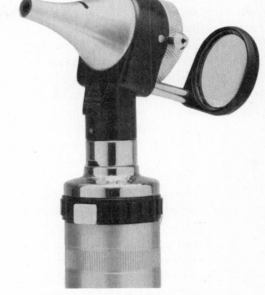

FIGURE 23.4 OTOSCOPE HEAD
Courtesy of Burton Division/Cavitron Corp.,
Van Nuys, California, and American Hospital
Supply Corp., McGaw Park, Illinois

observation of the color and condition of the conjunctiva.

(5) *Nose* With the patient's head tilted slightly backward, each inner nostril is inspected using a *nasal speculum* (Figure 23.2). Some examiners use the light from the *ophthalmoscope* instead of room light or a flashlight. The nares are inspected for color and condition of the mucosa, bleeding, and the presence of foreign bodies or masses.

(6) *Ears* With the head turned, each ear is examined with the *otoscope* for evidence of excess cerumen (earwax), growths, or redness (Figures 23.3 and 23.4). The eardrum (tympanic membrane) is assessed for signs of swelling or color change and for being intact. The area around the outer ear is palpated for tenderness. To test for hearing, a *tuning fork*

is struck and held an equal distance from each ear (Figure 23.5). This is to test air conduction. The struck tuning fork is then placed on each mastoid process, just below and behind the ears, and on the center top of the cranium to test for the bone's conduction of sound. A more definitive hearing test may be performed using electronic equipment.

(7) *Mouth* With a *flashlight* and *tongue blade,* the back of the throat is examined for swelling, redness, bacterial or viral patches, and the position and size of the uvula. When the patient says "Ah," the tonsils are checked. The teeth are inspected for looseness and the presence of caries. The mucosa of the inner mouth are observed for color and the presence of lesions. The patient is asked to clench the teeth and smile, which helps the physician assess bite and facial musculature. The color and smoothness of the lips are noted.

b. *Arms, hands, and fingers* The patient is asked to extend both arms out in front of the body. The musculature is examined for asymmetry and palpated for turgor. The arms, hands, and fingers are ranged to assess agility. The skin is observed for lesions, spotting, and general color. Joints are palpated and observed for nodules and enlargements. The hands and fingers are observed for color and palpated for temperature. The hands are observed for any tremors. Any deviation of alignment of the fingers is noted. The nails are observed for hardness and general condition. The grip of each hand is tested.

c. *Back* The patient is placed either in the prone position or sits in bed with the back facing the examiner. After the back is exposed, the skin is examined for spots or lesions. The curvature of the spine is noted, and the vertebral column is palpated. With the *stethoscope,* the examiner listens to the lower lobes of the lungs.

d. *Chest* A male patient will have the gown removed. Because a female patient may feel modest about exposing the breasts, her gown can be untied and parted for the chest examination. If more exposure is needed, the gown can then be dropped to the waist. With either a male or female patient sitting and facing the examiner, the levels of the shoulders are observed for equality. The pectoralis muscles of each side of the chest are observed for symmetry as the patient presses the palms together and lifts the hands over the head. Any abnormal dimpling, color, or discharge of the nipples is noted.

A female patient is then asked to lie in the supine position. Each breast is examined, and a *small folded towel* is placed under its outer side. With the flat of the fingers, each breast is palpated for masses or lumps from the nipple outward and then around the periphery.

e. *Heart* With the patient in the supine position, the neck veins are palpated for normal filling and the cardiac margins (outline of the heart) are percussed. A *stethoscope* is used to listen to the heart sounds. Then the gown is replaced.

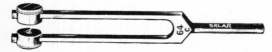

FIGURE 23.5   TUNING FORK
*Photograph courtesy of Sklar Manufacturing Co.,
Long Island, New York, and American Hospital
Supply Corp., McGaw Park, Illinois*

f. *Abdomen* The patient remains in the supine position. The abdomen is observed for general contour, distention, and asymmetry. The skin is grasped between the fingers to test for turgor. A *stethoscope* is used to listen to bowel sounds. The area is then palpated and percussed for areas of tenderness, for the presence of fluid, and for the loss of normal dullness of tone. With the patient breathing deeply and with the knees flexed, the abdomen is palpated for organs and masses. On expiration, the examiner's fingers can feel for the position of abdominal structures.

g. *Legs, feet, and toes* With the patient still in the supine position, each leg is palpated for muscle bulk, and observed for color, temperature, and skin condition. Each foot is dorsiflexed to check for calf pain and the possible presence of thrombophlebitis (Homan's sign). Pedal pulses are taken on each foot and compared. The ankles are palpated with the fingers to assess for edema. Strength is tested by having the patient press the sole of the foot against the examiner's palm. The joints are inspected for enlargement.

h. *Reflexes* The examiner, depending on the situation, may test only a few of the more prominent reflexes, or may proceed with an abbreviated neurological exam. Many of the measurements of neurological functioning will have been tested when the other systems or areas were examined. For example, an examination of the optic discs with the ophthalmoscope can reveal a neurological deficit or disease. Or, if the examiner wanted to check the cranial nerves, this was probably accomplished during the examination of the face by having the patient protrude the tongue, smile, and resist supraorbital pressure. (For a detailed description of a com-

plete neurological examination, refer to a medical-surgical text or a neurological nursing text.)

Reflexes are usually recorded with the following symbols: 0 (no response), 1+ (hypoactive), 2+ (normal), 3+ (more hyperactive than normal), 4+ (very hyperactive). If you are recording for the examiner, use this coding or the one designated by the examiner.

(1) *Corneal reflex (blink)* When the cornea is touched with a *soft small wad of cotton*, the patient should blink.

(2) *Biceps reflex* The examiner places his or her thumb on the biceps tendon, which is located just above the antecubital fossa. The striking of the thumb should produce flexion of the forearm.

(3) *Triceps reflex* While supporting the upper arm and allowing the forearm to hang freely at a right angle from the body, the *reflex hammer* (Figure 23.6) is struck directly on the triceps tendon, just above the elbow. Extension of the forearm should occur.

(4) *Brachioradial reflex* The striking of the radius slightly above the wrist with the *reflex hammer* should produce flexion and supination of the forearm.

(5) *Knee reflex* The patient's leg must be relaxed and hanging freely or supported on the hand. When the patellar tendon, which is just below the knee, is struck

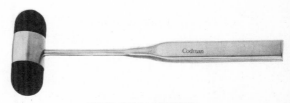

FIGURE 23.6 REFLEX HAMMER
Courtesy Codman & Shurtleff, Inc.

with the *reflex hammer,* extension of the lower leg should occur.

(6) *Ankle reflex* The foot is held in a position of dorsiflexion by the examiner. When the Achilles tendon at the back of the ankle is struck with the *reflex hammer,* plantar flexion of the foot should occur.

(7) *Babinski reflex* Using the end of the *reflex hammer* or the sharper edge of a *tongue blade,* the sole of the foot is stroked from heel to toe. The normal (negative) response is plantar flexion (the toes bending downward).

(8) *Skin sensation* The examiner may choose to test sensation by using a *pinwheel* that can be rolled over broad skin areas (Figure 23.7). The patient, without looking at the *pinwheel,* is asked whether the sensation is sharp or dull.

i. *Genitalia*

(1) *Male patients* Male patients are are examined in the standing position, if at all possible, so that the inguinal ring can be palpated for herniation. The foreskin of the penis is retracted and inspected for irritation, ulceration, and the presence of lesions. The testes are palpated to assess for size, position, and the presence of masses.

(2) *Female patients* Female patients are examined in the lithotomy position with the knees flexed. Drape the patient as you would for catheterization, using a *clean sheet or bath blanket.* Cover both legs exposing only the perineum.

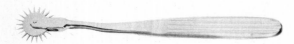

FIGURE 23.7 PINWHEEL
Courtesy Codman & Shurtleff, Inc.

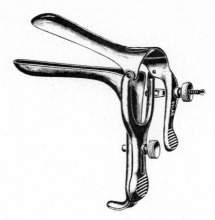

FIGURE 23.8   VAGINAL SPECULUM
Photograph courtesy of Sklar Manufacturing Co., Long Island, New York, and American Hospital Supply Corp., McGaw Park, Illinois

An examination table with stirrups is preferred, but the patient can be examined in bed. Provide a *gooseneck lamp.* The examiner puts on *clean gloves* and *lubricates* the outside of a *vaginal speculum* (Figure 23.8). The inside is not lubricated because the presence of the lubricating jelly interferes with the accuracy of the Papanicolaou (Pap) test. This test is done by obtaining secretions on a *swab* from the cervical os. The secretions are put on a *glass slide* and sent to the lab to be examined for the presence of abnormal cells. After the cervix is inspected with the speculum, the speculum is withdrawn and the examiner *lubricates* the index and middle fingers of one hand. By inserting these fingers into the vagina and pushing downward on the patient's abdomen with the other hand, the examiner can palpate the uterus and ovaries. These organs are assessed for location, size, outline, masses, and tenderness.

j. *Rectum* A female patient is usually examined after the genital exam is completed. With a *lubricated gloved* hand, the examiner inserts the middle finger and palpates for size of lumen, masses, internal hemorrhoids, and tenderness. The anal area is evaluated for the presence of external hemorrhoids. The same exam is performed on the male patient, either with the patient bending over the side of the bed or positioned in lithotomy with the penis and testes held aside. The knee-chest position can also be used. In the male exam, the prostate gland is also assessed for size and tenderness.

9. Return the bed to the low position, and help the patient to a position of comfort.
10. Provide a period of rest. Undergoing a complete physical examination is both an anxiety-producing and tiring procedure, especially for an ill person.
11. Dispose of the equipment properly. Wash, soak, or disinfect each item used according to the policy of your facility. If a Pap specimen was taken, label it and send it to the lab.
12. Wash your hands.
13. Record the procedure. The examiner may have a form on which you should record findings, or they should be recorded on an admission or progress note sheet in standard sequence. You should also make a brief notation on the nurses' notes. For example:

> Physical exam performed by Dr. Harris. Resting comfortably. Pap smear to lab.
>
> S. Lane, SN

Diagnostic and Therapeutic Procedures

A patient's signed permission is essential before diagnostic and therapeutic procedures are performed to legally protect the physician and the hospital. In some facilities, the more general consent-for-medical-treatment form, signed on admission, suffices. In other facilities, each procedure requires an individual consent. Know the policy of the facility in which you practice.

GENERAL PROCEDURE

1. Wash your hands.
2. Obtain the proper set for the procedure to be done. Most sets come in sterile packs and are disposable. Read the outside label to check which items are included, so that you can supplement if necessary. Sometimes you will have to provide sterile gloves, skin disinfectant solutions, or local-anesthetic agents.
3. Explain to the patient why the procedure is being done and how it is done. Very often, the physician assumes this responsibility and you need only clarify. On occasion, however, the physician will not have explained the process, in which case you should tell the patient in clear but general terms the steps in the procedure and how he or she might assist.
4. Close the door of the room and pull the bed curtains to provide privacy.
5. If room light is insufficient, obtain a gooseneck lamp.
6. Assist the patient to the proper position:
   a. *Thoracentesis* The patient must be upright, so that the pull of gravity will consolidate the chest fluid in the lower portion of the affected lung. Three methods can help the patient maintain this position.
      (1) Pad the back of a straight chair. Have the patient straddle the chair leaning the arms on the padded back.
      (2) Have the patient sit upright in bed and lean forward, resting on the overbed table.
      (3) Have the patient sit on the edge of the bed, leaning over the overbed table.
   b. *Paracentesis* Have the patient void, so that the bladder will not be perforated during the procedure. Place the patient in the upright position to consolidate the fluid in the lower portion of the abdomen. The patient, if able, can sit facing the physician in a chair or sit on the edge of the bed,

legs over the side and back on a rest. Use a wooden backrest padded with pillows or an ordinary cardboard box padded with pillows. Either device helps the patient to sit upright without tiring.

c. *Lumbar puncture (spinal tap)* The correct position for this procedure is very important and often is essential to its success. With the bed in the high position (the examiner sits facing the bed) place the patient in the side-lying position. Flex the legs and neck, bowing the back toward the physician. This position widens the intervertebral spaces. Do not use a pillow under the head because the height interferes with the equal level of flow of the spinal fluid during the puncture. You may want to stand facing the patient on the opposite side of the bed to offer support and to help hold the patient in position, by placing your hands at the back of the knees and neck.

d. *Liver biopsy* Place the patient in the dorsal recumbent position to flatten the liver tissue.

e. *Bone marrow biopsy* If a sternal puncture is to be done, place the patient in the dorsal recumbent position. If the iliac crest is to be tapped for marrow, the prone position is appropriate.

f. *Proctoscopy or sigmoidoscopy* Position the patient on a Ritter table, which is similar to the standard examining table except that it "breaks" at the hips with a kneeling platform at the end. This allows the patient to be placed in the knee-chest position with support. If a Ritter table is not available, place the patient in the knee-chest position near the end of the bed.

7. Assist the physician as directed:

a. *Thoracentesis* Open the set and provide sterile gloves. You may be requested to pour antiseptic solution over sterile cotton balls or flats (2 ×

2 gauze squares) for cleaning the area. After cleaning, a small area is anesthetized at the level of the seventh intercostal space. A 16- or 17-gauge needle attached to a 50-cc syringe with a stopcock is introduced, and the fluid removed. A small dressing is applied.

b. *Paracentesis* Open the pack and supply sterile gloves. You may be requested to pour the antiseptic solution as in step a, above. A small area is anesthetized 1 to 2 inches below the umbilicus. A trocar is introduced through a small stab wound; then a connecting catheter drains the fluid. A small dressing is applied.

c. *Lumbar puncture* Open the set and provide sterile gloves. You may be requested to pour the antiseptic solution as in step a, above. The area, usually between the third and fourth lumbar intervertebral space, is anesthetized. The spinal needle is introduced until spinal fluid appears in the syringe. A stopcock and manometer are attached. The pressure is read, specimens are obtained, and the needle is removed. Carefully number specimens by the sequence in which they were collected. A small dressing is applied. Usually, the patient is instructed to stay flat for six to eight hours until the fluid has been replenished. This measure can prevent spinal headache.

d. *Liver biopsy* Open the pack and supply sterile gloves. You may be requested to pour antiseptic solution as in step a, above. A small subcostal area is anesthetized. The patient should be instructed to hold his or her breath for the ten seconds needed to insert the needle. The needle is rotated to gather the tissue and withdrawn. Pressure is exerted to stop the bleeding, and a small dressing is applied.

e. *Bone marrow biopsy* Open the pack

and supply sterile gloves. You may be requested to pour antiseptic solution as in step a, above. A small area in the midsternum or over the iliac crest is anesthetized. A short large-gauge needle with a stylet is inserted. There may be a crunching sound as it punctures the bone tissue. The stylet is removed, a syringe is attached, and 1 to 2 ml bone marrow are aspirated. The needle is removed, pressure is applied to stop the bleeding, and a small dressing is applied. The patient may feel discomfort when the bone marrow is aspirated.

f. *Proctoscopy and sigmoidoscopy*
The scope is lubricated and inserted through the anus. Proctoscopes are shorter than sigmoidoscopes, and therefore the area visualized is more limited. More scopes have indwelling lighting, and many sigmoidoscopes have suction (Figure 23.9). If suction is available, attach tubing to wall suction or a suction machine. Provide long swabs and slides if a specimen is needed. A biopsy may also be done. Once the scope is removed, the anal area is cleaned with gauze squares.

8. Throughout all of these procedures, give the patient psychological support. If a patient is uncomfortable, assure him or her that it will only be for a short period of time. Let the patient know what is about to take place, and give clear instructions of ways the patient can help. All this adds to his or her psychological comfort. Remember that

patients feel less anxious if they know what is going to happen and what they should do. ("Please try not to move for the next few minutes so that we can get the test over with quickly.") Also, you may want to hold the patient's hand for reassurance.

9. You must observe the patient for untoward signs or reactions to the procedure. Many times the physician is preoccupied with performing the test, and it is you, the nurse, who can see early signs of impending problems. During any procedure, check the patient's pulse and respiration two or three times. Notify the physician promptly of any unusual signs.

a. *Thoracentesis* If the patient becomes pale, has sudden pain, coughs, or shows signs of dyspnea or diaphoresis, the needle could be irritating or possibly puncturing the pleura. Usually, the procedure is stopped or the needle is withdrawn slightly.

b. *Paracentesis* Particularly observe the patient for hypovolemic shock, as the fluid from the body's vascular system is channeled into the abdominal area to replace the sudden withdrawal of fluid in the procedure. Primary symptoms are a drop in blood pressure, dyspnea, diaphoresis, and pallor. Hypovolemic shock usually occurs only in patients having very large amounts of fluid withdrawn.

c. *Lumbar puncture* A skillfully performed lumbar puncture should not produce abnormal signs or symptoms. However, be alert for indications of pain radiating to a leg, sharp back pain, or sudden numbness or tingling of the feet or legs.

d. *Liver biopsy* The patient having a liver biopsy may have been given doses of vitamin K for several days before the test to prevent bleeding at the site. Take the patient's vital signs two or three times during the

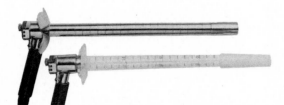

FIGURE 23.9 SIGMOIDOSCOPE
Photograph courtesy of Welch Allyn, Inc., Skaneateles Falls, New York, and American Hospital Supply Corp., McGaw Park, Illinois

hour after the test to determine if
the patient is hemorrhaging, but
complications are uncommon.

e. *Bone marrow biopsy*   Except for
mild tenderness at the site of the
bone marrow biopsy, complications
are rare. Watch for bleeding or the
formation of a hematoma.

f. *Proctoscopy or sigmoidoscopy*
These procedures should not cause
problems, but, as always, you should
closely observe any patient who is
undergoing a procedure. In the rare
instance of perforation of the colon,
the patient may experience sudden
abdominal pain.

10. Record test findings as appropriate.
Accurately measure the fluid aspirated
from the chest or abdomen. Both the
initial reading and the final reading of
spinal fluid pressure should be recorded.

11. Take specimens from all fluids aspirated.
The physician, after the initial pressure
has been recorded during the lumbar
puncture, will let the spinal fluid drip
into three small test tubes. These must
be labeled number 1, number 2, and
number 3 as they are collected. The
first may be slightly blood-tinged because of the trauma of the tap, but the
second and third tubes should be clear.

Observe all fluids for *clarity, color,*
and *viscosity.* Any specimen collected
should be sent to the lab promptly, so
that it does not change in character and
can be tested accurately.

12. Return the patient to a position of
comfort. Remember that the patient
who has had a lumbar puncture may be
ordered to remain flat for one to
twenty-four hours.

13. Provide a period of rest. Each of these
procedures is taxing, primarily because
of emotional stress. Also, the removal of
large amounts of fluid from the chest or
abdominal cavity, because of the shift
in fluid distribution, can cause weakness
and fatigue.

14. Dispose of the equipment correctly. The
packs used for thoracentesis, paracentesis, and lumbar puncture are covered
loosely with the outer wrap and dis-
posed of in a wastebasket. Liver biopsy sets are also usually disposable.
The trocar and glass syringe used in a
bone marrow biopsy and the scopes
used in a proctoscopy or sigmoidoscopy
should be washed after use and sterilized, usually in the central supply department.

15. Wash your hands.

16. Record the procedure and any pertinent
data.

COMMONLY PERFORMED DIAGNOSTIC PROCEDURES

	Asepsis	Position	Specific Observations or Concerns	Specimen	Recording
Thoracentesis	Sterile	Sitting upright	Pallor, sudden pain, cough, dyspnea, diaphoresis	Abnormal chest fluid	Thoracentesis performed by Dr. Kraft. 450 ml serosanguinous fluid removed. Specimen to lab. Resting comfortably. D. Chaney, SN
Paracentesis	Sterile	After voiding, sitting upright	Signs of hypovolemic shock: fall in blood pressure, dyspnea, diaphoresis, pallor	Abnormal abdominal fluid	Paracentesis performed by Dr. Kraft. 1200 ml cloudy fluid obtained. Specimen to lab. Resting comfortably. D. Chaney, SN
Lumbar puncture	Sterile	Side-lying, with neck and legs flexed	Sharp back pain, pain radiating to legs, or numbness or tingling in feet or legs; have patient lie flat six to eight hours afterward	Cerebrospinal fluid	Lumbar puncture performed by Dr. Kraft. Initial pressure 140 mm. Final pressure 90 mm. Three specimens clear fluid to lab. Appears comfortable. D. Chaney, SN

	Asepsis	Position	Specific Observations or Concerns	Specimen	Recording
Liver biopsy	Sterile	Dorsal recumbent	Have patient hold breath for ten seconds during puncture; check vital signs during procedure; watch for internal bleeding or bleeding from site	Liver tissue	Liver biopsy performed by Dr. Kraft. Specimen to lab. Small amount of bleeding from site. Dressing applied. D. Chaney, SN
Bone marrow biopsy	Sterile	Dorsal recumbent	Bleeding from site or hematoma formation	Bone marrow	Bone marrow biopsy performed by Dr. Kraft. Specimen to lab. Appears to be resting comfortably. D. Chaney, SN
Proctoscopy or sigmoidoscopy	Nonsterile	Knee-chest	Sudden abdominal pain or shock symptoms from perforation (rare)	Small fragments of lesions in colon if present	Sigmoidoscopy performed by Dr. Kraft. Biopsy specimen to lab. Appears to be resting comfortably. D. Chaney, SN

PERFORMANCE CHECKLIST

Assisting with a physical examination	Unsatisfactory	Needs more practice	Satisfactory	Comments
1. Wash your hands.				
2. Gather equipment.				
3. Explain procedure to patient.				
4. Provide for patient's privacy.				
5. Raise bed.				
6. Help patient into clean gown, ties toward front.				
7. If patient is able, assist to sitting position on side of bed.				
8. Assist physician as follows: a. Head and neck (1) At appropriate times, hand physician lighted ophthalmoscope to examine eyes; nasal speculum for nose; and otoscope for ears.				
(2) Have tongue blade and flashlight ready for examination of mouth and throat, and stethoscope for listening to neck veins.				
b. Arms, hands, and fingers (1) Have sufficient room light.				
c. Back (1) Remove gown from male patient; lift gown at back for female patient.				
(2) Provide stethoscope.				
d. Chest (1) Remove gown from male patient; untie gown to expose chest for female patient.				
e. Heart (1) Position patient in dorsal recumbent position.				
(2) Provide stethoscope.				
(3) Replace gown.				
f. Abdomen (1) Position patient in supine position.				
(2) Provide stethoscope.				
g. Legs, feet, and toes (1) Keep patient in supine position.				

	Unsatisfactory	Needs more practice	Satisfactory	Comments
h. Reflexes (neurological examination) (1) Position patient for reflex being noted.				
(2) Provide percussion hammer.				
i. Genitalia (1) Position male patient in standing position; female patient in lithotomy position.				
(2) For female patient, provide gooseneck lamp, gloves, vaginal speculum, lubricating jelly, long swabs, and glass slide.				
j. Rectum (1) Position male patient over side of bed or in knee-chest position; female patient in lithotomy position.				
(2) Provide clean glove and lubricating jelly.				
9. Lower bed and help patient to comfortable position.				
10. Provide rest period.				
11. Dispose of equipment properly.				
12. Wash your hands.				
13. Record procedure.				
Assisting with diagnostic and therapeutic procedures				
1. Wash your hands.				
2. Obtain proper set for procedure to be done.				
3. Explain procedure to patient.				
4. Provide for privacy.				
5. Secure adequate lighting.				
6. Assist patient to appropriate position. a. Thoracentesis: patient straddles straight chair, leaning over back, or sits up in bed leaning on overbed table, or sits at edge of bed leaning over overbed table.				
b. Paracentesis: patient sits up in armchair, or sits up in bed with legs over side.				
c. Lumbar puncture: patient in side-lying position with neck and legs flexed and back bowed.				
d. Liver biopsy: patient in dorsal recumbent position.				

	Unsatisfactory	Needs more practice	Satisfactory	Comments
e. Bone marrow biopsy: patient in dorsal recumbent position for sternal puncture, and in prone position for iliac puncture.				
f. Proctoscopy or sigmoidoscopy: patient in knee-chest position on examining table or Ritter table.				
7. Assist examiner as directed.				
8. Give psychological comfort to patient throughout.				
9. Observe patient.				
10. Record quantity of fluids aspirated from chest or abdomen and pressure levels of lumbar puncture.				
11. Collect specimens, label them, and make pertinent observations.				
12. Return patient to comfortable position.				
13. Provide rest period.				
14. Dispose of equipment correctly.				
15. Wash your hands.				
16. Record procedure and pertinent data.				

QUIZ

Short-Answer Questions

1. What are two important functions of the nurse when assisting with a physical examination or a diagnostic procedure?

   a. _____

   b. _____

2. What is the best position for a patient having a physical exam?

   _____

3. An ophthalmoscope is used to examine the _____ .

4. An otoscope is used to examine the _____ .

5. Heart sounds should be heard with the patient in the _____ position.

6. What do we call the test for abnormal cells of the cervix and vagina?

   _____

7. Why is lubricating jelly not used on the inside of a vaginal speculum?

   _____

8. A pinwheel is used to test _____ .

9. What is the proper term to describe the reflex if the toes bend downward when the sole of the foot is stroked? _____

10. The procedure used to aspirate accumulated fluid in the abdominal cavity is called _____ .

11. Specimens of fluid should be observed for what three characteristics?

    a. _____

    b. _____

    c. _____

Module 24 Applying Bandages and Binders

MAIN OBJECTIVE

To correctly apply commonly used bandages and binders.

RATIONALE

Although the application of bandages and binders does not require sterile technique, it does require skill on the part of the nurse in order to be effective. There are a variety of reasons for applying either a bandage or a binder. Some protect an underlying wound or dressing, while others provide pressure, warmth, support, or immobilization. Wrapping and securing an abdominal binder is very different from wrapping and securing a bandage on a swollen ankle.

It is important first to assess the needs of patients and then to select the material that best fulfills those needs. Physicians may order a specific type of bandage to be used or may give only a general order for bandaging.

PREREQUISITES

Successful completion of the following modules:

VOLUME 1
Assessment
Charting
Medical Asepsis
Basic Body Mechanics

SPECIFIC LEARNING OBJECTIVES

	Know Facts and Principles	Apply Facts and Principles	Demonstrate Ability	Evaluate Performance
Bandages				
1. Types and methods used in application	State common types of roll bandages and five methods of applying them	Given a patient situation, determine appropriate type of bandage and method of application	In the clinical setting, choose appropriate bandage and method of application	Evaluate own performance using Performance Checklist
2. Procedure	Explain procedures for applying bandages	Given a patient situation, explain rationale for selection of appropriate bandage and method chosen for application	Replace existing bandage or apply new bandage correctly with supervision	Evaluate own performance with instructor
3. Charting	State information to be recorded		Chart on patient's record	Review notes with instructor
Binders				
1. Types	State types of binders most commonly used	Given a patient situation, select appropriate binder	In the clinical setting, select appropriate binder and method of application	
2. Procedure	Explain selection of binder and method for applying	Given a patient situation, state rationale for choice of binder and principles to be observed in application	In the clinical setting, replace or apply binder correctly	Evaluate own performance with instructor

3. *Charting*	State information to be recorded	Chart on patient's record	Review notes with instructor
Arm sling			
1. *Type*	State size and material used for adult sling		
2. *Procedure*	Explain selection of sling and method for applying	Given a patient situation, select appropriate sling	
		Using Performance Checklist, correctly apply arm sling	Evaluate own performance with instructor
3. *Charting*	State information to be recorded	Chart on patient's record	Review notes with instructor

LEARNING ACTIVITIES

1. Review the Specific Learning Objectives.
2. Look up the module vocabulary terms in the glossary.
3. Read through the module.
4. In the practice setting:
   a. Become familiar with the materials and available types of bandages and binders.
   b. With a partner, practice bandaging, demonstrating each of the methods introduced using the Performance Checklist.
   c. Reroll the bandages and have your partner apply the bandages to you, using the described methods.
   d. Together, evaluate each other's performance of steps b and c.
   e. Again with your partner, apply the straight abdominal binder and the scultetus binder using the Performance Checklist.
   f. Have your partner apply these binders to you.
   g. Apply an arm sling to your partner.
   h. Have your partner apply an arm sling to you.
   i. Together, evaluate each other's performance of steps e–h.
5. In the clinical setting:
   a. Consult with your instructor about opportunities to apply bandages and binders to appropriate patients.
6. Evaluate your performance with your instructor.

VOCABULARY

Ace bandage
bandage
binder
circular bandage
double T-binder
figure-8 bandage
Kling bandage
net binder
recurrent bandage
reverse spiral
roller bandage
scultetus binder
sling
spiral bandage
straight abdominal binder
T-binder

APPLYING BANDAGES AND BINDERS

Most bandages are of a gauze material; binders are often made of muslin. Bandages and binders can be used to protect underlying tissues or secure underlying dressings. Although dressings are usually sterile, bandages or binders are not always sterile if there are underlying sterile dressings to protect the wound. To secure an underlying dressing, it is important to wrap in a manner that will be tight enough to hold yet loose enough not to constrict the body part in any way. You will learn the proper tension with practice. To keep a dressing clean, adequately cover all edges and corners with the bandage or binder.

When you apply any bandage or binder, you must take certain precautions. Avoid bandaging over wrinkled dressings, which can produce pressure on the wound or skin. Approximately 30 minutes after you have applied a bandage or binder, check the patient for comfort. A bandage or binder that is too tight can interfere with circulation, causing swelling, numbness, tingling, or color changes of the distal area. Most bandages are applied on parts from distal to proximal, to facilitate venous return.

Elastic bandages are used to provide constant pressure over an area or to support an injured joint. On a lower extremity, they also facilitate venous return.

Applying Bandages

TYPES OF BANDAGES

There are a variety of bandages that can be used for wrapping limbs. *Roller gauze* is available in ½-inch, 1-inch, and 2-inch widths. This material does not stretch and is quite strong. Roller gauze is used to hold dressings in place and as a dressing on fingers and toes. It is available in both sterile and nonsterile forms.

Kling bandage is a gauzelike bandage that is flexible and somewhat stretchable. It is commonly available in 3-inch and 4-inch widths, and is used on extremities, the head, and the torso. It can be part of the primary dressing or used to hold other dressings in place. Kling bandage is also available in both sterile and nonsterile forms. When applying a Kling bandage, keep feet or hands in a functional position while they are wrapped.

Another type of roller bandage is the *elastic,* or *Ace, bandage.* (On an extremity, elastic hose or elastic sleeves can be used instead of an Ace bandage.) To wrap a leg, keep the part in a horizontal position for at least 15 minutes before bandaging to ensure equal circulation. Secure the bandage by wrapping it under the instep of the foot. Wrap from distal to proximal; this, as well as the elastic quality of these bandages, promotes venous return.

All bandages should be placed over clean dry surfaces to prevent the harboring and growth of microorganisms. Change them frequently to keep them clean. Pad bony prominences to prevent pressure.

METHODS OF APPLICATION

There are five general methods of applying roll bandages: circular, spiral, reverse spiral, figure-8, and recurrent fold. The circular-turn bandage is used to secure a dressing or to cover a confined area of an extremity; the spiral and reverse spiral begin distally on an extremity and wind proximally, to cover a wider area with comfort. The figure-8 bandage is used over a joint to provide easy flexion. To bandage distal portions of extremities or a stump that has not been casted, the recurrent-fold technique is most appropriate.

Before you begin to apply any type of roll bandage, firmly roll the bandage. Always unroll it with the rolled-up portion on top (Figure 24.1).

A bandage can be secured with a strip of cloth or paper tape placed over the loose end and fastened to the bandage, not to the skin. If the material is porous, use a metal clip with sharp small teeth on the under surface. This last is commonly used with Ace bandages.

Circular With the roll on the inner aspect, unroll the bandage either toward you or

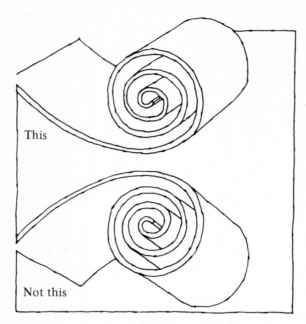

FIGURE 24.1   UNROLLING A BANDAGE

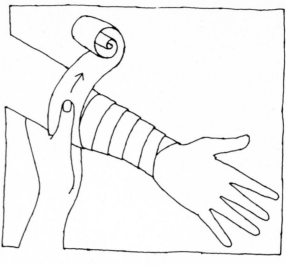

FIGURE 24.3   SPIRAL WRAP

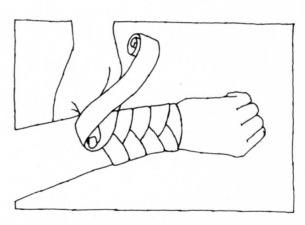

FIGURE 24.4   REVERSE-SPIRAL WRAP

laterally, holding the loose end until it is secured by the first circle of the bandage (Figure 24.2). Two or three turns may be needed to adequately cover an area. Hold the bandage in place with tape or a clip.

Spiral   Begin with the circular method. After securing with one or two complete overlaps, place the bandage to overlap a half or two thirds of the width, moving evenly up the extremity (Figure 24.3). Tape or clip the bandage in place.

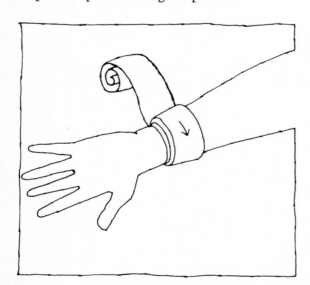

FIGURE 24.2   CIRCULAR WRAP

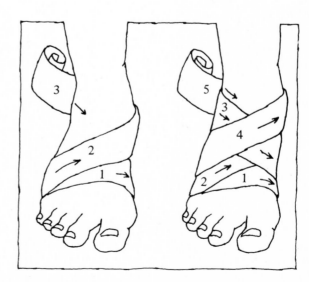

FIGURE 24.5   FIGURE-8 WRAP

Reverse Spiral Begin as you would for the spiral bandage. When the end is secured by the first turn, hold your thumb on the bandage as it approaches the side nearest you, and fold under, reversing the direction downward (Figure 24.4). Repeat this step with each turn, overlapping as before. Once the necessary area is covered, secure the bandage with tape or a clip.

Figure-8 This bandage is used most often on a joint. Make the first turns over the joint, securing with the overlap. Make the next turn higher (superior) to the joint. Make the following turn lower (inferior) to the joint (Figure 24.5). Continue working in this manner, one turn above and one below. The figure-8 pattern allows the joint to maintain its mobility without dislodging the bandage. Secure the bandage with tape or a clip.

Recurrent Fold Hold the end of the bandage in place with one circular turn. Then bring the roll downward, over the end of the finger, toe, or stump, and back up behind. Then, make a fold and bring the roll back downward again. Each turn is folded alternately to right and left of the center initial fold (Figure 24.6). Keep your fingers in place at the top to secure the bandage until a circular turn or two can be taken to complete the bandage (Figure 24.7). Clip or tape in place.

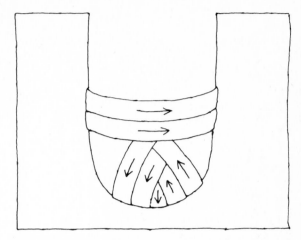

FIGURE 24.7   ANCHORING A RECURRENT-FOLD BANDAGE

SPECIFIC BANDAGING PROCEDURES

Wrapping an Ankle and Lower Leg Secure the bandage around the instep with a single circular wrap. Form a figure-8 around the ankle itself. Then, wrap as far up the leg as is necessary with a spiral wrap. To continue the wrap above the knee, use a reverse spiral just below the knee to secure the bandage firmly.

Stump Wrapping Surgeons may prefer one specific method of wrapping a stump over the others. Frequently, a recurrent bandage is placed on the stump first, and then a spiral is started at the distal end of the stump

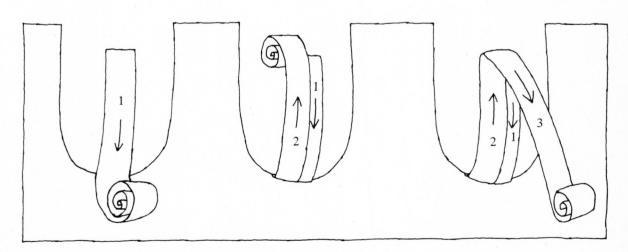

FIGURE 24.6   RECURRENT FOLD

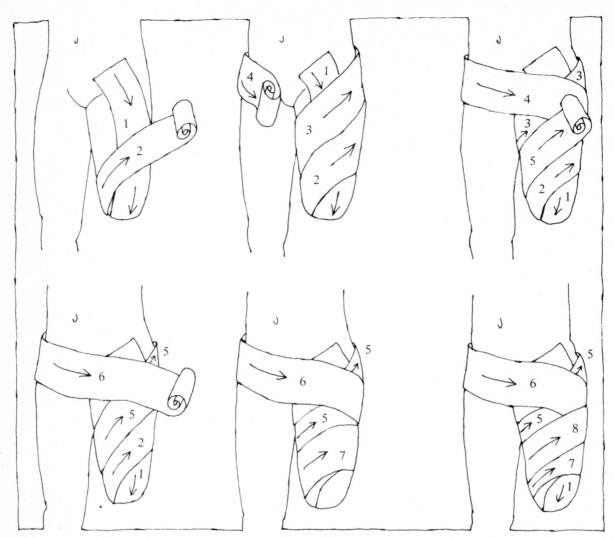

FIGURE 24.8   BANDAGING AN ABOVE-THE-KNEE AMPUTATION
Courtesy University of Washington Department of Prosthetics-Orthotics

moving up to the thigh (Figure 24.8). It is important that pressure be even with slightly more pressure at the most distal portion of the stump, both to enhance return circulation and to produce a smooth, even stump. Some surgeons prefer that a figure-8 bandage be wrapped from the stump up and around the hip and waist.

Applying Binders

TYPES OF BINDERS

Binders are generally used on the trunk of the body to hold dressings in place or to support tissues. They can be placed around the chest, the abdomen, or the pelvic area.

Most are made of a muslin material, although *elastic-net binders* are being used more frequently. They offer the advantages of being easily washed and quickly dried, of affording air circulation, and of stretching to conform to the shape of the part being bound.

Abdominal binders that are not made of net are usually straight and can be fashioned from any strong material, for example, a drawsheet or bath blanket. The *scultetus* ("many tailed") *binders* are nothing more than straight binders with tails of fabric at each end. These are interlaced upward to give strength and added support to the abdomen, especially after abdominal surgery.

T-binders are designed to hold perineal dressings or packs in place. Single T-binders are used for female patients; double T-binders are used for male patients so that the testicles are not unduly constricted.

Slings—or what are in effect arm binders— are used to rest the arm in a right-angle position. These are often made from bright patterned material that has been cut in a triangular shape.

METHODS OF APPLICATION

Straight Abdominal Binder   Place the patient in the supine position. Position the binder smoothly underneath the patient. Overlap the ends across the patient's abdomen, and secure them with several safety pins (Figure 24.9).

Scultetus Abdominal Binder   Place the binder underneath the supine patient, being careful to check for underlying wrinkles. Lace the lower tail in a slightly oblique direction

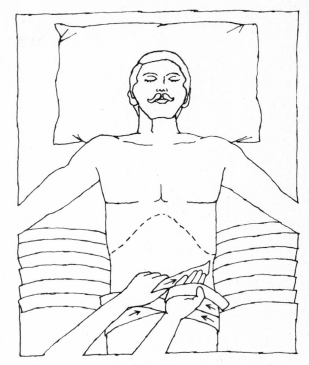

FIGURE 24.10   SCULTETUS ABDOMINAL BINDER

upward on the abdomen. Lace the tail on the opposite side in a similar way. Proceed to lace in this interlocking fashion until all the tails have been neatly and securely placed (Figure 24.10). If a tail is too long, fold the excess end smoothly back. Using two safety pins, fasten the last two tails at the ends, either pinning them horizontally or crossing them downward diagonally. For the post-partum patient, a scultetus binder may be applied starting at the top tails.

T-Binder   After selecting the appropriate binder for the patient (Figure 24.11), place it underneath the patient smoothly with the waistband at waist level and the tails down-ward in the midline in the back. Bring the waist tails around the patient and overlap. Bring the center tail or tails upward between the patient's legs and over perineal dressings, taking care to touch only the outside of dressings that should be kept in place. Make sure the two tails of the double T-binder are on either side of the scrotum and penis. Secure the ends with safety pins.

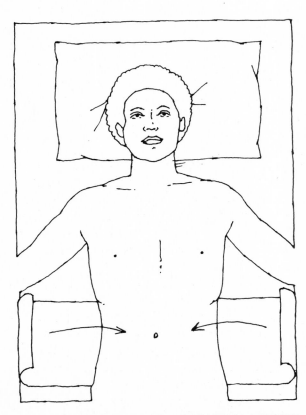

FIGURE 24.9   STRAIGHT ABDOMINAL BINDER

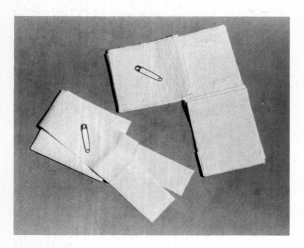

FIGURE 24.11   T-BINDERS

Arm Sling   To make an arm sling from muslin, fold or cut (for less thickness) a 36-inch square of fabric diagonally. There are two methods used for applying slings:

1. With the patient facing you, place one end of the triangle over the unaffected shoulder and the long straight border

under the hand on the injured side. Loop upward, positioning the other end of the triangle over the affected shoulder. Tie or pin the ends to one side. Never secure a sling at the back of the neck where pressure could be exerted. Fold the corner flat and neatly at the elbow, and pin. Check the position: the hand should be supported in the sling (Figure 24.12).

2. With the patient facing you, place the sling across the body and underneath the arms, as shown in Figure 24.13. Bring the corner of the sling that is under the unaffected arm to the back. Bring the lower corner up over the affected shoulder to the back, and tie. Fold the sling neatly at the elbow, and pin. Check the position: the hand should be supported in the sling.

Method 2 is preferred over method 1 because method 1 can pull or strain the neck muscles, even when it is tied at the side

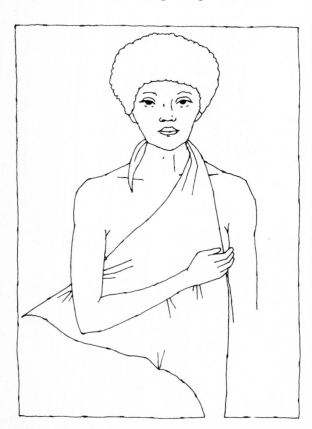

FIGURE 24.12   ARM SLING—METHOD 1

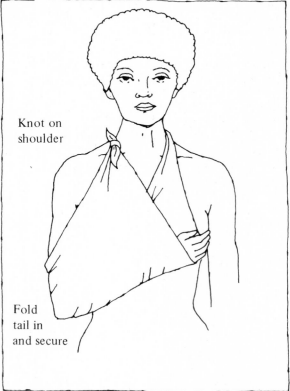

Knot on shoulder

Fold tail in and secure

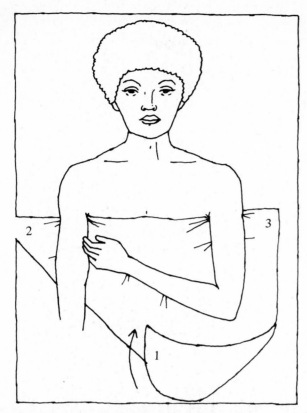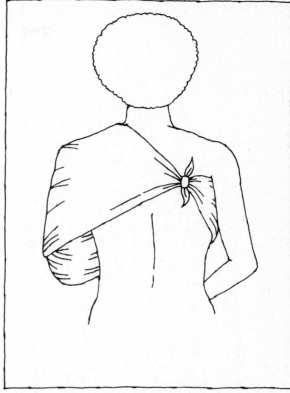

FIGURE 24.13   ARM SLING—METHOD 2

of the neck. Method 2 allows the entire shoulder to bear the weight of the immobilized arm.

Charting

Whenever a new bandage or binder is applied or whenever one is replaced, make a brief note on the patient's record. For example:

Sterile dressing held in place with figure-8 bandage.   J. Smith R.N.

or

Scultetus binder applied.   R. Jones R.N.

PERFORMANCE CHECKLIST

Applying bandages	Unsatisfactory	Needs more practice	Satisfactory	Comments
1. Assess method used for existing bandage (if there is one).				
2. Determine bandage needed and method to be used.				
3. Gather materials.				
4. Explain procedure to patient.				
5. Remove old bandage (if present).				
6. Discard, or reroll for reuse.				
7. Wash your hands.				
8. Using chosen method, apply new bandage.				
9. Check for comfort and effectiveness.				
10. Wash your hands.				
11. Chart.				
Applying abdominal binders				
1. Obtain appropriate binder.				
2. Remove soiled or used binder (if present), and save pins.				
3. Have patient lift midsection and place binder smoothly under patient, or turn patient side to side to place binder underneath.				
4. Straight binder: a. Bring ends upward around trunk.				
b. Overlap on abdomen.				
c. Secure with pins.				
5. Scultetus binder: a. Begin with lower tails and lace each at slightly upward angle over abdomen.				
b. Secure with pins.				
6. Check for comfort and effectiveness.				
7. Wash your hands.				
8. Chart.				

Applying T-binders

	Unsatisfactory	Needs more practice	Satisfactory	Comments
1. Obtain appropriate T-binder.				
2. Remove soiled or used T-binder (if present), and save pins.				
3. Have patient lift midsection or turn patient side to side, and place binder smoothly under patient with waistband at proper level and tail or tails downward at midline.				
4. Bring waist ends upward and around patient's abdomen.				
5. Bring lower tail or tails between patient's legs, over dressings.				
6. Secure with pin or pins.				
7. Check for comfort and effectiveness.				
8. Wash your hands.				
9. Chart.				

Applying an arm sling: Method 1

	Unsatisfactory	Needs more practice	Satisfactory	Comments
1. Remove soiled or used arm sling (if present).				
2. With patient facing you, place end of triangle over shoulder on unaffected side.				
3. Bring long straight side down smoothly under hand of affected side.				
4. Loop sling up around arm, placing other end of triangle over shoulder of affected side.				
5. Tie or pin ends to one side, not directly behind neck.				
6. Pleat or fold sling at elbow, and pin.				
7. Check for proper position and comfort.				
8. Wash your hands.				
9. Chart.				

Applying an arm sling: Method 2	Unsatisfactory	Needs more practice	Satisfactory	Comments
1. Remove soiled or used arm sling (if present).				
2. With patient facing you, place sling underneath arms, across body.				
3. Bring corner at unaffected side to back.				
4. Bring lower corner on affected side up over affected shoulder to back.				
5. Tie.				
6. Pleat or fold sling at elbow, and pin.				
7. Check for proper position and comfort.				
8. Wash your hands.				
9. Chart.				

QUIZ

Short-Answer Questions

1. List three reasons for the application of bandages.

    a. _____

    b. _____

    c. _____

2. List five methods for applying bandages.

    a. _____

    b. _____

    c. _____

    d. _____

    e. _____

3. The figure-8 method would most commonly be used to bandage

    _____ .

4. Bandages should be applied on extremities in a direction from

    _____ to _____ .

5. Abdominal binders are used primarily for what two purposes?

    a. _____

    b. _____

6. T-binders are available in two types depending on whether the

    patient is _____ or _____ .

Multiple-Choice Questions

_____ 7. The recurrent-fold method would be used to bandage

    a. the arm.
    b. the elbow.
    c. a joint.
    d. a fingertip.

_____ 8. The arm sling is not tied behind the neck primarily because it

    a. obstructs the blood flow.
    b. does not hold firmly.
    c. places strain on neck muscles.
    d. compresses nerves.

Module 25 Applying Heat and Cold

MAIN OBJECTIVE

To apply heat and cold appropriately, with emphasis on comfort and safety for patients.

RATIONALE

Applications of heat or cold are commonly ordered procedures and may be carried out in many different ways using a variety of equipment. It is essential that the nurse be aware of the indications and rationale for the application of heat and cold, as well as of safe and effective methods of application, in order to carry out the procedure in a way that meets the needs of patients.

PREREQUISITES

Successful completion of the following modules:

VOLUME 1
Assessment
Charting
Medical Asepsis
Bedmaking
Hygiene

VOLUME 2
Sterile Technique (optional)

SPECIFIC LEARNING OBJECTIVES

	Know Facts and Principles	Apply Facts and Principles	Demonstrate Ability	Evaluate Performance
1. *Physiological responses to application of heat*	State three responses of body to application of heat. State four indications for local application of heat.	State rationale for application of heat in a given situation. Given a patient situation, discuss expected responses to application of heat.		
2. *Physiological responses to application of cold*	State three responses of body to application of cold. State five indications for local application of cold.	Given a patient situation, state rationale for application of cold. Given a patient situation, discuss expected responses to application of cold. Explain effect of cold on already edematous area.		
3. *Safety*	State five precautionary measures to use in applying heat and cold. List signs and symptoms of harmful responses to applications of heat or cold.	Given a patient situation in which heat or cold is to be used, state appropriate safety measures	In the clinical setting, use appropriate safety measures when applying heat or cold	Evaluate with instructor using Performance Checklist. Assess patient's responses at frequent intervals to evaluate effects of therapy.
4. *Application of dry heat*	State four methods used to apply dry heat. Describe the general procedure for applying dry heat. Describe procedure for placing heat cradle.	Given a patient situation, select appropriate method of applying dry heat. Given a patient situation, discuss rationale for applying dry heat. Given a variety of patient situations, identify appropriate uses of heat cradle.	In the clinical setting, choose appropriate method for applying dry heat. In the clinical setting, correctly apply dry heat. In the clinical setting, correctly place heat cradle.	Evaluate choice with instructor. Evaluate with instructor using Performance Checklist

5. *Application of moist heat*	State three methods commonly used to apply moist heat	Given a patient situation, select appropriate method of applying moist heat	In the clinical setting, choose appropriate method for applying moist heat	Evaluate choice with instructor
	Describe procedures for application of warm moist compress, soak and sitz bath	Modify individual procedure based on patient situation	In the clinical setting, correctly apply warm moist compress, soak, and/or sitz bath	Evaluate own performance with instructor using Performance Checklist
6. *Application of moist cold*	State four methods used to apply moist cold	Given a patient situation, select appropriate method of applying moist cold	In the clinical setting, choose appropriate method for applying moist cold	Evaluate choice with instructor
7. *Application of dry cold*	Describe general procedure for applying dry cold	Given a patient situation, discuss rationale for applying dry cold	In the clinical setting, correctly apply dry cold	Evaluate with instructor using Performance Checklist
8. *Procedure for cooling sponge bath*	Describe procedure for cooling sponge bath	Given a patient situation, decide whether cooling sponge bath is appropriate	Correctly administer cooling sponge bath	Evaluate with instructor using Performance Checklist
9. *Charting*	State appropriate items to be charted in nurses' notes	Given a patient situation, simulate appropriate charting	In the clinical setting, chart appropriately with regard to application of heat and cold	Evaluate with instructor

LEARNING ACTIVITIES

1. Review the Specific Learning Objectives.
2. Read the section on heat production, heat loss, and hypothermia (in the chapter on neurological function) in Ellis and Nowlis, *Nursing: A Human Needs Approach,* or comparable material in another textbook.
3. Look up the module vocabulary terms in the glossary.
4. Read through the module.
5. With a partner in the practice setting:
   a. Prepare a hot water bottle and correctly apply it to your partner's shoulder.
   b. Reverse roles, and repeat step a.
   c. Evaluate each other's performance.
   d. Prepare a warm moist compress and apply it to the inner aspect of your partner's forearm, protecting the bed and the "patient" from the moisture. Do this as a clean procedure.
   e. Reverse roles, and repeat step d as a *sterile* procedure.
   f. Evaluate each other's performance.
   g. Prepare, apply, and secure an ice collar, cap, or glove to your partner's knee. Have your partner move around to see if the pack stays in place.
   h. Reverse roles, and repeat step g.
   i. Evaluate each other's performance.
6. In the clinical setting:
   a. Seek opportunities to observe the use of a heat cradle and a water-flow heating pad with control unit.
   b. Apply hot and cold treatments with supervision.

VOCABULARY

constriction
dilation
edema
inflammation
metabolism
oxygenation
suppuration

APPLYING HEAT AND COLD

The policies regarding the application of heat and cold vary from institution to institution. In some facilities, a physician's order is required; in others, nurses are allowed to administer heat and cold independently in order to provide comfort. Particularly in this last instance, you must know the physiological responses and appropriate uses of heat and cold.

Physiological Responses to Heat

When heat is applied to an area of the body, the blood vessels in that area *dilate* (expand), causing *increased blood circulation* and, therefore, *enriched oxygenation* to the tissues involved, which results in *improved tissue metabolism.*

Heat can be used to relieve pain from muscle spasms and affected joints. *Heat also reduces swelling* (and accompanying discomfort) by increasing circulation (fluid is more easily absorbed from the affected area). Increased circulation also eliminates any toxic waste products that have accumulated in the area of swelling or edema. *Heat relaxes muscles.* And, finally, *heat can promote healing* by increasing oxygenation of the tissues and by promoting suppuration in cases of infection.

Physiological Responses to Cold

The application of cold *constricts* blood vessels in the area. This slows circulation, which may reduce hemorrhage and/or oozing and decrease pain. The local application of cold may also reduce inflammation and prevent the formation of edema.

Frank hemorrhage from an external wound and internal oozing near the site of a fracture, as examples, may both be reduced by the application of cold and the subsequent constriction of blood vessels. Applying cold immediately following a sprain or contusion aids in preventing the accumulation of fluid in the area. However, applied to an already edematous area, cold slows the reduction of edema, because the decrease in circulation retards the reabsorption of fluid into the tissues. Preventing edema assists in decreasing pain. Pain also decreases by the anesthetic effect of cold directly on the skin, for example, when applied to a burned or inflamed area.

Safety

To safely apply heat and cold, you should be aware of the following precautions:

1. Patients vary in their ability to tolerate heat and/or cold. Factors that affect tolerance include age (the very young and the elderly are more susceptible to negative effects of heat and cold therapies), presence of circulatory or neurological deficiencies, the level of consciousness, and the condition of the skin in the area to be treated. The patient's diagnosis is also a factor to be considered, as is the particular type of heat or cold application. In any event, assess the patient carefully before you proceed with any treatment.

2. Temperature receptors in the skin adjust rapidly to mild stimulation. This adaptability explains why a sensation of either warmth or coolness dissipates in a short time. Explain this phenomenon to the patient, so that he or she does not increase or decrease the temperature of a treatment to an unsafe level.

3. Any time you apply heat or cold, check the affected area at frequent intervals (at least every 20 minutes). Increased pain and swelling, decreased sensation, mottling, and/or extreme redness may indicate that you should stop the treatment.

4. Moisture conducts heat better than air, so take special care when you apply moist heat or cold. Injury is more likely to occur in these situations. Because air is a poor conductor, it is used to insulate certain applications of heat and cold. For example, cover a hot water bottle or an ice cap with a cloth before

you apply it. The air between the cloth and the bag provides insulation.

5. The length of time the body is exposed to the application of heat or cold, as well as the size of the skin area being treated, affects the ability of the body to tolerate the treatment. The shorter the exposure time and the smaller the area being treated, the better the tolerance.

Methods of Applying Dry Heat

The heat cradle, heat lamp, water-flow heating pad with control unit, electric heating pad, hot water bottle or bag, and disposable heat pack are all methods of applying dry heat. All of these vehicles—with the exception of the heat cradle and heat lamp—use a similar procedure.

WATER-FLOW HEATING PAD WITH CONTROL UNIT

This device consists of a rubber pad with distilled water circulating through it. It is connected to a control unit that heats the water to a preset temperature and maintains it there. The temperature is usually set in the central supply department. A newer model of this device has a pad made of soft absorbent material on the inside surface and waterproof material on the outside (Figure 25.1). The absorbent material can be used to apply moist heat, and the device is disposable.

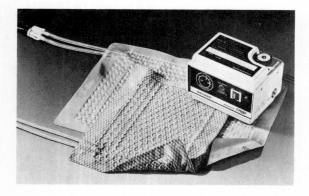

FIGURE 25.1   WATER-FLOW HEATING PAD WITH CONTROL UNIT
Courtesy Gaymar T. Pump & T. Pad, Gaymar Industries, Orchard Park, New York

ELECTRIC HEATING PAD

Electric heating pads are commonly used in the home and are still used in health care agencies, although many facilities no longer use them for safety reasons. The wires that provide the heat are usually covered by rubber or plastic, but sometimes may be covered only by fabric. In any case, do not use electric heating pads in the presence of moisture because of the danger of electric shock.

HOT WATER BOTTLE

The hot water bottle (bag) is another common device for the application of dry heat (Figure 25.2). Even though it is no longer used in some health care agencies, you should be familiar with its proper use. There are a few principles that are essential to its safe use.

1. Measure the temperature of the water *with a thermometer.* The maximum for an adult is 125° F; for an infant, 115° F. If a bath thermometer is not available, place the filled bag against the inner

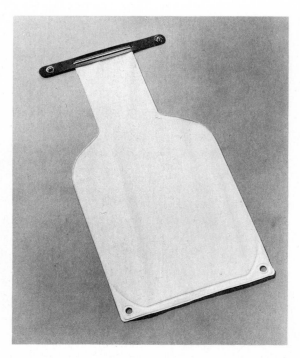

FIGURE 25.2   HOT WATER BOTTLE
Courtesy Searle Medical Products USA Inc.

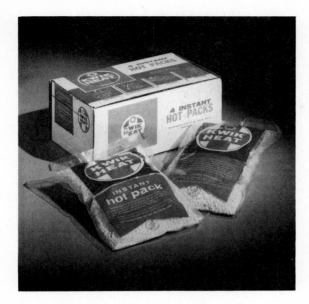

FIGURE 25.3   DISPOSABLE HOT PACKS
Courtesy Dyna Med Inc., Carlsbad, California, and Kay Laboratories

surface of your forearm. Except in special circumstances, what feels comfortable to you will probably be safe and comfortable for a patient.

2. Fill the bottle only half to two thirds full. Then fold or twist the bag to remove any air before you insert the stopper or fold the bag and clamp it

shut. This makes the bag lighter and easier to apply to a given surface because it will conform to the shape of that surface.

3. Cover the bottle with a cloth before you place it in contact with the skin.

DISPOSABLE HOT PACK

Disposable hot packs (Figure 25.3) are available commercially and are used in a variety of settings. They are especially useful in emergency rooms. They come in a number of sizes and shapes, and deliver a specific amount of heat for a specified length of time as indicated by the manufacturer's instructions. *Be certain to read these instructions carefully.* To use, strike the package, which creates a chemical reaction that releases the heat. Disposable hot packs are both safe and convenient when used properly.

HEAT CRADLE

A heat cradle is a metal frame, with a light socket in the center or at one end, that can be placed over the patient (Figure 25.4). The bulb used should be no larger than 25 watts and should be positioned no closer than 18

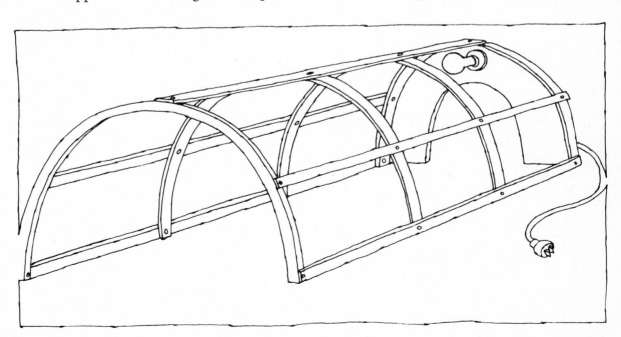

FIGURE 25.4   HEAT CRADLE

inches from the site to be treated. Place top linen over the cradle to keep the patient warm.

HEAT LAMP

A heat lamp is usually a portable floor lamp with a flexible neck (gooseneck). The bulb used should be no larger than 25 watts and should be positioned no closer than 18 inches from the site to be treated. If a larger bulb is used, it should be placed a greater distance from the patient.

GENERAL PROCEDURE

1. Secure the heating device you want to use. Water-flow heating pads and electric heating pads are often found in the central supply department; hot water bottles and disposable hot packs usually are found on the unit.
2. Wash your hands.
3. Explain to the patient what you plan to do.
4. Provide for the patient's privacy and warmth.
5. Fan-fold the top covers to the foot of the bed, if necessary.
6. Expose the area to be treated, uncovering as little of the rest of the body as possible. If a moist pack and/or sterile dressing is involved, follow step 6 in the procedure for placing a heat cradle, on this page.
7. Completely cover the heating device with a soft cloth cover, making sure the cover is as free of folds and wrinkles as possible. Some disposable hot packs come with a special outer covering.
8. Place the heating device over the area to be treated, molding it to that area as necessary or as possible. Tie it in place with clean cloth or roller gauze.
9. Return to the patient at frequent intervals (at least every 20 minutes), to check for adverse reactions and to see that the heating device has remained in place.
10. Remove the heating device at the end of the specified time.

11. Examine the treated area.
12. Leave the patient comfortable and dry.
13. Wash your hands.
14. Chart the treatment, including the length of time applied and the patient's response.

PROCEDURE FOR PLACING A HEAT CRADLE

1. Secure a heat cradle. They are often kept in the central supply department of the hospital.
2. Wash your hands.
3. Explain the procedure to the patient.
4. Provide for the patient's privacy and warmth.
5. Fan-fold the top covers to the foot of the bed, and place the heat cradle over the area to be treated.
6. Expose and/or dress the area to be treated according to the physician's order. You may need to apply a moist dressing and/or use sterile technique, depending on the situation. If moisture is involved, be sure to protect the bedding with plastic covered by a towel or a Chux. Be sure the patient is comfortable and in good alignment.
7. Replace the top covers over the heat cradle. The sheet should not come too close to nor be in direct contact with the lightbulb.
8. Keeping the cord off the floor, plug it into the outlet nearest the bed. Turn the bulb on. Do not use larger than a 25-watt bulb, and keep it a minimum of 18 inches from the patient. (If a larger bulb is used, place it a greater distance away from the patient.)
9. Return to check the patient at least every 20 minutes. Depending on the situation (elderly patient, presence of moist dressing), you may wish to check more often.
10. Remove the heat cradle at the end of the treatment. Occasionally, the cradle is left in place to keep bed linen off a specific area; in this case, you need only turn off the bulb and disconnect the cord.

11. Leave the patient comfortable and dry.
12. Wash your hands.
13. Chart the treatment, including the length of time applied and the patient's response.

PROCEDURE FOR PLACING A HEAT LAMP

1. Secure a heat lamp. They are often kept in the treatment room or utility room on the unit.
2. Wash your hands.
3. Explain the procedure to the patient.
4. Provide for the patient's privacy and warmth.
5. Fan-fold top linen as necessary to the foot of the bed.
6. Expose only the area of the body to be treated, keeping the rest of the body covered appropriately.
7. Plug the cord into the outlet nearest the bed and turn on the bulb. Usually, no larger than a 25-watt bulb is used, and it is kept a minimum of 18 inches from the patient.
8. Return to check the patient at least every 10 minutes because it is possible for a patient to move closer to the bulb in your absence. A heat lamp treatment usually lasts 20 minutes.
9. At the end of the treatment, remove the lamp.
10. Apply any topical medication and/or dressing ordered.
11. Replace any top linen removed earlier.
12. Wash your hands.
13. Chart the treatment, including the length of time applied and the patient's response.

Methods of Applying Moist Heat

Compresses, soaks, and sitz baths are commonly used to apply moist heat. A *compress* is a wet dressing that is applied to an area to provide moisture. It may be either hot or cold. A *soak* is used to apply moisture through immersion of a body part. A *sitz bath* is a way of providing a soak to the perineal and rectal areas.

PROCEDURE FOR APPLYING A WARM MOIST COMPRESS

1. Wash your hands.
2. Secure the material to be used for the compress. Use sterile material (including sterile basin, sterile solution, and sterile gloves) and technique as necessary. Often a washcloth is used when a small unsterile compress is needed; a towel can be used for a larger area.
3. Obtain a water-flow heating pad or other heating device to maintain the heat of the compress if necessary. Do not use an electric heating pad.
4. Explain to the patient what you plan to do.
5. Provide for the patient's privacy and warmth.
6. Expose the area to be treated, uncovering as little of the rest of the body as possible. Assess the area.
7. Moisten the compress in hot water and wring it out, so that it remains moist but doesn't drip. Apply it to the area to be treated, cover it with plastic, and then cover with further insulation, such as a towel.
8. Place a water-flow heating pad or other heating device on the outside to maintain the heat if necessary.
9. Hold the compress in place with ties.
10. Return to the patient at frequent intervals to check for adverse reactions and to see that the compress has remained in place.
11. Remove the compress at the end of the specified time.
12. Examine the treated area.
13. Leave the patient comfortable, warm, and dry.
14. Wash your hands.
15. Chart the treatment, including the length of time applied and the patient's response.

PROCEDURE FOR ADMINISTERING A SOAK

1. Obtain a basin. If a wound is involved, the basin and solution have to be sterile.
2. Wash your hands.

3. Explain to the patient what you plan to do.
4. Provide for the patient's privacy and warmth.
5. Fill the basin half full with water, saline, or the medicated solution that has been ordered. The temperature of the water or solution is usually 105° F–115° F, unless otherwise ordered.
6. Place the body part to be treated into the basin, making sure that the rest of the body is in good alignment and that there is no pressure on the part from the edge of the basin. Often, you will have to pad the edge of the basin with a towel to prevent pressure.
7. Check the patient at least once during the treatment. A soak usually is 15 to 20 minutes long.
8. Remove the body part from the basin and pat it dry gently, using sterile towels or gauze if necessary.
9. Examine the part carefully and reapply a dressing if indicated.
10. Leave the patient comfortable, warm, and dry.
11. Remove the basin to a dirty utility area.
12. Wash your hands.
13. Chart the treatment, including the length of time applied and the patient's response.

PROCEDURE FOR ADMINISTERING A
SITZ BATH

A sitz bath is a method of administering a soak to the pelvic area. Some facilities have special tubs designed for the purpose; portable chairs and disposable equipment that can be used on a toilet are also available (Figures 25.5 and 25.6). Sometimes, a patient is merely placed in a bathtub that has been filled with enough water to reach the umbilicus. Unless otherwise specified, the temperature of the water should be 105° F–115° F, and the treatment should last 15 to 20 minutes.

1. Gather the equipment. In addition to the equipment for the bath itself, you will need a bath blanket and at least one

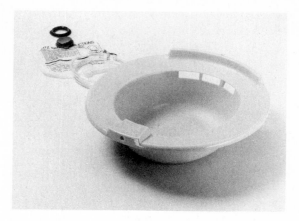

FIGURE 25.5   DISPOSABLE SITZ BATH
Courtesy Searle Medical Products USA Inc.

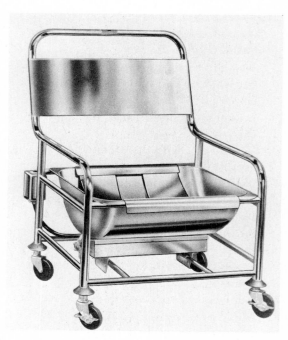

FIGURE 25.6   PORTABLE SITZ BATH CHAIR
Courtesy Ille, division of Market Forge

towel. Place the bath blanket over the patient's shoulders to provide warmth; use the towel for drying the patient at the end of the treatment. You may need additional towels to pad the tub or chair to relieve pressure or to assist with body alignment.
2. Wash your hands.
3. Explain to the patient what you plan to do.

4. Assist the patient to the tub room or bathroom. If a long distance is involved, you may want the patient to push a wheelchair. Then, if at any point he or she feels weak or tired, immediate transportation will be available.
5. Fill the tub or chair with enough water to cover the umbilicus. The water should be between 105° F and 115° F.
6. Provide for the patient's privacy and warmth.
7. Remove the patient's clothing and any dressing in place. Assess the area.
8. Assist the patient into the tub or chair, padding as necessary to prevent pressure and to provide for good body alignment.
9. Check the patient at least once during the treatment. If the patient's condition warrants (first post-op day, extremely fatigued or weak patient), stay in the room for the first five minutes or for the entire treatment.
10. Assist the patient out of the tub or chair.
11. Help dry the patient.
12. Examine the treated area and reapply the dressing if necessary.
13. Help the patient dress.
14. Assist the patient back to the room.
15. Leave the patient comfortable, warm, and dry.
16. Care for the equipment according to the procedure in your facility.
17. Wash your hands.
18. Chart the treatment, including the length of time applied and the patient's response.

Methods of Applying Dry Cold

Ice collars, ice caps, ice gloves, and disposable cold packs are all devices for the application of dry cold. Again, the procedure is similar no matter which device is used.

ICE COLLAR

An ice collar is a rubber or plastic bag, long and narrow in shape, that is designed for use around the neck but can be used for other small areas of the body as well (Figure 25.7).

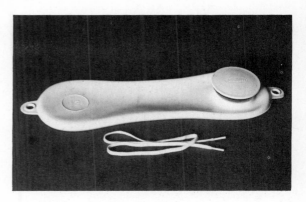

FIGURE 25.7   ICE COLLAR
Courtesy American Hospital Supply and Abbot Labs

ICE CAP

An ice cap is a large rubber or plastic bag that is designed for use over a large body area. Fill the bag (ice bag or ice collar) half to two thirds full with crushed ice, remove excess air by folding or twisting the bag, and insert the stopper. A rubber glove can also be used to apply dry cold. Close it by tying a knot in the open end.

DISPOSABLE COLD PACK

Disposable cold packs are used in the same way as are disposable hot packs. They come in a variety of sizes and shapes (Figure 25.8), including a shape similar to an ice collar, and deliver a specific amount of cold for a specified length of time as indicated by the manufacturer's instructions. *Be certain to read these instructions carefully.* To use, strike

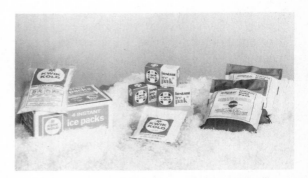

FIGURE 25.8   DISPOSABLE COLD PACKS
Courtesy Dyna Med, Inc., Carlsbad, California, and Kay Laboratories

the package, which creates a chemical reaction that releases the cold. Disposable cold packs are both convenient and safe when used properly.

GENERAL PROCEDURE

1. Obtain the device you want to use. In some facilities, they are stored in small numbers in the nursing unit. In other facilities, they are stored only in the central supply department.
2. Wash your hands.
3. Explain to the patient what you plan to do.
4. Provide for the patient's privacy and warmth.
5. Expose the area to be treated, uncovering as little of the rest of the body as possible to avoid chilling the patient.
6. Completely cover the ice collar or cap with an appropriate soft cloth cover. Be sure the cover is as free of folds and wrinkles as possible. Certain disposable plastic ice collars and bags come with a soft outer covering that makes another covering unnecessary. Disposable cold packs may also come with such a covering.
7. Place the ice collar or cap over the area to be treated, molding it to the area as necessary or possible.
8. Tie it in place, if possible, with clean cloth or roller gauze.
9. Return to the patient at frequent intervals to check for adverse reactions (numbness, mottled skin), to see that the device has remained in place, and to see if the ice has melted. For best results, leave the device in place no longer than one hour. Remove the device for at least one hour before reapplying it.
10. Remove the device at the end of the specified time.
11. Examine the treated area.
12. Leave the patient comfortable and dry.
13. Wash your hands.
14. Chart the treatment, including the length of time applied and the patient's response.

Cooling Sponge Bath

Occasionally, sponge baths are ordered to help reduce a patient's elevated temperature. In the past, alcohol was added to the bath water because it evaporates quickly, removing heat rapidly. This is no longer done in most facilities for a variety of reasons, including the potential adverse effects of inhaling alcohol fumes and the extreme drying effect on the skin.

PROCEDURE

1. Obtain a baseline body temperature before giving a sponge bath. In fact, the decision to give a cooling sponge bath usually is made only after a temperature is taken. If no temperature is recorded, take the patient's temperature and record it before you begin.
2. Gather the necessary equipment. You will need a basin, several washcloths (at least four), several towels, and a bath blanket.
3. Wash your hands.
4. Explain to the patient what you plan to do.
5. Close the windows and doors, and pull the bed curtains shut.
6. Remove the bedspread and blanket, position the bath blanket, and remove the top sheet as described in Module 6, Bedmaking, Occupied Beds, step 4, page 68.
7. Fill the basin with cool water. Temperatures lower than 65° F are likely to be uncomfortable for an alert patient, but the physician's order or your facility's procedure may require a lower temperature. In any case, never use water cooler than 50° F.
8. Wet three washcloths, wring them out so that they are wet but not dripping, and place them in the axillae and groin. Check them every five minutes to see whether they should be changed. They will probably warm up quickly in these vascular areas of the body.
9. Bathe each extremity for approximately

three minutes, depending on how the procedure is tolerated. This is more easily done with two people.

10. Dry each extremity.
11. Have the patient turn over.
12. Bathe the back and buttocks for approximately five minutes. Again, the length of time will be dictated somewhat by how well the patient tolerates the procedure.
13. Dry the back and buttocks.
14. Remove the washcloths from the axillae and groin, and dry those areas.
15. Check the patient's temperature to evaluate the effect of the bath. Stop the bath before the patient registers a normal temperature because the body continues to cool even after the bath is finished. If the patient is not cool enough, you may have to repeat the procedure.
16. Replace the top linen and remove the bath blanket as described in Module 6, Bedmaking, Occupied Beds, steps 21 and 22, page 69.
17. Return the equipment to the designated area.
18. Wash your hands.
19. Chart the patient's temperature, both before and after the bath, as well as his or her other responses.

PERFORMANCE CHECKLIST

General procedure for applying dry heat	Unsatisfactory	Needs more practice	Satisfactory	Comments
1. Secure appropriate heating device.				
2. Wash your hands.				
3. Explain procedure to patient.				
4. Provide for patient's privacy and warmth.				
5. Fan-fold top covers to foot of bed.				
6. Expose only area to be treated.				
7. Cover heating device, if necessary.				
8. Place and mold heating device over area to be treated, and secure.				
9. Return to check patient every 20 minutes.				
10. Remove device at end of specified time.				
11. Examine treated area.				
12. Leave patient dry and comfortable.				
13. Wash your hands.				
14. Chart.				

Applying a heat cradle				
1. Secure heat cradle.				
2. Wash your hands.				
3. Explain procedure to patient.				
4. Provide for patient's privacy and warmth.				
5. Fan-fold top covers to foot of bed and place heat cradle over area to be treated.				
6. Expose only area to be treated.				
7. Replace top covers over cradle.				
8. Plug cord into nearest plug.				
9. Return to check patient every 20 minutes.				
10. Remove cradle at end of treatment if appropriate.				
11. Leave patient comfortable and dry.				
12. Wash your hands.				
13. Chart.				

Placing a heat lamp	Unsatisfactory	Needs more practice	Satisfactory	Comments
1. Secure heat lamp.				
2. Wash your hands.				
3. Explain procedure to patient.				
4. Provide for patient's privacy and warmth.				
5. Fan-fold top linens to foot of bed, if necessary.				
6. Expose only area to be treated.				
7. Plug cord into nearest outlet and turn on bulb.				
8. Return to check patient every ten minutes.				
9. Remove heat lamp.				
10. Apply topical medication and/or dressing if ordered.				
11. Replace top linen.				
12. Wash your hands.				
13. Chart.				
Applying a warm moist compress				
1. Wash your hands.				
2. Obtain material to be used for compress.				
3. Obtain heating device to maintain heat of compress if necessary.				
4. Explain procedure to patient.				
5. Provide for patient's privacy and warmth.				
6. Expose only area to be treated.				
7. Moisten, wring out, and apply compress, covering with plastic and towel.				
8. Place heating device over outside to maintain heat if ordered.				
9. Secure in place with ties.				
10. Return to check patient at frequent intervals.				
11. Remove compress.				
12. Examine treated area.				
13. Leave patient comfortable, warm, and dry.				
14. Wash your hands.				
15. Chart.				

	Unsatisfactory	Needs more practice	Satisfactory	Comments
Administering a soak				
1. Obtain basin.				
2. Wash your hands.				
3. Explain procedure to patient.				
4. Provide for patient's privacy and warmth.				
5. Fill basin half full with water (105° F–115° F).				
6. Place body part to be treated in basin, checking for body alignment and pressure.				
7. Check patient at least once during procedure.				
8. Remove body part from basin and dry.				
9. Examine and reapply dressing as needed.				
10. Leave patient comfortable, warm, and dry.				
11. Remove basin.				
12. Wash your hands.				
13. Chart.				
Administering a sitz bath				
1. Gather equipment.				
2. Wash your hands.				
3. Explain procedure to patient.				
4. Assist patient to the location for the bath.				
5. Fill tub or chair with enough water (105° F–115° F) to cover umbilicus.				
6. Provide for patient's privacy and warmth.				
7. Remove patient's clothing and any dressings.				
8. Assist patient into tub or chair.				
9. Check patient at least once during treatment.				
10. Assist patient out of tub or chair.				
11. Help patient dry.				
12. Examine treated area and reapply dressing as indicated				
13. Help patient dress.				
14. Assist patient back to room.				
15. Leave patient comfortable, warm, and dry.				

	Unsatisfactory	Needs more practice	Satisfactory	Comments
16. Care for equipment.				
17. Wash your hands.				
18. Chart.				
Applying dry cold				
1. Obtain device to be used.				
2. Wash your hands.				
3. Explain procedure to patient.				
4. Provide for patient's privacy and warmth.				
5. Expose only area to be treated.				
6. Cover device with soft cloth cover if necessary.				
7. Place device over area to be treated, molding if necessary.				
8. Secure in place with ties.				
9. Return to check patient at frequent intervals.				
10. Remove device.				
11. Examine treated area.				
12. Leave patient comfortable and dry.				
13. Wash your hands.				
14. Chart.				
Administering a Cooling Sponge Bath				
1. Check for or take patient's temperature.				
2. Gather equipment.				
3. Wash your hands.				
4. Explain procedure to patient.				
5. Close windows and doors, and screen patient.				
6. Remove top linen and place bath blanket.				
7. Fill basin with cool water.				
8. Wet, wring out, and place three washcloths at axillae and groin.				
9. Bathe each extremity for three minutes.				
10. Dry each extremity.				
11. Have patient turn over.				

	Unsatisfactory	Needs more practice	Satisfactory	Comments
12. Bathe back and buttocks for five minutes.				
13. Dry back and buttocks.				
14. Remove washcloths from axillae and groin, and dry.				
15. Check patient's temperature.				
16. Replace top linen and remove bath blanket.				
17. Care for equipment.				
18. Wash your hands.				
19. Chart.				

QUIZ

Multiple-Choice Questions

_____ 1. Indications for the local application of heat include which of the following?
(1) relief of pain; (2) reduction of edema; (3) reduction of suppuration;
(4) promotion of healing

    a. 1 and 4
    b. 1, 2, and 4
    c. 2, 3, and 4
    d. All of the above

_____ 2. Indications for the local application of cold include which of the following?
(1) reduction of hemorrhaging; (2) relief of pain; (3) prevention of edema;
(4) treatment of edema

    a. 1 and 4
    b. 1, 2, and 3
    c. 1, 3, and 4
    d. All of the above

_____ 3. Factors affecting the tolerance of an individual to heat or cold include
(1) age; (2) level of consciousness; (3) condition of skin; (4) diagnosis.

    a. 1 and 3
    b. 1, 3, and 4
    c. 2, 3, and 4
    d. All of the above

_____ 4. The bulb in a heat cradle is generally no larger than a

    a. 15-watt bulb.
    b. 25-watt bulb.
    c. 40-watt bulb.
    d. 60-watt bulb.

_____ 5. A sitz bath is generally administered over

    a. 5 to 10 minutes.
    b. 15 to 20 minutes.
    c. 30 to 40 minutes.
    d. An hour.

_____ 6. During a cooling sponge bath, washcloths are placed in which area of the
body? (1) the forehead; (2) the back of the neck; (3) axillae; (4) the groin

    a. 1 and 2
    b. 1, 2, and 3
    c. 3 and 4
    d. All of the above

Module 26 Cardiopulmonary Resuscitation

MAIN OBJECTIVE

To recognize the need for and to perform cardiopulmonary resuscitation (CPR) on individuals of all ages.[1]

RATIONALE

The nurse is expected to carry out efficient and effective cardiopulmonary resuscitation, whether on the street or in a health care agency. The nurse must be able to perform this lifesaving procedure as a member of a team or alone on individuals of all ages. At least once a year, a refresher course must be taken to maintain expertise.

PREREQUISITES

Successful completion of the following modules:

VOLUME 1
Assessment
Charting

[1] Material in this module, including Figures 26.3 through 26.7, conforms to the American Heart Association recommendations as of July 1979.

SPECIFIC LEARNING OBJECTIVES

	Know Facts and Principles	Apply Facts and Principles	Demonstrate Ability	Evaluate Performance
1. *Airway*	State usual method for opening airway. State method used in case of cervical injury. State method used to remove foreign bodies.	Given a patient situation, identify appropriate method for opening airway and/or removing foreign bodies	Open airway on mannequin using both methods described	Evaluate with instructor and lab partner
2. *Breathing*	Describe usual method for rescue breathing. Describe alternative methods used in special situations.	Given a patient situation, identify appropriate method of rescue breathing	Demonstrate mouth-to-mouth and mouth-to-nose breathing	Evaluate effectiveness by checking chest for movement
3. *Circulation*	State where to palpate carotid pulse. State when precordial thump is appropriate. State where to apply compression on adults and children. State distance sternum must be moved for effective compression		Give precordial thump correctly. Apply compression in appropriate location. Move sternum appropriate distance when doing cardiac compression.	Evaluate by checking for adequate compression on mannequin gauge, if available
4. *One rescuer*	State ratio of breaths to compression for one rescuer		Perform CPR alone on mannequin	Evaluate with instructor using Performance Checklist

5. *Two rescuers*	State ratio of breaths to compression for two rescuers	Perform two-person CPR with partner on mannequin	Evaluate with instructor using Performance Checklist
6. *Age considerations*	State differences in procedure for adults, small children, and infants	Perform CPR on infant mannequin incorporating techniques that differ from adult procedure	Evaluate with instructor using Performance Checklist
7. *Charting*	State two items of particular importance to be observed and recorded when CPR is carried out	Observe and record accurately during real or simulated CPR	Evaluate own performance with instructor

LEARNING ACTIVITIES

1. Review the Specific Learning Objectives.
2. Read the section on basic life support (in the chapter on circulation) in Ellis and Nowlis, *Nursing: A Human Needs Approach,* or comparable material in another textbook.
3. Look up the module vocabulary terms in the glossary.
4. Read through the module.
5. In the laboratory, practice with a Resusci-Annie or similar mannequin under the supervision of your instructor.
   a. Establish an airway on the adult mannequin.
   b. Breathe 12 times per minute into the adult mannequin, watching for the rise and fall of the chest wall and allowing for "exhalation."
   c. Practice closed-chest massage on the adult mannequin at a rate of 60 per minute (as would be done with two rescuers) and 80 per minute (as would be done with one rescuer), compressing the sternum 1½ inches to 2 inches each time.
   d. Establish an airway on an infant mannequin.
   e. Breathe 20 times per minute into the infant mannequin, using only the amount of air your cheeks can hold for each breath.
   f. Practice closed-chest massage on the infant mannequin at a rate of 100 per minute, using only the tips of your index and middle finger to compress the sternum ½ inch to ¾ inch.
6. With a partner, practice CPR on both adult and infant mannequins, using the Performance Checklist as a guide. Take turns doing the breathing and the closed-chest massage. Have your instructor evaluate your performances.
7. With your partner as observer and evaluator, practice CPR alone on both the adult and infant mannequins, using the Performance Checklist as a guide. When you are satisfied with your performance, trade places and have your partner demonstrate CPR on the adult and infant mannequins with you observing and evaluating. When you are both satisfied with your performances, have your instructor evaluate them.

VOCABULARY

airway
cardiac arrest
carotid pulse
precordial thump
respiratory arrest
sternum
trachea
tracheostomy
xiphoid process

CARDIOPULMONARY RESUSCITATION

Cardiopulmonary resuscitation is a process of rescue breathing and chest compression that is provided to a person whose heart has stopped beating and who has stopped breathing. No matter where this person is, he or she needs *immediate* assistance to restore breathing and circulation. If there is more than a 4-minute delay, the potential for permanent brain damage is great. CPR may be needed anywhere: in the home, on the street, in the health care agency. Eventually, you may be involved, not only in performing the skill, but in teaching it to other professionals and lay people as well.

Basic CPR is as easy to remember as ABC: Airway, Breathing, and Circulation.

Airway

1. When you find a person in a state of collapse, grasp the shoulder firmly, shake, and shout, "Are you all right?" If there is no response, follow steps 2–4 to be sure that the airway is open.
2. Position the person flat on the back. If you must roll the person over, try to move the entire body at once, as a single unit.
3. Tilt the patient's head back with one hand on the forehead, while you lift the chin with your other hand to clear the tongue out of the airway. (This is the chin-lift method of opening the airway.)
4. Place your ear close to the patient's mouth and do three things:
   a. *Look* at the chest and the stomach for movement.
   b. *Listen* for breathing sounds.
   c. *Feel* for air against your cheek (Figure 26.1).

   Sometimes by establishing an airway, the person begins to breathe spontaneously. But, if you cannot see chest movement, hear breathing sounds, or feel air on your cheek, the patient is not breathing and you must provide rescue breathing.

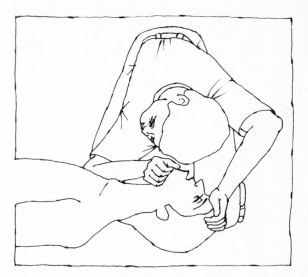

FIGURE 26.1   CHECKING FOR BREATHING
Note that the patient's head is tilted back.

Breathing

1. Using the hand that is on the patient's forehead, occlude the nostrils while you keep the head tilted back. Continue to lift the chin with your other hand, to maintain the airway (Figure 26.2).
2. Place your mouth over the patient's mouth, make an airtight seal, and give *four, quick, full breaths*. If the patient's chest rises and falls, showing that air has entered, proceed to step 5 below; if not, continue with steps 3 and 4.
3. If you feel resistance when you try to breathe into the patient's mouth, and the patient's chest wall does not rise and fall as you breathe, there may be an obstruction. Turn the patient onto his or her side, open the mouth, and check for foreign bodies. Scrape out vomitus with your hand or with a hankerchief. If you can see a foreign object in the throat, try to remove it. If it is *deep* in the throat, roll the patient toward yourself and deliver four blows to the back, between the shoulder blades, with the side of your hand. Then reposition the patient on his or her back. If the patient is still obstructed, put your hands on the lower half of the sternum (in the

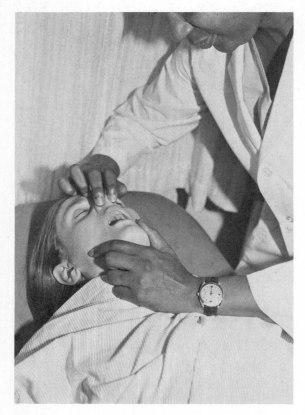

FIGURE 26.2   OCCLUDING THE NOSTRILS
Courtesy Lawrence Cherkas

same position you will use for chest
compression, Circulation, steps 2–4,
page 405) and exert four downward
thrusts. (This is the chest-thrust method
of removing a foreign body from the
airway.) There may be enough air
present to dislodge the foreign body.
An infant can be picked up and turned
head down over one arm, while you
deliver a quick blow between the shoulder blades with the other hand. When
you think you have cleared the obstruction, again attempt rescue breathing.
Even if the obstruction cannot be completely cleared, you can try to breathe
past the obstruction, perhaps inflating
only one lung.
4. If for some reason mouth-to-mouth
breathing is not desirable or possible
(For example, in the presence of vomiting or injury to the mouth or jaw),
mouth-to-nose breathing can be done

by closing the mouth with the palm of
one hand and breathing into the nose.
The position of the head would be the
same as for mouth-to-mouth breathing.
Mouth-to-stoma breathing is possible if
the patient has a permanent tracheostomy. In this case, there would be no
need to tilt the head back to open the
airway as you would for mouth-to-
mouth and mouth-to-nose breathing.
5. Feel for the carotid pulse by locating
the larynx (voice box) and sliding your
fingers off into the groove beside it.
You should feel for the pulse on *your*
side of the patient (Figure 26.3) to
avoid compressing the other carotid
artery with your thumb. If you locate a
pulse, perform rescue breathing at a
rate of 12 breaths per minute, recheck-
ing the pulse after each 12 breaths. If
you cannot locate a pulse, you will have
to provide artificial circulation in addition to rescue breathing.

Circulation

1. Kneel at the side of the patient, directly
beside the patient's chest. It is best for
the patient to be on a hard surface. In a
health care agency, you would have a
cardiac board to slip under the patient.
But do not waste time; if you can't
reposition the patient quickly and easily,
get on with the compression.
2. Locate the lower margin of the patient's
rib cage on the side nearest you. Run

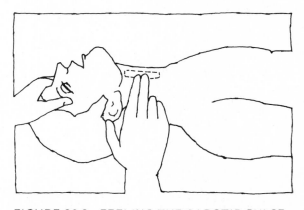

FIGURE 26.3   FEELING THE CAROTID PULSE

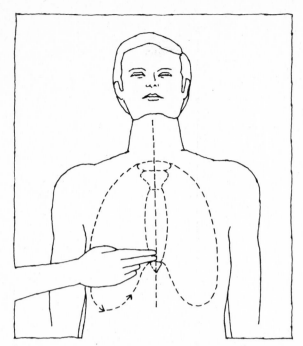

FIGURE 26.4   LOCATING THE LOWER MARGIN OF THE RIB CAGE

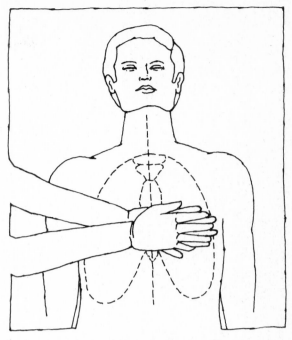

FIGURE 26.5   HANDS IN PLACE FOR CHEST COMPRESSION

your fingers up along the rib cage to the indentation where the ribs meet the sternum. Keeping one finger on the indentation, place another immediately above it, on the lower end of the sternum (Figure 26.4).

3. Place the heel of your other hand just above that finger, at right angles to the sternum. *Note:* The location of the xiphoid process is irrelevant if this method is used.

4. Remove your fingers from the indentation and place that hand on top of the one already in position. Your hands should be parallel and directed away from you (Figure 26.5). Keep your fingers up off the chest wall to avoid fracturing a rib. This may be easier for you to do if you interlace your fingers (Figure 26.6).

5. With your shoulders directly above the patient's chest, compress downward, keeping your arms straight. You should feel the sternum of an adult move 1½ to 2 inches with each compression (Figure 26.7). You must allow equal time for relaxation, but do so without

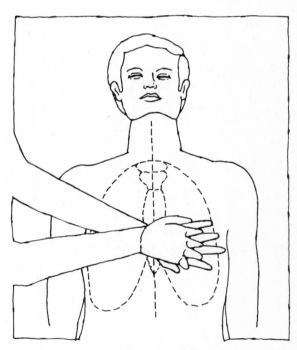

FIGURE 26.6   HANDS IN PLACE WITH FINGERS INTERLOCKED

changing the position of your lower hand. Your motion should be a rhythmical 50 percent down and 50 percent back up. Avoid quick ineffective jabs to

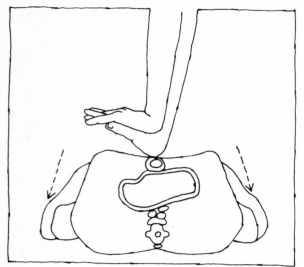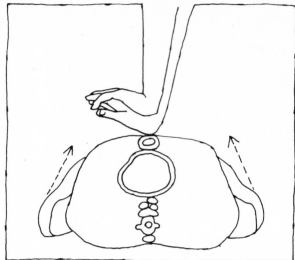

FIGURE 26.7 CORRECT COMPRESSION FOR AN ADULT

the chest. Also avoid bouncing compressions because they are less effective and more likely to cause injury. A definite hesitation at the end of each chest compression is recommended to achieve maximal arterial flow.

Precordial Thump

Use a precordial thump *only* in the event of a witnessed cardiac arrest; that is, when you are there and can deliver the thump within one minute of the cardiac arrest. Immediately after positioning the patient on his or her back, identify the middle of the sternum and, using the bottom of your fist, deliver a sharp blow to that area. The shock of the blow can cause the heart to start beating again. Immediately check the carotid pulse, and, if it continues to be absent, begin CPR.

One-Rescuer CPR

If you are the only rescuer present, you are responsible for both rescue breathing and cardiac compression. The proper ratio is 15 compressions to 2 quick breaths, at a rate of 80 compressions per minute. You must maintain this rate to compensate for those compressions lost when you take time out to do the breathing. Move smoothly from one function to the other, keeping a steady rhythm. Say "One and two and . . ." to yourself to maintain the correct rate.

Two-Rescuer CPR

When there are two rescuers, it is best to position yourselves on opposite sides of the patient. Rescuer 1 should compress the sternum at a rate of 60 compressions per minute, while rescuer 2 interposes a breath after every fifth compression. Rescuer 2, the breather, should be in position and ready to breathe at the time of the fourth compression. Breathing must be done between compressions, or else the chest compression will restrict air entry into the chest. Say "One one-thousand, two one-thousand . . ." aloud to help both rescuers maintain the rate and ratio.

When either of the rescuers gets tired, rescuer 1 (the compresser) calls for a change of tasks by saying, "*Change* one-thousand, two one-thousand, three one-thousand, four one-thousand, five one-thousand." Rescuer 2 breathes after "five one thousand" as rescuer 1 moves up and checks the carotid pulse for five seconds. Rescuer 2 gets in position to compress the sternum and *waits*. If the carotid pulse is absent, rescuer 1 says, "Resume CPR," and rescuer 2 immediately begins compression. Rescuer 1 breathes as soon as possible, and rescuer 2 restarts the compression count at "one one-thousand" immediately after the breath.

Terminating CPR

CPR is terminated when *one* of the following occurs:

1. Breathing and a spontaneous heartbeat are detected.
2. An advanced life support team arrives to take over the patient's care.
3. A physician pronounces the patient dead and states that CPR can be discontinued.
4. The rescuer(s) reaches a state of physical exhaustion and there is no replacement(s). This is the most difficult reality for a rescuer to face, but there are limits to your own physical endurance. Fortunately, this doesn't happen very often.

Cervical Neck Fractures

If a patient has been in an accident (an automobile crash, a fall) and you suspect that there may be a cervical (neck) fracture, do not open the airway using the chin-lift method. Instead, keep the head in a flat position. Grasp the jaw at the angle and pull the lower jaw forward, so that it is higher than the upper jaw. (This is called *displacement of the mandible*.)

Infants and Small Children

Although the basic procedure is similar, there are some important differences to keep in mind when you administer CPR to an infant or small child.

AIRWAY

Be careful not to push the infant's head too far back. Because of the extremely pliable neck and trachea, you can easily occlude the breathing passage in this manner.

BREATHING

Cover both the mouth and nose of the child with your mouth, and breathe once every three seconds (Figure 26.8). You should use

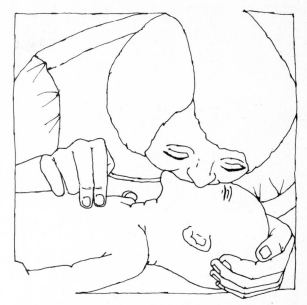

FIGURE 26.8 BREATHING FOR AN INFANT

only the amount of air in your cheeks because it takes much less volume to inflate small lungs.

CIRCULATION

You need only one hand to provide compression. Place the other hand under the child's back to provide support. For an infant, use only the tips of your index and middle fingers to compress the chest at midsternum, at a rate of 80 to 100 times a minute. You should feel the sternum move ½ to ¾ inch (Figure 26.9).

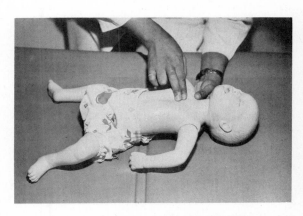

FIGURE 26.9 CORRECT COMPRESSION FOR AN INFANT
Courtesy Lawrence Cherkas

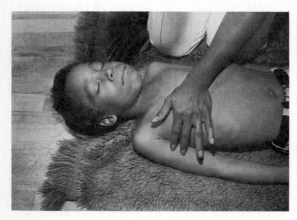

FIGURE 26.10   CORRECT COMPRESSION FOR A CHILD
Courtesy Lawrence Cherkas

For a small child, use only the heel of one hand to compress the chest at mid-sternum, 80 to 100 times a minute (Figure 26.10). You should feel the sternum move ¾ to 1½ inches, depending on the size of the child. For both infants and small children, interpose a breath after every fifth chest compression. The same person can both breathe and compress for an infant at a 1-breath-to-5-compressions ratio.

CPR in the Health Care Facility

Acute health care facilities follow a specific procedure whenever resuscitation is needed.

1. The person who discovers the victim's collapse is expected to call for assistance, either by telephone or by actually calling to someone at the desk. To simplify matters and to avoid alarming other patients, the call is made with a designated code. The code number differs from facility to facility, but code 99 and code 199 are used in many places.
2. The discoverer initiates CPR following the procedures above.
3. The person who responds to the call for help gathers the emergency equipment (cardiac board, a breathing bag, oxygen setup, emergency meds, and the like) and brings it to the location of the victim's collapse.
4. The second person then assists as necessary. This might include placing the cardiac board and participating in two-person CPR.
5. Most facilities designate a team of specially trained personnel (including a physician) to respond to all codes. The team arrives bringing special life support equipment such as defibrillator and emergency drugs. When the team arrives, it takes over care completely. The first persons with the victim relinquish care to the team. They can stay to provide assistance if that is part of the facility's procedure, or they may return to their other duties.
6. If sufficient personnel are available, someone should reassure any family members present as well as any patients in the immediate area.

Recording

Certainly, the initiation of CPR is of primary importance, but also important is the nurse's responsibility to maintain a record of all activities. Whenever you find yourself an "extra" during CPR, you can fulfill an important function by observing and recording, in particular the times of initiation and discontinuation of CPR.

PERFORMANCE CHECKLIST

	Unsatisfactory	Needs more practice	Satisfactory	Comments
One-rescuer CPR				
1. Shake and shout, "Are you all right?"				
2. Turn patient on back.				
3. If witnessed arrest *only,* palpate carotid pulse and, if absent, give precordial thump.				
4. Establish airway: look, listen, and feel.				
5. If patient does not begin to breathe, give four, quick, full breaths, using mouth-to-mouth breathing. a. If chest rises and falls, continue with step 6.				
b. If chest does not move, clear the obstruction and then continue.				
6. Palpate carotid pulse. If absent, begin chest compression.				
7. Kneel beside patient's chest.				
8. Position hands correctly on patient's chest.				
9. Compress downward, keeping arms straight and moving sternum 1½ to 2 inches.				
10. Interpose 2 quick breaths after each 15 chest compressions, at a rate of 80 compressions per minute.				
Two-rescuer CPR				
1. Use Performance Checklist for one-rescuer CPR through step 6.				
2. Have one rescuer breathe while the other compresses chest.				
3. Breather should interpose 1 breath between each 5 chest compressions, at a rate of 60 compressions per minute.				
4. Rescuer 1 calls for change and compresses through the count of "five one-thousand."				
5. Rescuer 2 breathes after "five one-thousand."				
6. Rescuer 1 moves up and checks carotid pulse for 5 seconds.				
7. Rescuer 2 gets in position to compress and waits.				

	Unsatisfactory	Needs more practice	Satisfactory	Comments
8. If carotid pulse is absent, rescuer 1 says, "Resume CPR," and rescuer 2 immediately begins compression.				
9. Rescuer 1 breathes as soon as possible.				
10. Rescuer 2 restarts compression count immediately after breath.				
CPR for infants and small children				
1. Airway a. Do not push infant's head too far back.				
2. Breathing a. Cover both mouth and nose of victim with your mouth.				
b. Breathe once every three seconds.				
c. For infants, use only the amount of air in your cheeks.				

3. Circulation
  a. Infants:
    (1) Use tips of middle and index fingers of one hand.				

(2) Position midsternum.				
(3) Compress at rate of 80 to 100 times per minute.				
(4) Move sternum ½ to ¾ inch.				
b. Small children: (1) Use heel of one hand.				
(2) Position midsternum.				
(3) Compress at rate of 80 to 100 times per minute.				
(4) Move sternum ¾ to 1½ inches, depending on size of child.				

QUIZ

Short-Answer Questions

1. What is the *first* step you should take when you see a person collapse?

   _____

2. When should a precordial thump be delivered? _____

3. What are two methods of clearing the airway and removing an obstruction?

   a. _____

   b. _____

4. How do you position the victim's head if a cervical (neck) injury is

   suspected? _____

5. How can you quickly locate the carotid pulse? _____

6. Where should the chest be compressed? _____

7. How many chest compressions per minute should be performed in the following situations:

   a. One-rescuer CPR _____

   b. Two-rescuer CPR _____

   c. CPR for an infant _____

   d. CPR for a small child _____

8. What is the ratio of breaths to chest compression in one-person CPR?

   _____

9. What is the ratio of breaths to chest compressions in two-person CPR?

   _____

Glossary

abduction The act of drawing away from the median line or center of the body.

Ace bandage A brand name that is commonly used as a synonym for a heavy, elastic roller bandage.

adduction The act of drawing toward the median line or center of the body.

ADL Activities of daily living.

affected Involved, such as the part of the body involved with pain or disease.

agility The state of being nimble or of moving with ease.

airway (1) The passageway by which air circulates in and out of the lungs. (2) A device used, generally when a patient is not breathing normally, to prevent the tongue from slipping back and occluding the throat.

alignment Arrangement of position in a straight line. Used to refer to body parts being positioned so that they are in correct relationship, with no twisting.

alveoli Air sacs of the lungs, at the termination of a bronchiole.

ambulate To walk from place to place.

amoeba Any of various protozoans of the genus *Amoeba* and related genera, occurring in water, soil, and as internal animal parasites, characteristically having an indefinite, changeable form and moving by means of pseudopodia.

anal sphincter The two ringlike muscles that close the anal orifice. One is called the *external anal sphincter;* the other, the *internal anal sphincter.* The actions of both sphincters control the evacuation of feces.

anatomical position A body position in which body parts are in correct relationship to one another and in which correct function is possible.

aneroid manometer An air pressure gauge that indicates blood pressure by a pointer on a dial.

anorexia Loss of appetite.

antecubital space A depression in the contour of the inner aspect of the elbow; also called *antecubital fossa.*

apical Pertaining to the apex.

apical pulse A term used to denote the hearing of the heartbeat through a stethoscope held over the apex of the heart.

apnea The absence of respiration.

arrhythmia Any irregularity in the force or rhythm of the heartbeat.

ascending colon The portion of the colon on the right side of the abdomen that extends from the junction of the small and large intestine to the first major flexion near the liver.

ascitic fluid An abnormal accumulation of serous fluid in the abdominal cavity; also called *ascites.*

asepto syringe A medical instrument that is used to aspirate and instill a fluid. The tip is graduated in size so that it fits into tubings of various sizes; the rounded bulb is used to create suction to fill the barrel and pressure to expel the fluid.

aspirate To remove gases or fluids by suction.

assessment The process of gathering data and analyzing it to identify patient's problems; the first step in the nursing process.

asymmetry   Lack of balance or sameness.

autopsy   An examination of the body after death to determine the cause of death and to further scientific investigation.

axilla   The armpit.

bacteria   Single-celled plantlike micro-organisms that can cause disease.

bandage   A strip of fabric or other material that is used as a protective covering for a wound or to wrap a part of the body.

barrier   (1) Anything that acts to obstruct or prevent passage. (2) A boundary or limit.

base of support   That which makes up the foundation of an object or person and supports the weight.

bedboard   A thin board, often hinged for easy use and storage, that is placed underneath a mattress when a firmer sleeping surface is wanted.

bedpan   A metal or plastic receptacle for the excreta of bedridden persons.

bell   On the stethoscope, the cone-shaped head that is most often used for listening to heart sounds.

binder   A type of bandage, worn snugly around the trunk or body part, that provides support.

body language   Conveying thoughts or meanings through the posturing or positioning of the body.

body mechanics   The analysis of the action of forces on the body parts during activity.

bone marrow   Soft material that fills the cavities of bones.

bounding pulse   A body pulse that strikes the fingers with excessive strength.

brachial artery   An artery that supplies blood to the shoulder, arm, forearm, and hand.

bradycardia   An abnormally slow heartbeat, usually defined as below 60 beats per minute.

bruit   An abnormal sound that results from circulatory turbulence.

burp   To cause to belch, especially a baby after feeding.

cane   A rehabilitative device used as an aid in walking.

canthus   The corner at either side of the eye, formed by the meeting of the upper and lower eyelids. *Inner canthus* is the corner next to the nose; *outer canthus* is the corner to the outside of the face.

cardiac arrest   The cessation of heart action.

caries   The decay of bone or tooth.

cariogenic   That which contributes to the formation of dental caries.

carotid artery   Either of the two major arteries in the neck that carry blood to the head.

carotid pulse   The wave of blood felt as it passes through the carotid artery.

catheter   A slender flexible tube, of metal, rubber, or plastic, that is inserted into a body channel or cavity to distend or maintain an opening; often used to drain or to instill fluids.

Celsius   A temperature scale, devised by Anders Celsius, that registers the freezing point of water at 0° C and the boiling point at 100° C, under normal atmospheric pressure; also called *centigrade*.

center of gravity   A point in an object or person at which gravitational pull functions as if the entire weight of the object or person were at that single point.

centigrade   See *Celsius*.

cerebrospinal fluid (CSF)   The serumlike fluid that bathes the lateral ventricles of the brain and the cavity of the spinal cord.

cerumen   A yellowish waxy secretion of the external ear; earwax.

chart   The official, legal record of health care.

Cheyne-Stokes   A cyclic pattern of respirations that gradually increase in depth followed by respirations that gradually decrease in depth, with a short period of apnea before the next cycle begins.

circular bandage   A bandage that is wrapped in circular fashion around a body part.

circumcise   To surgically remove the prepuce (foreskin).

circumduction   A circular movement of the eye or of a body part.

clove hitch   A knot that consists of two turns, with the second held under the first.

colic   Severe paroxysmal abdominal pain in infants, that usually results from the accumulation of gas in the alimentary canal.

concurrent   Happening at the same time or place.

condiments   Seasonings for food.

constriction   A feeling of pressure or tightness.

contaminate   To introduce microorganisms to an object or person.

contracture   A shortening of a muscle that causes distortion or deformity of a joint.

contraindicate   To indicate the inadvisability of an action; for example, in treatment.

coroner   A public officer whose primary function is to investigate by inquest any death thought to be of other than natural causes.

cradle   A frame shaped like an inverted baby's cradle, which is used to protect the lower extremities from the pressure of bed linen or to supply electrical heat.

cradle cap   Yellowish oily scales on the scalp of an infant that result from the accumulation of sebaceous secretions.

cranium   The portion of the skull that encloses the brain.

crutch   A staff or support that is used by the disabled as an aid in walking; usually has a crosspiece that fits under the armpit and often is used in pairs.

crutch palsy   A weakness or paralysis of the hands caused by damage to the brachial nerve plexus through leaning on the crosspiece of crutches.

culture and sensitivity (C&S)   A laboratory test in which a swab or smear is placed in a nutrient medium to observe for growth of microorganisms. If microorganisms do grow, the culture is then tested with various antibiotics to determine whether the microorganisms are sensitive to the effects of these antibiotics. If the microorganism is destroyed, it is termed *sensitive* to the antibiotic. If the microorganism is not destroyed, it is termed *resistant*.

cytology   A laboratory test in which cells are examined microscopically.

data   Information, especially material that is organized for analysis or used as a basis for decision making.

defecation   The act of expelling the contents of the bowel.

descending colon   The portion of the colon on the left side of the abdomen that extends from the major flexion at the spleen to the point where the colon again flexes into the sigmoid portion.

diaphoresis   Perspiration, especially copious or medically induced perspiration.

diaphragm   (1) A muscular membranous partition that separates the abdominal and thoracic cavities and that functions in respiration. (2) On a stethoscope, the flat, drumlike head that is used most often for listening to blood pressure, the lungs, and bowel sounds.

diarrhea   Pathologically excessive evacuation of watery feces.

diastolic blood pressure The lowest pressure reached in the arteries during the heart's resting phase.

dilation The condition of being enlarged or stretched.

distal In anatomy, located far from the origin or line of attachment.

distention Bloat and turgidity from pressure within; usually refers to the stomach, bowel, or bladder.

diuresis The increased production of urine.

diuretic A drug that increases the production of urine.

dorsalis pedis artery An artery located on the top of the foot, used for palpating the pedal pulse.

dorsal recumbent position Person lies on back with knees bent.

dorsiflexion Bending or moving a part in a backward direction.

double T-binder A binder with two tails that is used to hold a dressing in place on the perineum of a male patient, so that the testicles are not restricted.

droplet nuclei Microscopic particles that, when surrounded by moisture, become airborne.

dysphagia Difficulty in swallowing.

dyspnea Difficulty in breathing.

edema An excessive accumulation of serous fluid in the tissues. *Dependent edema* is fluid that has accumulated in the lower areas of the body due to gravity, *periorbital edema* is a fluid that has accumulated in the soft tissue around the eyes, and *pretibial edema* is fluid that has accumulated over the tibia.

electroencephalogram A record of brain waves measured on the electroencephalograph.

electrolyte A substance that dissociates into ions in solution; in the body, electrolytes are critically important chemicals.

emulsify To combine two solutions that do not normally mix into one liquid, resulting in a suspension of globules.

ethnic Characteristic of a religious, racial, national, or cultural group.

euthanasia Peaceful death. *Positive euthanasia* indicates taking action to facilitate death in a terminally ill patient, *negative euthanasia* indicates withholding treatment in order to allow a natural death to occur.

eversion Turned in an outward direction.

excretion The process of eliminating waste matter, such as feces, urine, or sweat.

expectorate To eject from the mouth; spit.

extension The act of straightening or extending a limb.

external rotation Moving a body part outward on an axis.

Fahrenheit A temperature scale that registers the freezing point of water at 32° F and the boiling point at 212° F, under normal atmospheric pressure.

fan-fold To fold or gather in accordion fashion; for example, the top linen of a bed toward the bottom or one side.

febrile Having an elevated body temperature.

feces Waste excreted from the bowels.

femoral artery Either of the two large arteries that carry blood to the lower abdomen, the pelvis, and the lower extremities.

fever Abnormally high body temperature.

figure-8 bandage A bandage that is wrapped around a body part in a figure-8 configuration.

flaccid Lacking firmness; soft and limp; flabby.

flatus Gas generated in the stomach or intestines.

flexion Bending of a joint.

flow sheet A schematic representation of a sequence of operations or events.

fontanel Any of the soft membranous intervals between the incompletely ossified cranial bones of fetuses and infants.

footboard A board or small raised platform against which the feet are supported or rested.

footdrop The abnormal permanent extension of the foot that results from paralysis or injury to the flexor muscles.

forensic medicine The legal aspects of medical practice.

foreskin The loose fold of skin that covers the glans of the penis; the prepuce.

Fowler's position The patient is in bed on his or her back with the head elevated approximately 60°. Traditionally, knees were also elevated, but this is seldom done today. The degree of elevation of the head can vary: in *semi-Fowler's position* the head is at a 30° angle from the horizontal; in *high Fowler's position,* the head is as close to 90° as possible.

fracture pan A container of metal or plastic with a lower edge, or lip, than a conventional bedpan; used for purposes of excretion by bedridden person, often with fractured hips or in casts.

friction The rubbing of one object or surface against another.

funeral director A licensed person who is responsible for a body from the time of death until ultimate disposition; *mortician.*

gait A way of moving on foot; a particular fashion of walking, running, or the like.

genital Pertaining to the reproductive organs.

genital area The body area that contains the reproductive organs.

gooseneck lamp An adjustable lamp with a slender flexible shaft.

graphic Represented by a graph; often used to refer to the record of temperature, pulse, and respiration.

gravity The force exerted by the earth on any object, tending to pull the object toward the center of the earth.

guaiac A natural resin that is used as a reagent to test for blood in specimens.

Harris flush A term used to refer to a return-flow enema.

Hematest A brand name for a product that is used to test for the presence of blood in fecal specimens; commonly used to refer to the test itself.

Homan's sign A pain in the dorsal calf when the foot is forcibly flexed that can indicate thrombophlebitis.

horizontal Parallel to or in the plane of the horizon.

hyperalimentation The intravenous introduction of nutrients into a large vein, usually the subclavian.

hypertonic Having a higher osmotic pressure than body fluid.

hypotonic Having a lower osmotic pressure than body fluid.

hypovolemic shock A state of shock that is caused by an abnormally low volume of body plasma.

hydraulic Moved or operated by a fluid, especially water under pressure.

incubate To warm (eggs), as by bodily heat, so as to promote embryonic development and the hatching of young; to brood.

inflammation Localized heat, redness, swelling, and pain as a result of irritation, injury, or infection.

infused Put into or introduced.

infusion The introduction of a solution into

a vessel; commonly, the introduction of a solution into a vein.

ingested   See *ingestion.*

ingestion   The taking in of food by swallowing.

instillation   The process of pouring in drop by drop; commonly used to indicate a slow process of introducing fluid.

intermittent   Stopping and starting at intervals.

internal girdle   Those muscles of the abdomen, back, and hips that provide support to the abdominal contents and the pelvis.

internal rotation   Moving a body part inward on an axis.

inversion   Turning in an inward direction.

isolation   To separate or place in quarantine.

Kling bandage   A brand name that is commonly used as a synonym for a loosely knit, lightweight, stretch roller bandage.

Korotkoff sounds   The characteristic sounds, produced by the pressure of blood entering the artery during systole, that are heard on auscultation of an artery after it has been occluded.

Kussmaul's respirations   Deep rapid respirations, often seen in states of acidosis or renal failure.

labia   The lips or folds of tissue that surround the female perineum.

legibility   Able to be read or deciphered.

lesion   A wound or injury in which tissue is damaged.

lithotomy position   Person lies on back with legs flexed and spread apart.

liver biopsy   The excision of microscopic liver tissue for examination.

lumbar puncture (LP)   The insertion of a needle into the spinal canal for purposes of withdrawing spinal fluid or instilling contrast-dye materials; also called a *spinal tap.*

lumbosacral   Pertaining to the lumbar and sacral regions of the spinal column.

macerate   To soften by soaking.

macular   A skin rash consisting of separate, circular flat reddened spots.

manometer   An instrument that measures the pressure of liquids and gases.

medical asepsis   The technique designed to prevent the spread of microorganisms from one person (or area) to another.

medical examiner   An appointed public official, usually a forensic pathologist, whose function it is to investigate deaths that result from traumatic causes (homicide, suicide, accident) and sudden natural deaths in the absence of medical attention.

metabolism   The complex of physical and chemical processes involved in the maintenance of life.

microorganism   An animal or plant of microscopic size, especially a bacterium or protozoan.

midclavicular line   An imaginary line running vertically through a midway point of the clavicle or collarbone.

military (24-hour) clock   A system for noting time in which the time after midnight begins the cycle, and the time is noted consecutively for 24 hours: hours before 10:00 a.m. are noted with a zero before the hour; minutes after the hour are noted immediately after the numbers for the hour. For example, fifteen minutes after 1:00 a.m. would be noted 0115; the hours after noon are numbered 13, 14, and so on, so 15 minutes after 1:00 p.m. would be 1315.

minibottle   A small container for intravenous-infusion solutions.

mitered corner   A method of folding a sheet or blanket to achieve a smooth squared covering over the corner of the mattress.

morgue   A place in a health care facility

where the bodies of deceased patients are temporarily detained pending release to a mortician, coroner (medical examiner), or other authorized person.

mortician   A funeral director and embalmer who is responsible for the care and disposition of a deceased person.

nares   The openings in the nasal cavities; the nostrils.

narrative charting   The traditional style of recording data on a patient's chart.

nasal speculum   An instrument that is used to dilate the nostrils for purposes of inspecting or treating the nasal passages.

net binder   A tube made of netlike material that is used to secure dressings to the body.

nursing history   The initial data gathered through interview by the nurse.

objective   Based on observable phenomena.

ophthalmoscope   An instrument that consists of a light and a disc with an opening through which the interior of the eye is examined.

opposition   Positioned opposite one another; for example, the thumb to the fingers.

orthopnea   A situation in which a person has difficulty breathing and is relieved by sitting upright or standing.

otoscope   An instrument, for inspecting the ears, that consists of a light and a cone.

ova   The female reproductive cells of animals; eggs. Microscopic examination of stool is often done to identify the ova of intestinal parasites.

oxygenation   Treating, combining, or infusing with oxygen.

palpation   Examining or exploring by touch.

paracentesis   The insertion of a trocar into the abdominal cavity for the removal of excess fluid.

paralysis   Loss or impairment of the ability to move or have sensation in a bodily part as a result of injury to or disease of its nerve supply.

parasite   Any organism that grows, feeds, and is sheltered on or in a different organism while contributing nothing to the survival of its host.

parenteral fluid   Fluid given directly into tissues or blood vessels.

patellar tendon   A continuation of the quadriceps tendon that leads from the patella to the tibia.

pathogenic organism   A microorganism that causes disease.

pectoralis muscles   Four muscles of the chest.

pedal pulse   A pulse wave that can be felt over the arteries of the feet.

penis   The male organ of copulation and urinary excretion.

perineum   The portion of the body in the pelvic area that is occupied by urogenital passages and the rectum.

periphery   The outermost part or region.

peristalsis   Wavelike muscular contractions that propel contained matter along the alimentary canal.

peritoneal dialysis   Removing waste products from the body by the instillation and removal of dialyzing solution through the peritoneal cavity.

piggyback   An intravenous-infusion setup in which one bottle is attached to the tubing of the primary bottle through a short tubing.

pinwheel   A wheellike instrument with sharp points that is used to test peripheral sensation of the body.

planning   The second step in the nursing process, in which information is reviewed and synthesized in order to form goals and a plan of action.

plantar flexion   Bending the foot so that the toes point downward.

popliteal artery   The major artery that extends from the femoral artery down behind the knee.

postmortem examination   See *autopsy.*

precordial thump   A blow delivered to the lower sternum to trigger a change in the cardiac conduction pattern and to restore normal cardiac rhythm.

preformed water   The water content of ingested liquids and foods.

problem-oriented medical record (POMR)   A system of keeping medical records that is organized according to patients' problems.

proctoscope   An instrument that dilates the anus for purposes of inspecting or treating the lower intestine.

profuse   Plentiful, overflowing, copious.

pronation   Turning the palm or inner surface of the hand or forearm downward.

prone   Lying with the front or face downward.

protein   An organic compound of living matter that contains amino acids as its basic structural unit.

proximal   Near the center part of the body or a point of attachment, or origin.

ptosis   Paralytic drooping of the upper eyelid caused by nerve failure.

pulse deficit   The difference in rate between apical and radial pulses.

pulse pressure   The difference between systolic and diastolic blood pressure readings.

pureed   Strained, as in food.

pyrexia   Fever.

quad cane   A cane with a 4-legged base for stability.

radial artery   The artery that descends from the brachial artery along the radius of the arm.

radial deviation   Bending the hand on the wrist in the direction of the thumb.

recurrent bandage   A bandage that is wrapped in such a way that it recurs, or folds over, on itself.

referral   A specific plan for directing a patient or client to other health care resources.

reflex contraction   An involuntary response of muscle contraction.

reflex hammer   A small rubber-headed hammer that is used to test body reflexes; also called a *percussion hammer.*

regurgitate   To vomit.

remittent   Increasing and decreasing in measurement.

renal calculi   Kidney stones.

repose   A body position that appears peaceful.

respiratory arrest   The sudden cessation of breathing.

respite   An interval of rest or relief.

resuscitate   To revive or restore to life.

reverse spiral   A bandage that is applied, usually on a limb, in a circular fashion with a reverse fold.

rhythm   A variation of energy occurring in a regular pattern.

rigor mortis   Muscle stiffening after death.

roller bandage   Bandaging material that has been rolled to provide for easier application; commonly used to refer to rolls of gauze.

rotation   A circular movement around a fixed axis.

scultetus binder   A heavy fabric binder that is held to the body by the interwrapping of cloth tails in an oblique fashion across the abdomen.

semi-Fowler's position See *Fowler's position*.

sensory deprivation A lower level of sensory input than that required by an individual for optimal functioning.

sigmoid flexure The distal portion of the colon, which appears as an S-shaped curve preceding the rectum.

sigmoidoscope A tubular instrument with a light that is used to dilate the anus for inspection and treatment of the sigmoid.

Sim's position A side-lying position with the top leg flexed forward.

sling A device that suspends and supports a body part.

smegma A thick whitish substance, composed of epithelial cells and mucus that is found around external genitalia.

sordes Accumulation of dried secretions and bacteria in the mouth caused by not eating, mouth-breathing, and inadequate oral hygiene.

sphincter A circular muscle that controls an internal or external orifice.

sphygmomanometer An instrument that measures blood pressure in the arteries.

spiral bandage A bandage that is applied, usually on a limb, in a circular ascending fashion.

stab wound A direct scalpel puncture into skin or membrane.

stereotype A presumed form or pattern that is attributed to a group and generalized to an individual.

stertorous Respirations having a heavy snoring sound.

sternum A long flat bone that forms the midventral support of most of the ribs; the breastbone.

stethoscope An instrument that is used for listening to sounds produced in the body; also see *bell* and *diaphragm*.

stopcock A valve that regulates a flow of liquid through a tube.

straight abdominal binder A large cloth that is placed snugly around the lower part of the trunk to give support or to secure a dressing.

stylet A slender pointed instrument; a surgical probe.

subjective Personal; in assessment, refers to information from the patient's viewpoint.

supine Position lying flat on the back.

supination Turning or placing the hand and forearm so that the palm is upward.

suppuration The formation or discharge of pus.

sutures The thread, gut, or wire used to stitch tissues.

symmetry The equal configuration of opposite sides.

systolic blood pressure The highest pressure reached in the arteries, created by the contraction of the ventricles of the heart.

tachycardia An abnormally rapid heartbeat, usually defined as 100 beats per minute, in the adult.

T-binder A binder with a single tail that is used to hold a dressing in place on the perineum of a female patient.

temporal artery One of the two three-branched arteries that lie at the temple of the head.

thoracentesis The insertion of a trocar into the pleural space of the chest for the removal of abnormal fluid.

thready pulse A weak, faint pulse.

toe pleat A method of folding top bed linen to provide extra room for the feet.

tolerance In activity, the capacity to endure.

torsion The act or condition of being twisted or turned; the stress caused when one end of an object is twisted in one direction and the other end is held motionless or twisted in the opposite direction.

trachea A thin-walled tube of cartilaginous and membranous tissue that descends from the larynx to the bronchi, carrying air to the lungs.

tracheostomy A surgically devised opening into the trachea from the surface of the neck.

transverse colon The portion of the colon across the top of the abdomen from the hepatic flexure to the splenic flexure.

trapeze A short, horizontal bar suspended from a frame over the top of a bed. It is used by the patient to facilitate moving in bed and transfer.

tremor An involuntary trembling motion of the body.

trocar A sharp-pointed surgical instrument that is used with a cannula to puncture a body cavity for fluid aspiration.

trochanter The bony processes below the head of the femur; often used to refer to the greater trochanter, which is on the lateral aspect of the femur.

tuning fork A small two-pronged instrument that, when struck, produces a sound of fixed pitch; used to test auditory acuity.

turgor Normal tissue fullness in relationship to superficial body fluids.

ulnar deviation Bending the hand on the wrist in the direction of the fifth, or small finger.

umbilicus The navel.

urethral meatus The opening of the urethra onto the surface of the body through which urine is passed.

urinal A receptacle for urine that is used by bedridden patients.

urinalysis The chemical analysis of urine, which commonly includes color, clarity, pH, specific gravity, and checks for the presence of glucose, RBCs, casts, and WBCs.

urination The act of excreting urine.

uvula The small, conical fleshy mass of tissue that is suspended from the center of the soft palate above the back of the tongue.

vaginal speculum An instrument that is used to dilate the vagina for purposes of inspecting or treating the vaginal passages or to obtain a specimen for a culture or smear.

vital capacity The maximum volume of air that can be expired from the lungs after a maximal inspiration.

void The emptying of urine from the bladder through the urethra; to urinate.

vulva The external female genitalia, including the labia majora, the labia minora, the clitoris, and the vestibule of the vagina.

walker A rehabilitative device that is used to support a disabled person while standing or walking.

water balance The ratio of water taken into the body to water excreted.

weight-bearing The side on which the weight of the body can be placed while standing; *partial weight-bearing* indicates that an individual cannot stand solely on the affected limb and must have other means of support also.

xiphoid process The lower tip of the sternum.

Answers to Quizzes

Module 1

1. a. Oxygenation
    b. Respiratory
2. a. Comfort
    b. Neural
3. a. Oxygenation, and possibly activity and rest
    b. Respiratory, and possibly musculoskeletal
4. b
5. d
6. c
7. S
8. O
9. S
10. O

Module 2

1. b
2. c
3. a
4. a. Narrative
    b. Problem-oriented medical records
5. So that others may check the original data and make their own inferences
6. Depressed, upset
7. Error 175 ml SJ

    or

    wrong amount SJ
    clear yellow urine 175 ml
8. Persons involved in the patient's care; others—the patient, the patient's attorney, and so on—only as provided by regulations, laws, or court order

Module 3

1. c
2. d
3. d
4. b

Module 4

1. T
2. T
3. F
4. F
5. T
6. F

Module 5

1. Environment, emotions, physical disability, dentures
2. c
3. b
4. a
5. a
6. c
7. F
8. F
9. T
10. F

Module 6

1. b
2. d
3. a
4. c
5. b
6. 6, 8, 5, 2, 1, 4, 7, 3

Module 7

1. a. Good medical asepsis
    b. Psychological comfort
    c. Approximation of normal conditions

2. a. Bedpan
   b. Urinal
   c. Fracture pan
   d. Emesis basin
3. a. Pad the pan
   b. Warm it
4. a. Lifting the buttocks
   b. Rolling onto the pan
5. Any five of the following: amount; color; consistency; odor; blood; mucus; foreign matter
6. a. Postpartum patients
   b. Surgical patients
   c. Patients with catheters in place
7. Refer to Performance Checklist.

Module 8

1. c
2. b
3. d
4. F
5. F
6. T
7. F
8. T
9. F
10. T
11. T
12. F

Module 9

1. The thickest part is placed where the greatest absorbency is needed, and the infant has free movement of legs.
2. Urine or feces on the skin contributes to a variety of skin problems.
3. Close them and put them out of reach of the infant.
4. Diaper rash is a reddened rash throughout the diaper area; scald is a solid red, burn-type area.
5. Shake some onto the inner aspect of the forearm.
6. It will not slip and become tighter, cutting off circulation.

7. Any three of the following: avoid chilling; keep one hand on the infant; check water for correct temperature; place basin on a safe surface; put side rail or crib net in place when finished

Module 10

1. b
2. a
3. c
4. c
5. d
6. d
7. d
8. c
9. b

Module 11

1. a
2. c
3. c
4. b
5. a
6. c
7. d
8. a
9. a
10. b
11. a
12. d

Module 12

1. Not be working against the gravitational pull
2. a. Promotes physical progress
   b. Adds to patient's self-esteem
3. Dislocation of the shoulder
4. The patient's trunk
5. a. For patients' comfort and safety
   b. To see that there is no pressure on parts
6. a. Prevents pressure sores

b. Prevents joint contractures
c. Improves muscle tone and circulation
7. Trochanter or ankle roll
8. Flexed
9. a. Feet in space between mattress and footboard
   b. Roll placed under ankles
10. b
11. b

Module 13

1. a. To protect the patient
   b. To protect the staff
2. Wrist, mitt
3. Body, vest
4. a. For hygiene
   b. For exercise
5. d

Module 14

1. a. To maintain muscle tone
   b. To maintain joint mobility
   c. To prevent lengthy rehabilitation
2. Flexors
3. Active
4. Supination
5. Abduction
6. b
7. c
8. c

Module 15

1. Any four of the following: maintains and restores muscle tone; stimulates respiration; stimulates circulation; improves elimination; improves psychological well-being
2. Ease patient back onto bed or chair of origin.
3. Chair must be placed on left side; extra support may be needed; right leg must be braced with nurse's leg or knee while pivoting.

4. To provide a firm handhold and support for the nurse transferring the patient
5. To prevent dizziness

Module 16

1. Any four of the following: maintains muscle tone; restores muscle tone; stimulates respiratory system; stimulates circulatory system; improves psychological well-being; facilitates elimination
2. Falls
3. They give better support, are less likely to slip, and usually stay on better.
4. A transfer and ambulation belt; a cane; a walker; or crutches
5. Crutches should extend from the floor, about 6 inches out from the foot, to the side of the chest 2 inches under the axilla.
6. When the patient needs balance and support but can use both legs and both arms
7. The arms of the chair (or the bed), not the walker
8. Opposite the weak leg
9. Hold both in one hand.
10. Three-point gait

Module 17

1. c
2. An examination of the body after death
3. a. To determine exact cause of death
   b. To gather scientific knowledge
   c. To add to statistical data
4. Coroner is elected or appointed, not necessarily a physician; medical examiner is an appointed physician, usually holding a special degree in pathology.
5. See your county's requirements.
6. Any three of the following: rigor mortis; skin discoloration; skin indentation; cooling
7. To prevent discoloration and indentation of the underlying hand if folded over the chest

8. a. IVs
   b. Nasogastric tubes
   c. Urinary catheters
   d. Oxygen equipment
9. Any four of the following: clean the patient; place the patient in repose; straighten the unit; soften the lights; rearrange flowers; provide chairs

Module 18

1. a. Equipment with which to obtain the specimen
   b. Equipment in which to place the specimen
   c. Equipment with which to observe the patient's response
2. a. Privacy
   b. Lighting
   c. Positioning
   d. Draping
3. a. Right amount
   b. Right container
   c. Right time
   d. Right patient
4. Any five of the following: patient's name; identification number; age; room number; physician's name; date
5. 7/15/80 Coughed up approximately 15 ml thick, blood-tinged sputum, which was sent to lab for C&S. c/o fatigue after coughing. Resting in bed.
   S. Penobscot, RN
6. F
7. T
8. F
9. F

Module 19

1. Any four of the following: *cleansing*—to remove fecal material and clean the bowel; *medicated*—to allow medication to be absorbed; *oil retention*—to soften fecal material; *cooling*—for extremes of elevated temperature; *return flow*—to remove gas

2. a. Embarrassment
   b. Modesty
   c. Fear of discomfort
3. a. Color
   b. Respiratory rate
   c. Pulse
   d. Signs of excess fatigue
4. By lowering the fluid container below the level of the bowel
5. Slow fluid way down. If this doesn't stop cramping, stop the procedure altogether until cramps subside.

Module 20

1. 37° C, 98.6° F
2. Any four of the following: time of day; age; presence of infection; environment; exercise; emotions
3. Prevent injury to the mucosa
4. 8 minutes, 3 minutes, 10 minutes, only seconds
5. 3, 1, 2
6. 50, 100
7. Any four of the following: exercise; application of heat or cold; medications; emotions; blood loss
8. a. Radial
   b. Carotid
   c. Temporal
9. 16, 20
10. Any four of those listed in answer 7, as well as disorders of the respiratory tract

Module 21

1. c
2. c
3. b
4. a
5. a
6. c
7. 140 / 80 / 70

Module 22

1. a. To protect the patient
   b. To protect the environment

2. Strict isolation
3. Enteric isolation
4. Any three of the following: private room with running water; sign on door; stand outside door for equipment; laundry hamper inside room; wastebasket lined with plastic; thermometer and blood pressure equipment
5. No special precautions are used.
6. Thoroughly wash your hands, doing a complete scrub.
7. To protect the patient from infection
8. Sensory deprivation
9. Any three of the following: give her care first; answer her call light promptly; stop and visit often; find diversions for her

Module 23

1. a. Meeting the physical and psychological needs of the patient
   b. Gathering necessary equipment and assisting the physician
2. Sitting on the edge of the bed facing the physician
3. Eyes
4. Ears
5. Supine
6. Papanicolaou test (Pap smear)
7. It interferes with the Pap smear.
8. Skin (peripheral) sensation
9. Negative Babinski reflex
10. Paracentesis
11. a. Clarity
    b. Color
    c. Viscosity

Module 24

1. a. To provide support
   b. To protect wounds
   c. To protect and hold underlying dressings
2. a. Circular
   b. Spiral
   c. Reverse spiral

   d. Figure-8
   e. Recurrent fold
3. A joint
4. Distal, proximal
5. a. To hold layer dressings in place
   b. For support
6. Male, female
7. d
8. c

Module 25

1. b
2. b
3. d
4. b
5. b
6. c

Module 26

1. Shake the person and say loudly, "Are you all right?"
2. Only when you witness the arrest and can deliver the thump within one minute
3. Any two of the following: tilt head back and chin up; wipe out vomitus; reach in and remove object; turn victim on side and thump between shoulders; place both hands on lower half of sternum and push firmly
4. Flat with the neck straight
5. Locate the larynx (voice box), and slide your fingers to the hollow beside it.
6. 1½ inches above the xiphoid process
7. a. 80 per minute
   b. 60 per minute
   c. 80 to 100 per minute
   d. 80 to 100 per minute
8. 2 breaths to each 15 chest compressions
9. 1 breath to each 5 chest compressions